Food policy: integrating health, environment and society

Food policy: integrating health, environment and society

Tim Lang
Professor of Food Policy, City University, London, UK

David Barling
Senior Lecturer, Centre for Food Policy, City University, London, UK

Martin Caraher
Associate Dean and Reader in Food and Health Policy, City University, London, UK

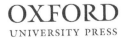
OXFORD
UNIVERSITY PRESS

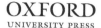

OXFORD

UNIVERSITY PRESS

Great Clarendon Street, Oxford OX2 6DP
United Kingdom

Oxford University Press is a department of the University of Oxford.
It furthers the University's objective of excellence in research, scholarship,
and education by publishing worldwide. Oxford is a registered trade mark of
Oxford University Press in the UK and in certain other countries

First published 2009
Reprinted 2012

British Library Cataloguing in Publication Data
Data available

Library of Congress Cataloging in Publication Data
Data available

ISBN 978-0-19-856788-2

Printed and bound by CPI Group (UK) Ltd, Croydon, CR0 4YY

Contents

Preface

The origins of this book lie in discussions begun when we started working on the basis of food policy together in the mid-1990s. For many years, with colleagues around the world, we have observed, researched and engaged with the unfolding world of food policy. We have done this as academics, as people engaged in real policy discourse and as ordinary citizens ourselves. This multiplicity of perspectives has fanned, rather than diminished, our interest in the subject.

Whether working with communities or governments, watching commerce or civil society, helping generate or respond to initiatives, being asked for evidence or interpretations, privately or publicly, it has been clear that new discourses and arguments have been bubbling up in the world of food policy, which too many books about food, let alone policies attempting to set frameworks for action, failed to make adequate sense of. It is many years since there was an academic attempt to outline what food policy is and could mean. The purpose of this book, therefore, is to try to fill that gap. It is intended to make sense of what is meant by food policy; to explore whether the term has any currency in current policy discourse; to assess whether current policies help or hinder what happens; to judge whether consensus can triumph in the face of competing bids for understanding; to consider what direction food policies are taking, not just in the UK where we work or locally where we live, but internationally and regionally; to assess who (and what) gains or loses in the making of those food policies; and, thus, to help identify a modern framework for judging how good or limited processes of policy-making are.

We are social scientists in a school of community and health sciences in a university located in one of the great cities of the world. The scope of the book, like all books, reflects both that and the training and worldview of its authors. By original training, we each brought different inputs to our deliberations: one political science, another environmental health and health promotion, and the third social psychology; but we have worked on food policy collectively for decades. Although living and working in a great metropolis, our upbringing and interests keep our eyes and hearts elsewhere too: Ireland, Wales, India and rural England. Our colleagues, Fellows and post-graduate programmes at the Centre for Food Policy at City University London, add a wealth of perspective by bringing together people from across the world and with diverse training across the natural and social sciences. Capturing that diversity is at the heart of our social science perspective on food policy and what our Centre and this book are about. The excitement of doing so keeps so many people around the world working together. This book is our London contribution to that shared endeavour, based on thinking done with people across Europe, North America, Australasia, Latin America and Africa over recent years.

Each of us has experience of the world of food policy-making. It is our privilege to have worked as consultants, advisers, observers, researchers and participants in various UN, international and European bodies and in national and community/local organizations and processes. Our focus is on public and civil society bodies, rather than on commerce, but our views and research have propelled us at times to the commercial heartlands and to those who shape current business models in the food sector. This has generated many vibrant and useful engagements with people and organizations throughout the food chain, for which we are very grateful.

The perspective taken here is that of the Centre where we work. It and we are unashamedly committed to the public good and to debating what that might mean. Of course, the public good means different things in different parts of the world. This is something the book does not skirt. Unlike the excellent work of, for example, the International Food Policy Research Institute, the Washington DC-based body, which is part of the global agriculture and development oriented Consultative Group on International Agricultural Research network, our Centre for Food Policy has championed the need to look at rich developed world food policies. As historic centres of power, wealth and influence, Western country food policies have not received their due share of scrutiny, yet their governments, companies and tastes have shaped and continue to shape how 'world' food systems are defined and perceived. If the West feels a food crisis, it is a 'crisis'. If the developing world has a crisis, it may too often be defined as 'normality'.

This book is about our view that food policy has to address the triple challenge of health, environment and social justice, or it is nothing. Where possible we have drawn on our diverse food-policy experience, not just our observations, research and reading in addressing that inquiry. We also have tried to refer to the many researchers and programmes around the world with whom we share this commitment to understand the world of food and food policy. Collectively we all bear a responsibility to speak out loudly and clearly about how we see events unfolding; about whether the dynamics shaping the current direction of travel are appropriate; about which criteria to deploy when judging what a sustainable food future could be; and whether institutions and policies are appropriate for that purpose. We hope our colleagues in this endeavour find the thinking presented here useful and a foil to their own.

David Barling, Martin Caraher, Tim Lang
Centre for Food Policy
City University London
July 2008

Acknowledgments

Like all books, this one owes an enormous debt to many people too numerous to list who have helped us with facts, figures and literature when working up to, and on, this book in the five years since inception. We leave it to them to judge whether our trips to give lectures and seminars in the name of exploring the issues, analyses and interpretations offered here were worthwhile! From our side, it is a privilege to know and work with so many colleagues in universities, organizations and civil society organizations around the world who share our commitment to improve understanding of what makes the world of food tick, and why bits don't.

We also owe a deep debt of gratitude to our band of Fellows, Research Assistants and students, past and present, at City University; they have provided a continuous testbed for our thinking. Wherever possible we have tried to cite all these people's work as acknowledgement of their collective input into the view of food policy presented here. Part of the joy of working on food policy over recent decades has been the rich camaraderie it inspires and the acuteness of the intellectual debates that it offers. Not everyone agrees, nor could they, but the commitment to clarification and progress is widely shared.

We also thank the many people in governments, civil society organizations and commerce who have sent us papers or patiently explained to us what they do and how they see the world of food policy. Obviously what we present in these pages is our own perspective but this owes an enormous debt to their kindness and thoughts over the years. Thanks also to the WHO, David Gordon, USDA and FAO for their help. We trust that the patience they have shown us as we try to understand this complex international, regional, national and local world of food is warranted. Food policy discussions are all the richer for the support of all of these people at home and abroad.

Like all authors, we have placed additional burdens on our friends, families and households when writing this. Rachel Barling, Maggie McNab and Liz Castledine put up with us as we wrote. Our thanks too go to the team at Oxford University Press: Helen Liepman, who first suggested the book after one of us gave a lecture at the Royal Society of Arts in London; Georgia Pinteau, who saw it to completion; and Richard Martin and Eloise Moir-Ford, who shepherded us along the path to print. A heartfelt thanks to Anna Stephenson Boyles for helping with references. We hope they all find this book enough to their liking.

London
July 2008

Abbreviations

AoA	Agreement on Agriculture (of the GATT)	EC	European Commission
		EEA	European Environment Agency
ASEAN	Association of South East Asian Nations	EFSA	European Food Safety Authority
BEUC	Bureau of European Consumers Unions	EP	European Parliament
		EU	European Union
BMI	Body Mass Index	FAD	Food Availability Decline
bn	billion	FAO	Food and Agriculture Organization (of the United Nations)
BRC	British Retail Consortium		
BSE	Bovine Spongiform Encephalopathy		
		FDF	Food and Drink Federation (UK food industry)
BST	Bovine Somatotrophin		
CAP	Common Agricultural Policy	FIAN	Food First Information & Action Network (USA)
CEC	Commission of the European Community (also EC)	FISS	Food Industry Sustainability Strategy (UK)
CFP	Common Fisheries Policy (EU)		
CGIAR	Consultative Group on International Agricultural Research	FIVIMS	Food Insecurity and Vulnerability Information and Mapping Systems
CHD	Coronary Heart Disease	FLO	Fairtrade Labelling Organization
CI	Consumers International (world body of consumer NGOs)	GAIN	Global Alliance for Improved Nutrition
CO_2	carbon dioxide	GATT	General Agreement on Tariffs and Trade
CO_2e	carbon dioxide equivalents		
Codex	Codex Alimentarius Commission (joint WHO/FAO body)	GBD	Global Burden of Disease
		GEF	Global Environment Facility
		gha/cap	global hectares per capita (person)
COPA-COCEGA	Organisation of EU farmers and agricultural co-operatives		
		GFSI	Global Food Safety Initiative
CSR	Corporate Social Responsibility	GHG	Greenhouse Gases
		GHGe	Greenhouse Gas equivalents
CVD	Cardiovascular disease	GM	Genetic Modification
DALY	Disability adjusted life year. This is the sum of life-years lost owing to premature death and years lived with disability adjusted for severity.	GMO	genetically modified organism
		gmp	greater warming potential
		HACCP	Hazards Analysis Critical Control Point
Defra	Department for Environment, Food & Rural Affairs (UK)	HGV	Heavy Goods Vehicle

IAASTD	International Assessment of Agricultural Science and Technology Development
IARC	International Agency for Research into Cancer
ICN	International Conference on Nutrition 1992
IDF	International Diabetes Federation
IFN	integrated farm management
IFPRI	International Food Policy Research Institute
IPR	Intellectual Property Rights
JECFA	Joint Expert Committee on Food Additives
Kcal	Kilocalorie
KVI	Known Value Items
LCA	Life Cycle Analysis
MAFE	Ministry of Agriculture, Fisheries & Food (UK)
Mercosur	Free trade agreement of Latin America
MoF	Ministry of Food (UK in World Wars I and II)
MS	member state
MSC	Marine Stewardship Conservation
Mt	million tonnes
NAFTA	North American Free Trade Agreement
NCD	non communicable disease
NFU	National Farms Union (UK)
NGO	Non-Governmental Organization
NIDDM	Non-insulin dependent diabetes mellitus
NZ	New Zealand
OECD	Organization for Economic Co-operation and Development
PSA	Public Service Agreement (a UK government policy tool)
RCT	Randomized Controlled Trials
RDC	Regional Distribution Centre
RUAF	Resource Centres on Urban Agriculture and Food
SAI	Sustainable Agriculture Initiative
SAP	Structural Adjustment Programme
SCN	Standing Committee on Nutrition (UN)
SPS	Sanitary and Phytosanitary Standards (part of 1994 GATT)
TBT	Technical Barriers to Trade (part of the 1994 GATT)
TNCs	Transnational corporations
TRIPS	Trade-Related Intellectual Property Rights
TUAN	The Urban Agriculture Network
UN	United Nations
UNCED	UN Conference on Environment and Development 1992
UNDP	UN Development Programme
UNEP	UN Environment Programme
USA	United States of America
WANAHR	World Alliance for Nutrition and Human Rights
WASH	World Action on Salt and Health
WFC	World Food Council (UN, 1974–96)
WFS	World Food Summit 1996
WFP	World Food Programme
WHO	World Health Organization (of the United Nations)
WHO-E	World Health Organization Regional Office for Europe
WIC	Women, Infants and Children (US welfare programme)
WIPO	World Intellectual Property Organization
WSSD	World Summit on Sustainable Development (2002)
WTO	World Trade Organization

Chapter 1

Introduction and themes

This chapter provides a background and introduction to the book. It outlines the perspective taken and key cross-cutting themes which inform the analysis of food policy presented here.

The perspective

It is hard, if not impossible, to be neutral about food. Food is essential for life yet contributes to premature death everywhere—even in rich societies. It brings pleasure and lubricates social interaction but carries risks and cements social divisions. Its production reflects a wondrous mix of natural and human actions, yet it results in increasingly well-documented social, health and environmental costs. This book is about how and whether food policy fully integrates three elements integral to its mix, namely human health, the environment, and social relations.

The book's thesis is that mounting evidence has suggested the need for a reconfiguration of policy, yet responses are patchy, tentative and inadequately integrated. After decades of experimenting with a system that 'mines' the earth, a more sustainable food system is urgently needed. For over half a century, an approach to food has been pursued that was designed to tackle public health problems associated with under-consumption, yet now faces a more complex co-incidence of under-, mal- and over-consumption. Power relations and fundamental inequalities within and between societies are being exposed.

Anyone committed to the clarification of food policy knows that these are interesting but sensitive times. Already at the end of the 20th century, the tectonic plates of food policy and global food supplies were rumbling. The slow but steady advance in absolute and per capita production was levelling off.[1, 2] Awesome evidence about unmet need was available. 'New' issues such as climate change and water shortage emerged alongside 'old' issues like energy supplies and fertilizer prices. Tensions and pressures, which have long been tracked, are re-emerging. The question troubling the food policy community is whether that movement will become more violent, reconfigure more fundamentally or tremble slightly and return to a more quiescent, uneasy state.

This book explores the present, past and possible futures for food policy and what shapes contemporary food policies. It also reflects on actions to improve those policies, documenting failings as well as successes. To learn about the present, we need to understand why policies got to this point and what drove them there. As with all policy work, food policies can be improved if lessons are learned and if there are structures that listen. Part of our original motivation for this book was to describe the interplay of global, national and personal food worlds in a way that might help people share our sense of urgency about the importance of food policy. Food production, distribution, cooking, consumption and waste disposal are not processes that just happen. Nor are they natural, even if the desire for food is. The world of food is populated by people, organizations and interests all doing things.

Throughout, we try to map the global situation and policy context within which regional, national and local policy responses are situated. Examples from around the world are deployed but often these also refer to the UK, not just because this is the authors' home base but because it is such a fascinating 'hotspot' for food policy. The UK's food policy history has run the gamut—from growing its own food to reliance on its colonies and now to Europe, from cheap to expensive food systems, from skilling up to de-skilling its people, from taking health seriously as a population issue to individualizing responsibility. As the first industrial nation, its people have been severed from the land arguably the longest of any mass population in the world. In a world that is characterized by rapid urbanization, growing population, ecological crisis, a mixture of extreme wealth and poverty, wide disparities of health, the UK's experience should be shared; in part it acts as a warning.

Although geographically an island, in food terms Britain is not, nor long has been. Like everywhere its diet and food system reflect the movement of plants, people, animals and power around the world. Today, although a centre of financial capital, it is just one of 27 member states of political Europe, jostling for attention within global policy structures such as the World Trade Organization (WTO). The juxtaposition of the local and global is central to how this book tackles its three substantive topics of health, environment and society. The issue explored here is how to make sense of these competing perspectives within complex multi-level frameworks of governance. It is a matter of debate whether food policy thinking is swimming or drowning in the process. Arguably there is a narrow dividing line between success and failure. If more people eat less, does that mean more people can eat more?

Working in food policy and observing its unfolding dramas, we are acutely aware of the various appeals to base food policy on science or market economics or social justice or ethics or culture … the list of 'essential solutions' offered to policy-makers is in fact very long. Our view here is that if any policy framework underplays what we believe to be the core issues of health, environment and society, they will be likely to add to, rather than replace, current confusions in food policy. There are already many signs of policy cacophony—competing powerful voices drowning out equally worthy positions when there is a case for integration and symphony. Actions to ensure decent, health-enhancing food supply and equitable consumption require integration and coherence rather than pursuit of 'silver bullets', mystery 'factor Xs' to resolve food policy's complexities.

The fact is that food policy covers immense and diverse terrain. Actions in the name of one sphere of interest can have a knock-on effect elsewhere. For instance, in a rush to compensate for fossil fuel reliance in the 2000s, rich Western Governments introduced biofuel schemes and subsidies, which merely brought to a head the simmering world food crisis.[3, 4] The fact that land is a site for competing interests for food, fuel, amenity, water, carbon sequestration, cultural identity, biodiversity and much more, had apparently been lost on the clever financial market-makers and policy advisers who shaped public policy... until reality hit back and food prices rocketed, putting an estimated 100 million more people on the planet into food insecurity.[5] For years, observers of food policy had been quietly warning that the food system is taut, highly stressed and lacking global resilience.[6-8] The rich might be being fed, indeed arguably over-fed, but the warning signs about simmering crisis have long been documented yet ignored, marginalized or downplayed by political processes. The challenge now is to articulate a way through this crisis without delaying big decisions that need to be faced. The challenge running throughout this book is how policy must help to create a food system that ticks all the policy boxes. Currently this is not the case.

The modern food system faces a serious dilemma. On the one hand, it has delivered unprecedented quantity and choice of food to hundreds of millions of people. On the other hand, evidence has mounted as to food's impact on health, the environment and social structures. Rightly, it claims this as a policy success.[9] How to conceptualize, resolve or manage this treble burden—health, environment and social behaviour—is the subject of this book. The dilemma has not been resolved, yet the need and pressures to deliver have grown. This situation has not been helped by policy-makers tacitly, if not overtly, handing responsibility to the food supply chain and some powerful interests.[10] The challenge we now face is how to encourage—speedily but sensibly—the production, distribution and consumption of a good, health-enhancing and environmentally principled diet. And who can do this when commercial and public policy signals have for years encouraged another direction for investment? Addressing such questions is why this book outlines existing societal and institutional processes within and surrounding 21st century food policy thinking.

Food policy is not owned intellectually or otherwise by any one academic constituency or intellectual tradition. The book ranges widely across different disciplinary legacies. Active engagement in the world of policy-making at all levels of governance suggests that this multi-disciplinary approach is appropriate. One cannot understand the drivers and dynamics at local, sub-national, national, regional or global levels from within any one particular disciplinary standpoint. A multiplicity of perspectives allows for a more comprehensive understanding; 21st century food policy has to improve knowledge integration.[11]

The scope here tends to be on the rich, developed countries, not because the food world should be permanently segmented into 'developed' *versus* 'developing' blocs, but because food policy tends to be shaped around rich world interests (see Preface). Indeed, an argument explored throughout this book is whether that fissure falsely narrows understanding of food policy in the 21st century. Our view is that the world of food supply chains and food decision-making now overlaps continents, in which case bi-polar distinctions like rich–poor, developed–developing, male–female, urban–rural, production–consumption etc., while hugely important, can restrict understanding if applied singly. Our approach, by contrast, has been to explore the diversity of tensions, not to champion (or indeed to challenge) only one over others. Instead of seeing developing countries as the policy problem—though real problems they of course have—this book's attention is more on developed countries as the problem, for it is they who drive the current unsustainable food systems.

Food policy-makers frequently have an understanding of policy architecture, institutions and actors, and of their themes, tensions and possibilities that is not widely broadcast. Policy 'insiders' know how processes really work and the trade-offs that go on. A glimpse of this reality is given when countries negotiate at big trade gatherings, which occasionally spill into the open, as they have over agricultural subsidies in the WTO Doha Round. Workings and final results, which are presented as seamless, rational products, may have been produced in a less linear and orderly mode than final statements indicate. There is often a gap between the official and actual passage of events. These insights deserve to see the light of day, to be scrutinized, theorized and held to account within democracies. Part of our motive for this book was to articulate such understandings and to place them at the heart of the modern discourse of food policy. This is why we depict policy as subject to power relations, conflicts as well as consensus, irrational alongside logical thinking, sectoral interest triumphing over the public good. This tapestry of interwoven interests deserves to be explored in the open, and much good policy thinking now bears, rather than disguises, these tensions.[12] To reflect on policy realities, enables better understanding of where the public and planetary good might lie.

Food policy is not a new subject. Part of the motivation for this book was to connect present dilemmas and understandings with those of the past. There is something thrilling as well as chilling about the weight and extent of contemporary challenges to food policy. To witness the frisson of fear about rising food commodity prices that ran through the world of food policy in the mid-2000s, much as it did in the early 1970s, is to raise a question: what has been learned? How did this energy-dependency go unchallenged? Whose interests triumphed to maintain the policy lock-in to an oil-based food system when this is recognized to be a finite resource, yet so critical for fertilizer-based productivity increases? What were the official institutions doing if not co-ordinating and engaging on fundamentals such as that? The idea for this book in fact began in the early 2000s when we were clear that food policy was moving into a period of great difficulty;[13, 14] it was finished at a time of worldwide awareness that this was indeed the case.[2, 11]

The food system is clearly under stress. There is widespread recognition in companies, ministries, universities and think-tanks that old policy mixes are not working sufficiently well to address the formidable challenges of the present century. New thinking is emerging and must do so on an accelerated basis. Companies that denied the public health crisis when it was articulated by public health specialists now cautiously, if still insufficiently, acknowledge it. Often this concern may appear paper thin, accused by critics of being more 'greenwash' than a real shift. But in some companies, concerns about unsustainability are being taken seriously and built into their business model.[15, 16] It helps when financiers see it as a deciding factor in company performance.[17]

There are grounds for sober optimism rather than despair about the future. The tectonic plates of food supplies may be shifting—due to price volatility, oil/energy, water, population, changed demand, climate change, rampant inequalities, rising healthcare costs (for those who can even afford it), and much more discussed in later chapters—but it is at least possible to chart what these tensions are and to indicate barriers and opportunities. From there being little action or policy debate, there is a now a general hum and, in some places, even signs of quiet symphony replacing cacophony.[18] This is helped by vociferous and questioning civil society organizations around the world, actively engaged in debating what directions might or should emerge.

The book proposes and concludes with the argument that a combination of factors—better understanding, a preparedness to think fundamentally, a clear set of principles, an articulate and engaged civil society, politicians and political classes prepared to think, a commercial sector where enough companies realize their long-term interests, and more—just might help shift food policies towards a happier mix than appears to be the case today. There is much rich work and understanding on which to draw. Ultimately, however, the transition from failing to sensible food policies, from localized experiment to population-wide involvement, from policy rumble to symphony is not an academic exercise. Although we outline theories and interpretations of what happens in the world of food policy, the ultimate test is reality. Daily, food policies are tested by the billions who live on the planet, and by the plant and animal species with whom humanity shares it. The mix is currently not a sustainable one. But it could be.

This book sets out to explore how and whether food policies address the needs of societies, the environment and human health satisfactorily, and it concludes by asking whether society is sufficiently clear about the criteria by which a decent food system might be judged. The huge international interest in these issues gives great hope. The test for this book is whether it helps the reader appreciate and also engage with the world of food policy, wherever you might be. The test for food policies is whether they can deliver a sane, safe, healthy, sustainable, productive and equitable food system. That responsibility falls on everyone but on some actors in the food system particularly heavily, hence the argument rehearsed here that food policy ultimately has to be part of the democratic process.

Our perspective is informed by and seeking to develop what is meant by sustainable development, a term that was promulgated by the 1987 Brundtland Commission. This proposed a now classic definition that sustainable development is 'meeting the needs of the present without compromising the ability of future generations to meet their own needs'.[19] Although firmly within that perspective, we here use a more focused term 'ecological public health', which we have championed before and which is explored in subsequent chapters.[18, 20–22] Sustainable development is a world-view, an holistic approach to how society, the economy and culture can be organized to protect planetary health. The focus here is on food, not all existence! The term 'ecological public health' is used to reformulate what is meant by health, seeing food as an intersection point for human, societal and planetary relations. The environment is the infrastructure and context within which humans live and eat. How humans eat has an impact on environment, simultaneously affecting population health.[23] The book proposes that 21st century food policy will inevitably reconfigure food systems as the interaction between material, biological, cultural and social worlds. This approach is very demanding. It requires the integration of knowledge across disciplines and across policy areas. As a result, the book ranges across many sources of knowledge and inputs, trying to pull out sources of conflict and consensus about food's role in human health, the economy, political processes, the environmental infrastructure of food, cultural confines and demands, and more. The approach taken is to conceive of food policy as the intersection of policy issues, which vary in strength, influence and constituency (see Fig. 1.1).

Food policy in the 21st century has to juggle competing demands from each of these sources. Evidence summarized here and elsewhere suggests that it will have to deliver a low-impact food system, to meet human social and cultural needs, to enhance biodiversity, to be socially just, to contain and reduce diet-related ill-health, and so on. Some argue that this can be done within existing capitalist economics; others that it requires a re-orientation of the rules. A land-use policy that focused, for example, just on biodiversity, without linkage to feeding people, might be good for ornithology but not mass urban populations. This complexity makes modern food policy particularly difficult yet interesting. It requires new public involvement in sifting the relationship between evidence and policy. This makes new demands on policy-makers as well as ordinary citizens.

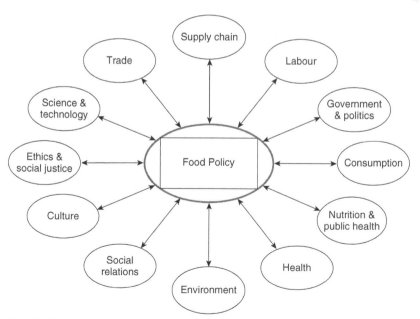

Fig. 1.1 Food policy as an intersection point of competing issues.

Cross-cutting themes

The book is structured around a number of core problems in food policy—governance, supply chain, nutrition and health, environment, behaviour and culture, social justice and poverty. When scrutinizing these in turn, a number of key cross-cutting themes are explored. Each proposes an argument or concern that is either already central to food policy discourse or looks set to be so.

Defining the remit of food policy

The notion and meaning of food policy itself needs to be redefined and classified for the 21st century. Historically, as later chapters show, food policy has tended to veer between concerns for agriculture (primary production), nutritional aspects of human health (consumption) and trade (international economics). Measured on their own terms, these foci are presently failing to be delivered adequately, let alone addressing the combined triple burden of modern forms of ill-health, environmental stress and social inequality. A new focus on food policy is required, which can address and re-shape the whole food system, from farm to consumption, not just a few sectors chosen for historic reasons. Already the need to shift from an 'old' to 'new' food policy has been articulated,[24] but the old–new distinction does not do justice to the enormity or extent of the policy challenge. The argument explored here is that modern policy-making faces considerable complexity as to how food should be, and is, grown, processed, distributed and consumed. A food policy framework that is 'fit for purpose' needs to be as sensitive to planetary and ecological demands as to social and human demands. Quite where food policy goes, needs to be kept open and constantly debated, not pigeon-holed.

The complexity of the health–environment–society interface

Re-thinking the health–environment–society interface has to be at the heart of any modern food policy.[25] The eco-health nexus on its own poses immense challenges and has considerable implications for defining what is meant by progress. Rich-country diets may have to be simpler, having gone in a century or two from restricted to excess without pausing at what might turn out to be more sustainable choice ranges. In an era when ill-health associated with overweight and obesity sits alongside 'classic' health outcomes (and policy imperatives) such as hunger and malnutrition,[26] the creation of better links between productive capacity and social capacity might move centre stage for food policy. Certainly, it will have to be more subtle and address questions about *how* food is derived and *whom* is fed. The environmental impact of food is almost certain to re-shape productive capacities on the land, and in turn have knock-on effects on social demand. Equally, social demands—from urbanizing cultures—will pose huge stress on food-productive capacity, not least in relation to labour. Food cultures are always dynamic but the political ramifications of altering food choice might threaten political obeisance to the notion of consumer rights. To developing countries already constrained by food poverty, such talk of choice might seem luxurious, but they too will be affected by a world that has to internalize environmental, health and social costs in food prices.

Already, there are signs of pressure for food policy to recognize the need to deliver low calorie, low carbon foods.[27, 28] The implications for rich societies suffering overweight and obesity will be different to those of developing countries burden by underweight, but with increasing incidence of overweight-related health problems too. How public policy addresses these complexities, while simultaneously responding to strong evidence about the social determinants of health and the existence of clear social gradients, remains to be seen. But they must, and in concert with powerful commercial forces too.[29, 30]

Power and conflicts of interest

Food policy is contested space. It covers a food world fissured by power relations and subject to tensions and sometimes outright battles between competing interests.[31] This is not to say that food is a Hobbesian world of warring factions that only can be tamed by an all-powerful authority. Patently this is not true; there can be consensus or, if not consensus, quiescence. The tectonic plates of food policy have not always ground together in the 20th century, not least due to the impact of technological and social advances. Food policy nevertheless can best be understood if the potential for contestation is recognized alongside asymmetries of power. Part of the struggle witnessed within and about food policies is the result of different interest groups seeking to influence policy frameworks and accepted understandings of food.

Our argument is that food policy is a constant 'juggle' of competing interests and perspectives. Food policy is made, not given. It is a social construct, not ordained by a pre-programmed, perpetual or externally affirmed human order. To understand this role of human agency in food policy, we have to unpick the different actors' class, sectoral and economic interests. Within food policy lies a web of social relations, actors and institutions. Permanence in these relations cannot be assumed. Within the supply chain, for example, giant retailers are currently on a trajectory of dominance, whereas in the past farming held centre stage. Who knows yet who will dominate the mid 21st century? The struggle within the food system to control food—as a primary source of money, power and influence—will continue to evolve. New food barons will replace current ones. New consciousness about the system among consumers will perhaps take food policy into uncharted terrain.

Multi-level and multi-sectoral food governance

Food policy needs to be understood through multi-level and multi-disciplinary analysis. This book explores five levels of governance: the global, supra-national regions, the national, sub-national regions and the local. The levels add both complexity and tensions to food policy-making. In the 20th century, power tended to rise up from the national to the global. In the UK, for instance, 19th century powers to ensure food was fit to eat were given 'downwards' to local authorities by the national state. With accession to the European Union in 1973, regional governance became more important, first for agriculture via the Common Agricultural Policy, then across quality issues with the creation of the European single market in 1987 and for safety after a wave of scandals in 2000. With the creation of the World Trade Organization under the 1994 General Agreement on Tariffs and Trade, the global level became immensely significant in arbitrating between different national and regional standards. In Europe and elsewhere there were also counter-trends in that national states gave new powers to sub-national bodies. Regions such as Tuscany in Italy and Wales and Scotland in the UK developed powerful sub-national food policies.[32, 33]

In the debate about globalization, an impression is sometimes given that nation states no longer have any influence over policy. While multi-level governance changes the distribution of power, considerable room for political manoeuvre still remains. State bodies that previously held sway at national level now have to operate within fast changing international forums. Local organizations, which have long had to deliver food interventions, may feel relatively powerless to do so but that status is malleable, a matter with significant implications for the democratic process and accountability about food systems.

Policy effectiveness and integration

Policy responses to problems may draw upon a variety of available policy instruments. These range across legislation, regulation, self-regulation, fiscal (tax) measures, education, labelling and advice. Such policy approaches vary from 'hard' to 'soft'; some are *dirigiste*, others appeal to self-regulation, letting industry police itself. A common criticism from health and environmental advocates is that food policy has relied excessively on soft approaches such as education and labelling. Policy effectiveness has to be judged against goals and urgency. The existence of a food problem does not mean it receives the requisite policy response. Some are ignored; others are weighed down by good intentions. This happened with the rush to biofuels by oil-dependent food economies in the 2000s.[34] Such crises expose lack of coherence in formal and official policies. It may make sense for Sweden to develop biofuels from its forestry, but not for the US or UK to turn edible corn or wheat into biofuels.[35, 36] Clearer criteria are required for what is sustainable. Rational coherence and integration of food policies may be more often aimed for than achieved.

The policy task is to find integrative processes and mechanisms to achieve rational coherence and integration. In times of war or crisis, governments tend to become more co-ordinated or at least more overtly than at other times. Generally, the level of policy integration depends how high up the political agenda food is. This is true for commercial interests as much as governments. In the world of the giant food retailers, for example, where profit margins can be tight but throughput immense, business drivers are more likely to be conventional features such as price, quality, appearance, regularity, rather than on social or ethical matters such as environmental impact or whether primary growers have been paid a fair price. 'Soft' features (seen as social responsibility matters) are often not deeply integrated into 'hard' commercial ones. But this can change, and has changed, due to public pressure and high profile campaigning.

The public interest problem

Defining and locating the public interest in food policy is a core problem. The era when food policy could focus on primary production and assume that public good flowed from that alone is probably closing; it was always inappropriately too narrow.[37, 38] The challenge for 21st century food policy is how to voice where the public interest lies and how best to narrow the gap between what is and what could be. Historically, food policy has tended to be seen as the preserve of governments. Today, however, the world of food is straddled by giant food and drink corporations who are equally, if not more, significant and *de facto* formulate their own food policies. With articulate and educated consuming publics, however, which have access to globalized media, there is now a triangular set of relationships: state, supply chain and civil society. The public interest is defined via this interaction.

Intriguing questions arise. Governments and food companies often voice strong commitment to consumer choice within markets, but are consumers really in command or merely selecting between goods whose style, cost, mode of production and features are set before the purchaser even sees them? Is Western-style consumer power more rhetorical than real? And is consumer power the same thing as the public interest? One theme in modern food policy discourse is whether the commercial focus on the 'consumer' is congruent with a 'citizen' approach historically associated with democracy. The former is appealed to through 'value-for-money'; the latter through 'values-for-money'. Sceptics argue that consumers are mere mouths, offered and consuming too often the cheapest, easiest, softest, sweetest and fattiest foods. Consumerists reject this as a caricature; one that leads public health and environmentalists into a patronizing position, that they know best. In such debates, civil society organizations have become increasingly active.

Levels of responsibility and morality

The allocation of resources leads to tensions between individual and collective responsibilities. This applies throughout the world of food, nowhere more than over health, environmental and societal matters. Where should policy attention lie? On reframing markets or encouraging individual consumers to act? Encouraging systemic change or niche markets? Part of the crisis of early 21st century food policy is the difficulty of allocating authority and institutional reach to address the new complexities raised here. Institutions and bodies inherited from the 20th century do not, so far, appear able to shape food policy to address the triple challenge coherently enough. At every level of food governance, there are deep fissures; at the global level, for instance, the Bretton Woods bodies of the International Monetary Fund (IMF) and World Bank are ill at ease with the UN bodies such as the Food and Agriculture Organization (FAO) and World Health Organization (WHO), the UN Environment Programme (UNEP) and UN Development Programme (UNDP). Across this institutional architecture, food policy is framed by moral and philosophical assumptions. Responsibility easily becomes a rhetorical notion, shrouded by defensiveness, legal constraint and cultural uncertainty.

Countries that espouse neo-liberal economics tend to emphasize the primacy of individual choice in food policies. They often prefer to advise or educate consumers to 'choose wisely', putting the onus of responsibility ideologically on choice, and existentially on the consumer. But is it reasonable to leave public health to individualized choice at supermarket check-out points? And how can environmental aspects of food production, about which consumers may barely be aware, be reflected or translated in food prices? Such questions are not just abstract dilemmas. They privately trouble retailers, growers and processors, too, not least since they know only too well the volatility of consumers and how finely tuned Western food supplies are, and therefore subject to risk. In the 21st century, major changes in supply are likely. Faced by rising populations, there are strong voices urging policy-makers to aim for food growth at all costs, using all technologies available. Environmental protection or worries about sustainability are 'luxuries' that need to be kept in check. Others urge caution, fearing a Gadarene rush into new energy-intensive systems. These are large-scale policy conflicts of perspective, now at the heart of the moral complexity of modern food systems. With such questions, food policy is being scrutinized through a moral filter.[39]

Narrowing the evidence–policy–practice gap

The relationship between evidence, policy and practice in food policy is often problematic. While few could resist the advantages of having good evidence to inform policy, this happy state of affairs is not always feasible. The history of food policy is replete with examples of where policy has been pursued despite evidence or in the face of evidence or denying evidence, and where evidence has been crying out for a policy response. So the ideal of evidence-based policy might be sound but the reality of the relationship between policy, evidence and what people do is more problematic.[40] Policy is made without perfect evidence, and on the basis of partial and biased evidence. The case for 'evidence-based policy' is frequently rehearsed and sometimes well made. Who could want policies to fly in the face of sound evidence? But caution is required as to how and how frequently this aspiration can be realized. An idealized conception of policy-making is given in Fig. 1.2. The question is how often this can be realized?[41] How much evidence of a health problem is needed before policy is re-cast? Are policies really based wholly on evidence? Could they always be?

Evidence-based practice is, for very sound reasons, essential for ever improving the quality of medical and environmental services. The 'gold standard' for evidence in medicine are randomized control trials (RCTs).[42] In the softer, messier world of food systems, RCTs may not be appropriate or even feasible. Policy does not necessarily work from evidence in the scientific sense but is shaped by philosophies, contingencies and practicalities. Evidence is framed by the questions asked and assumptions made, hence the realities of a desired evidence-based policy may be shaped by politics or conflicts of interests more than the call for an objective process might desire.[43] Experience of food and alcohol suggests how 'events' can drive policies.[44, 45] Sometimes, policies have to be made despite evidence deficits, driven by other reasons. There can also be a time-lag between policy and evidence. For example, in food safety crises, ministers have to act having good evidence of public concern but lacking good evidence about what is the best course of action scientifically, hence decisions being made that, retrospectively, appear crude.[46] 'Best evidence in the circumstances' is not necessarily evidence-based policy. Sometimes the world cannot wait for evidence.

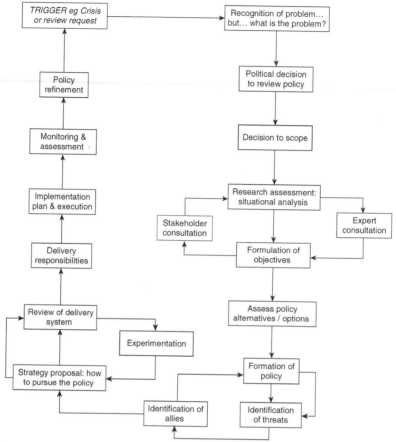

Fig. 1.2 An idealized cycle of continual policy-making improvement.

Risk, science and technology

Food policy has long struggled with the notion of risk and when to intervene in food markets. Throughout the 20th century, public scandals about food risks—from adulteration, toxins, new technologies—peppered public discourse. New laws and institutions were created to address whether food might contain residues or toxins, and to set tolerances and loads. Policy responses to risk debated how best to deliver prevention at source and openness of information.[47] Estimating risk was thus connected within policy-making to notions of proportionality and accountability. Risk became a core concern for food management, with social scientists arguing that societies are increasingly shaped around managing everyday risk, sometimes out of proportion to the real or statistical risks.[48, 49] In this process, the role of scientists and technology becomes problematic, seen on the one hand as purveyors of truth (liberators), on the other as shapers of reality (controllers).

Interventions based on risk assessment inevitably raise questions about who and what defines the risk, how inclusive the processes of defining risk are, and how risks are managed.[50] Western consumers worry about the quality of their diet, when the risks may be low compared to developing countries. Risks are far greater from diet-related degenerative diseases than from food-borne pathogens. But who is to say that consumers are wrong to worry? It is their food, their consumption. Risk, in short, is framed by social expectations, tolerances and exposure. Risk has become a key concern for food policy in relation to both public health and the environment. In response, new institutions have been created but within a fragmented architecture. The EU food institutions that address health risks, such as the European Food Safety Authority (EFSA), are not the same as those that address environmental risks, such as the European Environment Agency (EEA), yet consumers eat food that affects both. The evidence of the value of eating fish—for its omega 3 fatty acids—is overwhelming.[51] But the evidence of fish stocks reaching environmental limits is equally overwhelming.[52] So which risk is the consumer to respond to?

Political control and institutional suitability

Food is politically charged. Although not always a high-profile policy area, food policy has well-established institutional structures that are often being modified, particularly in response to crises or 'events'. Until the mid-20th century, as a general rule, such institutions tended to be at national or local levels, but gradually over the latter half of the century, new institutions were created and older ones thrown in flux. This was hastened by revised trade rules designed to facilitate cross-border food flows. Food policy is now embedded within more complex international structures, with parallel systems also existing in the commercial sector. Political hues vary as to whether these institutions favour mandatory or voluntary regulations. The commercial structures tend to prefer voluntary instruments and self-regulation rather than heavy-handed intervention and mandatory controls. Yet in war circumstances, governments will exert strong 'top down' controls, such as rationing, price control and quotas; the case for intervention has moral supremacy and new norms can emerge.

In the 21st century, these institutions will have to be engaged in 'squaring the circle' of raising production, while lowering food system's impacts on health, environment and social inequality. But are existing institutional structures and political accountability fit for purpose? The appropriateness and democratic accountability of food institutions becomes problematic. How can the institutional mix and historical legacy of political processes move fast but deftly enough to address the complexities already documented and accepted as unavoidable?

Outline of the chapter structure

These themes introduced above are picked up throughout this book, which is structured as a number of discrete areas, chosen for policy saliency. In each, problems are posed, evidence marshalled and the extent to which there are any policy responses, and how adequate these are, is considered. In Chapter 2, an overview of food policy is presented, suggesting various historical phases in policy and institutional development but giving especial attention to the 20th century and to developments since the great restructuring of world food systems after World War II; four phases in the development of food policy are proposed. Chapter 3 identifies some key concepts that aid understanding of the dynamics of public policy-making and the shift from governing to broader governance flows found in contemporary food policy. Chapter 4 reviews the impact food has on health, and considers the extent to which the picture of global nutrition is now fissured by under-, mal- and over-consumption; it asks whether this picture is helped or hindered by an intellectual fragmentation within nutrition science itself. Chapter 5 gives an account of the contemporary dynamics in food supply and considers the impact of the emergence of enormously powerful commercial forces and whether policy structures are sufficiently engaged. Chapter 6 reviews the evidence of food's reliance on environmental goods and ecosystem services, and considers how modern 'advanced' food supplies have measurable impacts on them. Chapter 7 focuses on the behavioural and cultural aspects of food, proposing that food behaviour is shaped by cultural contexts but that food cultures are dynamic. Chapter 8 investigates a core concern about social inequality in food consumption and considers whether the pursuit of food justice and rights has been an effective response to alarming evidence of social fissures. The final Chapter 9 responds to the collective case made in Chapters 1–8 for reconceptualizng food policy around ecological public health. It proposes that food policy gains renewed clarity of purpose if it adopts the perspective of ecological public health but that structural challenges are awesome. The themes introduced in this present chapter are woven throughout.

References

1. FAO. *State of food and agriculture 2007*. Rome: Food and Agriculture Organization, 2007.
2. World Bank. *World development report 2008: agriculture for development*. New York: World Bank, 2007.

3. von Braun J. *Agriculture for sustainable economic development: a global R&D initiative to avoid a deep and complex crisis.* Charles Valentine Riley Memorial Lecture. Capitol Hill Forum, Washington DC, February 28, 2008. Washington DC: International Food Policy Research Institute, 2008.

4. Evans A. *Rising food prices: drivers and implications for development.* Food Supply Project Briefings. London: Chatham House, 2008:11.

5. FAO. *World food security summit, June 3–5 2008.* Rome: Food & Agriculture Organization, 2008.

6. Brown LR. *Who will feed China? Wake up call for a small planet.* New York: WW Norton, 1995.

7. Brown L. *Outgrowing the earth: the food security challenge in an age of falling water tables and rising temperatures.* New York: WW Norton, 2004.

8. Brown AD. *Feed or feedback: agriculture, population dynamics and the state of the planet.* Utrecht: International Books, 2003.

9. Dyson J. *Population and food: global trends and future prospects.* London: Routledge, 1996.

10. Vorley B. *Food inc.: corporate concentration from farm to consumer.* London: UK Food Group, 2004.

11. IAASTD. *Global report and synthesis report.* London: International Assessment of Agricultural Science and Technology, 2008.

12. Sustainable Development Commission. *Green, healthy and fair: a review of government's role in supporting sustainable supermarket food.* London: Sustainable Development Commission, 2008.

13. Millstone E, Lang T. *The atlas of food: who eats what, where and why.* London: Earthscan, 2008.

14. Lang T, Heasman M. *Food Wars: the global battle for mouths, minds and markets.* London: Earthscan, 2004.

15. Porritt J. *Capitalism as if the world matters.* London: Earthscan, 2005.

16. Senge P, Smith B, Kruischwitz N, Laur J, Schley S. *The necessary revolution: how individuals and organizations are working together to create a sustainable world.* London: Nicholas Brealey, 2008.

17. Langlois A, Zuanic PE, Faucher J, Pannuti C, Shannon J. *Obesity: re-shaping the food industry.* London: JP Morgan Global Equity Research, 2006:112.

18. Lang T, Rayner G. Overcoming policy cacophony on obesity: an ecological public health framework for policymakers. *Obesity Reviews* 2007;**8**(Suppl.):165–181.

19. Brundtland GH. *Our common future: report of the World Commission on Environment and Development (WCED) chaired by Gro Harlem Brundtland.* Oxford: Oxford University Press, 1987.

20. Waltner-Toews D, Lang T. A new conceptual base for food and agriculture: the emerging model of links between agriculture, food, health, environment and society. *Global Change and Human Health* 2000;**1**(2):116–130.

21. Lang T, Barling D, Caraher M. Food, social policy and the environment: Towards a new model. *Social Policy & Administration* 2001;**35**(5):538–558.

22. Barling D, Lang T, Caraher M. Joined-up food policy? The trials of governance, public policy and the food system. *Social Policy & Administration* 2002;**36**(6):556–574.

23. McMichael AJ. *Human frontiers, environment and disease.* Cambridge: Cambridge University Press, 2001.

24. Maxwell S, Slater R. Food Policy Old and New. *Development Policy Review* 2003;**21**(5–6):531–553.

25. McMichael AJ. Integrating nutrition with ecology: balancing the health of humans and biosphere. *Public Health Nutrition* 2003;**8**(6A):706–715.

26. Gardner G, Halweil B. Underfed and overfed: the global epidemic of malnutrition. *Worldwatch paper 15.* Washington DC: Worldwatch Institute, 2000.

27. Tukker A, Huppes G, Guinée J, Heijungs R, de Koning A, van Oers L *et al.* *Environmental Impact of Products (EIPRO): analysis of the life cycle environmental impacts related to the final consumption of the EU-25.* EUR 22284 EN. Brussels: European Commission Joint Research Centre, 2006.

28. Cabinet Office Strategy Unit. *Recipe for success: towards a food strategy for the 21st century.* London: Cabinet Office, 2008.

29. Commission on Macroeconomics and Health. *Macroeconomics and health: investing in health for economic development.* Harvard University/Center for International Development/World Health Organization, 2002.

30. Commission on the Social Determinants of Health. *Achieving health equity: from root causes to fair outcomes.* Interim Statement from the Commission. http://www.who.int/social_determinants/resources/interim_statement/en/index.html. Geneva: World Health Organization, 2007.

31. Tansey G, Rajotte T (ed.) *The future control of food: a guide to international negotiations and rules on intellectual property, biodiversity and food security.* London & Ottawa: Earthscan & IDRC, 2008.

32. Morgan K, Marsden T, Murdoch J. *Worlds of food: place, power and provenance in the food chain.* Oxford: Oxford University Press, 2006.

33. Lochhead R. *A national food and drink policy.* Speech to Royal Highland Show, June 19, 2008. http://www.scotland.gov.uk/News/This-Week/Speeches/Greener/food. Edinburgh: Scottish Government, 2008.

34. OECD, FAO. *Agricultural outlook 2008–2017.* Rome & Paris: Organization for Economic Co-operation & Development and Food & Agriculture Organizationi, 2008.

35. Commission on Oil Independence. *Making Sweden an OIL-FREE Society.* Stockholm: Government Offices of Sweden, 2006.

36. Commission of the European Communities. *An EU strategy for biofuels.* Communication SEC (2006) 142. Brussels 8.2.2006. COM(2006) 34 Final. Brussels: Commission of the European Communities, 2006.

37. Dubos R. *Man adapting.* New Haven, Connecticutt: Yale University Press, 1965 (1980).

38. Dumont R, Rosier B. *The hungry future.* London: Deutsch, 1969.

39. Korthals M. *Before dinner: philosophy and ethics of food.* Dordrecht NL: Springer, 2004.

40. Sutton R. *The policy process: an overview.* Working paper. London: Overseas Development Institute, 1999.

41. Kelly MP, Speller V, Meyrick J. *Getting evidence into practice in public health.* London: Health Development Agency, 2004:12.

42. Cochrane Collaboration. *About the Cochrane collaboration.* www.cochrane.org Oxford: The Cochrane Collaboration, 2008.

43. Black N. Evidence based policy: proceed with care. *British Medical Journal* 2001;**323**:275–279.

44. Cannon G. *The politics of food*. London: Century, 1987.

45. Marmot M. Evidence based policy or policy based evidence? *British Medical Journal* 2004;**328**(7445):906–907.

46. Phillips (Lord), Bridgeman J, Ferguson-Smith M. *The BSE inquiry report: evidence and supporting papers of the Inquiry into the emergence and identification of Bovine Spongiform Encephalopathy (BSE) and variant Creutzfeldt-Jakob Disease (vCJD) and the action taken in response to it up to 20 March 1996*. London: The Stationery Office, 2000:16 volumes.

47. Trichopoulou A, Millstone E, Lang T, Eames M, Barling D, Naska A *et al. European policy on food safety*. Luxembourg: European Parliament Directorate General for Research Office for Science and Technology Options Assessment (STOA), 2000.

48. Beck U. *Risk society: towards a new modernity*. London: Sage, 1992.

49. Adams J. *Risk*. London: UCL Press, 1995.

50. van Zwanenberg P, Millstone E. *BSE: risk, science, and governance*. Oxford: Oxford University Press, 2005.

51. Nestle M. *What to eat*. New York: North Point Press (Farrar, Straus and Giroux), 2006.

52. Royal Commission on Environmental Pollution. *Turning the tide: addressing the impact of fishing on the marine environment, 25th report*. London: Royal Commission on Environmental Pollution, 2004.

Chapter 2

Defining food policy

Charting the terrain of food policy

It could be argued that food policy is not a discipline in and of itself but merely a subsection of other studies. This argument proposes that sufficient policy direction and understanding of food can be derived from, say, macro-economics or health or environmental studies. No special attention is needed under the general heading of 'food policy'. Indeed, many languages make little distinction between food policy and food politics. This argument is superficially seductive, not least because many disciplines and subjects cross-reference to issues covered in this book, invoking the term 'food policy'. Nevertheless, the case to see food policy as a topic in and of itself is strong. Its value lies in focusing attention on how policy addresses food from the field to the table, from inputs to outputs. By recognizing how policy affects food, improvements can be made and dynamics can be better understood.

One everyday answer to the question 'what is food policy?' is that food policy is to food what economic policy is to economics, foreign policy is to foreign affairs and social policy is to the shaping of society. Such an answer makes the point that, although food policy may lack the profile of those other policy spheres, food has a policy framework nonetheless. Actions shape food outcomes. This helps explain what food policy analysts do. They study the dynamics at work. Their findings cumulatively add to facts, theories and questions about what shapes the food system. The study of food policy is the pursuit of improved knowledge of how policy-making determines and responds to the food system.

To turn the above into everyday terminology, and echoing Harold Lasswell, we can define the study of food policy as of how policy-making shapes who eats what, when and how; and of whether people (and animals) eat and with what consequences. The remit of food policy ranges from how food is produced and grown, to how it is processed, distributed and consumed; from the structures that shape food supply, to those that determine health and environment; from the sciences and processes that unlock food's potential, to the formal governance and lobbies that seek to control it; from the impact the food system's dynamics have on society, to the way its demands are factored into policy-making itself. The value and purpose of studying food policy, therefore, is to help unravel the complex relations between food and these other domains of existence in order to make what is otherwise implicit (or hidden behind doors) more explicit, open and democratically accountable. In this vein, given the strong evidence about food's impact on human health and the environment—the focus of this book—food policy ought to be a key element that informs conventional thinking about public health and policy. This is sometimes not the case. Food has an impact on the material and ecological world; it is a commodity extracted from biological and physical processes. Vice versa, the ecological and material world shapes what foods are produced and their impact on humans and how they live and die. Food policy is thus about these complex webs of interaction and, centrally, about how policies—deliberate and unintended—affect food and its outcomes: who eats, what, when and how.

If this begins to sketch the domain of food policy, we should ask who makes these policies, and who studies them. There is no profession of food policy, or not in the conventional sense. There is no institutionally or legally recognized 'canon' of food policy such as those subscribed to by lawyers, doctors, social workers or engineers. Such professions have a corpus and ethos that oversee a knowledge base and have organizations that set professional standards, nationally or internationally, and that stipulate and monitor what is essential knowledge and best practice. Measured by such criteria, there is no food policy profession; yet, as we explore here, there is a deep and complex body of thinking about food policy, and it is a term that has long been in the public policy sphere. There are numerous reports, statements, suggested policy frameworks, institutions and standards, which collectively indicate the reality of food policies in everyday governance.

Companies, civil society and government all vie with the others' conception of what good food policies are. In addition to statutes, policy documents and aspirations, it also has to be recognized that many people hold down jobs, either with the term food policy in their job description or in its formal title. These are specialists, working mostly at the local or national levels for health or governments or companies whose job is to monitor, respond to or initiate policy positions. There are organizations, researchers, community workers and university specialists with food policy in their title; and, as many books and journals bear evidence, there is a body of thinking on food policy on which policy-makers draw. Sociologically, food policy may not have generated a profession but it does generate events. In short, it is meaningful to talk of food policy as a 'live' process. We can assert with confidence that food has been problematic for policy-makers for generations. It is not a hyped up, peripheral or passing concern; it has extensive historical roots. Issues of security of supply, quality, health, employment and agriculture have peppered policy-making and politics for generations.

Like all policy studies, there is a tension between trying to pin down and refine or define food policy, and retaining a breadth of perspective that does not rule out factors whose importance may vary, depending on the topic within food policy. Our position, academically and in this book, is to take the broad route, exploring food policy as the accumulation of a number of core themes and subject matter; shaped by different disciplinary inputs and insights; and as a tussle between traditions and schools of thought. We favour studying food policy from an inter-disciplinary approach, aware that this makes it more complex; but we do so mindful, firstly, that policy-makers in government and industry alike draw widely from different disciplines and, secondly, that the evidence-base for sound food policy (not always what finally emerges!) is inter-disciplinary.

In sum, our conception of food policy is broad. The need for food policy to take this panoramic view has been recognized by others.[1, 2] We argue that food policy today—and in the past—involves diverse actors and institutions, at local, national, regional and international levels, not all immediately apparent or open to scrutiny. Food policy is not ordained by the state necessarily, although the state has a considerable role and stake in policy frameworks. We propose that the best way to understand food policy is as contested terrain, where actions and implications are tussled among interest groups and social forces from the state, supply chain and civil society. Each of these three nodes of the food policy triangle is explored throughout this book. This explains why, in our conception, food policy is inevitably contested space; it is made not ordained; its possibilities are therefore open for negotiation. It may be imposed or inherited from the past, but it can be re-shaped, made more democratically accountable, and made appropriate for the times in which we live, a time of environmental and health threat, yet with great promise and opportunity.

Disciplinary traditions

Many disciplines offer insights and stake claims on food policy. Their different approaches add to the richness and complexity of understanding, now coming into formal policy-making discourse.[3, 4] The list of disciplinary input to food-policy thinking—in alphabetical rather than intellectual order—includes the following:

- *Agricultural scientists* work on food production, agricultural systems and rural livelihoods, trying to balance increased output with maintenance of the land's capacity. Their expertise has underpinned the farm revolution of the last century and a half but increasingly they pay attention to the social dimensions of primary food production.[5, 6]

- *Anthropologists* analyse food as culture, a set of meanings, shared or otherwise.[7, 8] Contemporary Western society's approach to food is deciphering, through its meals and consumption.[9–13]

- *Biologists and bio-chemists* explore food as a combination of chemical and biological features, which can be well or badly managed, yielding improvements or failures to achieve potential. From Justus von Liebig's creation of fertilizers and beef extract to Gowland Hopkins' discovery of vitamins and the 21st century mapping of the genome, biological science's contribution to food policy has been hugely influential.

- *Economists* build on the two century-old analysis and political arguments of Adam Smith and David Riccardo that food is a traded commodity where markets can either work well or be bent to suit vested interests.[14] Their focus is on making markets more efficient, mostly through price mechanisms,[15] but not always.

- *Environmental scientists*, rather like food policy, draw widely from difference disciplines, bringing a focus on food's reliance and impact on the environment. Its influence on food policy grew rapidly with concerns about climate change, biodiversity, conservation, water shortage and population growth. Notions of carrying capacity and ecological survival now have high policy currency,[16] as has the kudos of scientists pooling knowledge to lever governmental action and policy change.[17, 18]

- *Epidemiologists* bring a skills set to food policy from public health. They focus on the nature, causation and prevention of diseases, bringing a population rather than individual perspective. Epidemiological data on diet's impact on non-communicable diseases such as heart disease and some cancers have been hugely important and also threatening.[19, 20] Food policy in the second half of the 20th century was heavily influenced by the battles between epidemiological analyses – arguing that changes in diet was creating preventable disease patterns – and food supply chain commitments to producing more but cheaper.

- *Geographers* study how the spatial world is affected by human demands, through products, process and place.[21, 22] Their contribution is to explain the interactions between humans and the spatial environment, mapping how commodities are produced in global networks of supply chains.[23]

- *Historians'* chronicles of food events have helped sift contemporary rhetoric from events, taking a long view of events. Modern food-quality scandals, for instance, are nothing new.[24] Exposés of adulteration consistently reshaped policy for two centuries.[25, 26]

- *Home economists* have been tasked with helping populations translate circumstances into feasible diets.[27–30] Their focus is on the domestic aspects of food—cooking, household management, budgeting, and the panoply of quotidian choices which shape what is eaten, by whom and why.[31, 32]

- *Journalists* have recently produced some powerful critiques of current food systems and captured an important slice of public discourse about its direction and implications.[33–36] The media is immensely important in framing discussion, not least playing to politicians' sensitivities. The role of journalism as both spotlight and commentator on how food is made and delivered is very old. Upton Sinclair's classic *The Jungle*, an exposé of the Chicago meat business in the early 1900s led to a Presidential inquiry and the framing of the US Food and Drug Acts.[37] Frederick Accum's 1820 *Treatise on Adulteration* tried to do the same in the UK but failed.[38] Journalists' role has been to speak directly to the public, guardians of the tradition of *caveat emptor* - buyer beware!

- *Nutritionists* came of age in the mid-19th century and refined understanding of the role of particular nutrients—proteins, vitamins, macro-/micro-nutrients and so on.[39, 40] Transferring this science into policy has not always been seamless, with battles over whether diet is being distorted by production.[41, 42] Modern nutrition ranges from exploring diet and genetic pre-programming [43, 44] to concerns about social inequalities in consumption.[45]

- *Political scientists* explore how institutions and political processes shape policy outcomes and they explain the ideas and concepts that inform these processes, such as authority, legitimacy, accountability and democracy.[4] Questions about decision-making on food policy have led to consistent reform of the institutional architecture of food.[47, 48]

- *Philosophers* have the oldest disciplinary pedigree, two thousand years or more of viewing food as location for moral dilemmas and daily philosophical choices.[49, 50] Contemporary issues range from children's rights in food behaviour change, the morality of meat-eating[51, 52] and the application of biotechnology[53, 54] to nutrigenomics.[55]

- *Psychologists*, since Sigmund Freud and William James began unravelling cognition and learning, have both studied and been paid to help alter consumption and choice.[56, 57] Edward L. Bernays, Freud's nephew, helped shift US marketing from being based on a model of rational behaviour to one that tapped unconscious meanings.[58]

- *Public health specialists* used to have to be medical doctors but may have wider disciplinary origins. They do, however, have to have a formal training in public health. Their role in many countries is as guardians of the protection of public health, ie the prevention of disease and the promotion of health. Historically, food has been a big concern and they have taken a leading role – particularly at the local level – in limiting low food standards and in highlighting how poor diet lowered life expectancy.[59] They have championed public health considerations in market-dominated economies' approach to, for instance, the obesity epidemic.[60, 61]

- *Sociologists* have a long tradition of studying rural life and the class relations of the countryside;[62] and also of their transition to urban living.[63] Today, social determinants studied range from gender to social class, to age.[64, 65] They have helped develop cultural analysis of consumption,[66–68] health and healthcare,[69] gender and body attitudes,[70] and trust relationships. [71]

Even this brief overview of disciplinary input to food policy suggests that good policy on food can and should draw widely, with no special disciplinary core or heart. Food policy is as good as the sum of its disciplinary parts. Whatever one's disciplinary training, the panoramic has to be retained. Against this perspective, it could be argued that food policy will never come of age as a discipline if it retains this broad multi-disciplinary focus. Good policy, like cutting-edge science, goes the argument, comes from mining down into detail, not remaining broad. Further, food policy might only become a defined discipline if it develops clear intellectual boundaries. This argument might be persuasive if the intent of food policy was to create a defined profession, like lawyers or medicine. Our view is that this would perpetuate one of the major traps for food policies; by not being aware of the broad context and not being alive to competing bodies of evidence, food policies can have unintended consequences. Turning vast quantities of land to biofuels exacerbated the food crisis of 2006–08, for instance. Biofuels appeared a good solution to energy shortage but decision-makers failed to make the connection with food stocks and food security concerns.

The argument favouring ever more detailed specialism in food policy does not fit the realities of governance. A 2008 report on UK food-retailing governance found that the UK government had at least 100 points of policy entry into the food supply chain, involving at least 19 government ministries, agencies and bodies.[72] In such a policy world, co-ordination and coherence become problematic. The remit of food policy has to remain broad but draw together various disciplinary expertises. Failure to do this can lock policy into a state of 'cacophony', loud incoherent noise without clarity or harmony.[73, 74]

If food policy draws on diverse expertise and evidence, what is it that defines food policy *per se*?

Four phases in the evolution of modern food policy

Food policy has long historical roots as a discourse, although the modern use of the term 'food policy' starts to emerge in the academic and policy litera-ture, and in unfolding events, in a serious and consistent way from the early 1970s. In this section, we focus mainly on modern food policy, which we take to be from the mid-20th century on. In a special issue on food policy of the journal *Development Policy Review*, later a book, Simon Maxwell and Rachel Slater argued that the 1970s and 1980s saw the emergence of a distinctive dis-course of food policy.[75] They drew a distinction between 'old' (1970s) and 'new' (2000s) food policy, proposing that food policy had changed its focus from agriculture to processed foods; from home to outside foods; from rural to urban; from micro-nutrient deficiencies to fats and sugars; from peasants to the urban poor; from food-based welfare relief schemes to income transfers.[76] In this shift, the focus of food policy had moved from agriculture and health ministries to ministries of trade, from development to consumer affairs, from a farm to macro-economic perspective. While we agree with some of their analysis and that a new era is indeed emerging, not least since we have long proposed this ourselves around ecological public health,[77–80] we disagree with the implicit assumption that food policy only begins in the 1970s. On the contrary, the 1970s position was really an adjustment of a policy approach built upon foundations laid in the post-war period, itself a reaction to the pre-ceding era of 1930s Depression. It is more helpful, therefore, to depict the broad evolution of modern food-policy from the mid-20th century as in phases. The first three were responses to shock or perceived threat, and a fourth is now unfolding before the challenges about society, health and environment; we characterize this phase as food policy for ecological public health.

1940s and 1950s: food policy as agricultural productionism

World War II sparked a fundamental reconsideration of policy direction. Within governments, among companies and wider society, even in the midst of war, there was intense reflection about the need to learn from, and prevent, the chaos in food and agricultural markets in the pre-war period. The 1930s had seen a global agricultural depression and collapse of markets, famously captured for the USA by Steinbeck's *The grapes of wrath*, a period of rural decline accompanied by rising urban unmet need.[81] Throughout the Western and Colonial world, scientists had documented unmet need alongside under-performing agricultural output.[82] The policy approach of an entire generation of policy thinkers and scientists was shaped by this experience. Whether looking at how to improve upland hill grassland farming,[5] or African and Indian output,[83] or whether from politics of the Left,[84] or the Right,[85] the 1930s and 1940s created a broad consensus that a new policy direction, mechanics of governance and instruments of policy were required. A shared view was that land was being poorly used and human needs were unmet. New interventions and investment were required to compensate for policy and market failure. Scientists had shown that it was possible to produce more food, reduce waste and feed people better, but this required markets to be shaped and directed. A new global vision was articulated, in which regions of the world that could raise their productive capacity (then thought to be North America and Europe) would feed those that could not (the main concern was then on Asia).

A new productionist framework posited that science plus capital and skills could do this. The war effort had shown the potential and prepared the ground for policy shift.[86, 87] Peacetime world food-policy should learn from what wartime planning experience at national and international levels can suggested might be done.[88] The form this took would vary in different parts of the world, of course. Ironically, wartime measures such as rationing showed the health advantages of the unprecedented intervention. This required a re-balancing of the state and private sector; controls replaced 'free' markets; funding was available for Agriculture Ministries to enable longer term planning with confidence; extension systems were created to improve skills; consumers were appealed to by new cultural messages, ranging from appeals to grow your own food ('dig for victory') to cutting down on waste and eating more unrationed home-grown vegetables ('food wasted is another ship lost'). Unlike after World War I, when the belated and reluctant intervention had been quickly rolled back,[89] in the 1940s there was acceptance that a return to 'business as usual' would be politically and socially unacceptable. Crisis spawned a more socially inclusive, equitable and progressive ideological basis for policy. Post-war, the offer from science was once and for all to banish the fear raised a century and a half earlier by the Rev. Thomas Malthus in his *Essay on the principle of population*.[90] Malthus had proposed that while population could grow geometrically, food supply could only increase arithmetically; action was needed, therefore, to contain excess population growth, to keep it in line with promised food advances.

Malthus made his proposition just as European land-owners in fact entered a period of systematic experimentation, such as with drainage, new breeds and equipment. With European colonial expansion in the 19th century, his prognosis appeared unfounded. Empires could feed burgeoning industrial populations. Wars and economic slumps in the early 20th century showed that under-feeding was an economic issue, rather than a population issue. The eugenics movement had resuscitated Malthus, in the early 1900s, promoting the argument that it was the poor who bred most children, ate worst and threatened population decline of intelligence. The argument had considerable traction, for instance spawning the UK's Inter-departmental Committee on Physical Deterioration, which published a eugenics-influenced report in 1904,[91] but such views faded with the horrors of systematic ethnic cleansing under Hitler. The World War II pressure for a new pro-active policy ('what are we fighting for?') was thus not just a reaction to the shock of war but to a previous ideological dalliance with notions of naturally ordained societal limits. Things could be changed. At least, under the first phase of post-World War II food policy, this optimism after hard times was captured. The new food policy was unleashed secure in the potential of new scientific evidence about raising output. Children could be better fed. Farms could grow more. Health and life-expectancy could be altered.[92] Utilizing a more complex understanding both of natural systems and farm potential, and of how markets could be improved by social goals, productionist food policy could increase output and settle questions of poor health and welfare. This new food approach was bracketed with international commitments to improve welfare; in the UK this was heralded by Beveridge's vision for national insurance and the case for addressing his Five Giants: Want, Ignorance, Disease, Squalor and Idleness.[93] But globally not dissimilar thinking emerged.[94]

This background helps explain the commitment to productionism. It was food policy's contribution to a better world post-war. Progress would defeat pessimism. The lessons of the 1930s and 1940s would move human food supplies into a new era, which would provide food for health. Boyd Orr and Mackintosh, both leading public health specialists of the day (both Scots), published popular versions of these arguments in the middle of the war, with an eye on capturing political as well as public imagination.[95, 96] They and others proposed agricultural reform and a new emphasis on agricultural policy. This coming together of agricultural and social reform to meet health and welfare goals was best expressed in a privately run Commission of Inquiry in the late-1930s. Viscount Astor and Seebohm Rowntree, both wealthy men, one from finance, the other from chocolate, but both socially liberal, came together in 1934 to conduct an inquiry into changing primary food production in the UK.[97] They republished and edited their findings in 1938, 1939 and 1941,[98] tapping the public imagination that food output could be increased. They reflected a scientific consensus that policy structures, not nature, held back production.[99] The role of policy was to remove the blockages and chart a different course. In Canada and the USA, similar sentiments were captured in new policies.[94] If the UK could increase its self-sufficiency from a mere 30% in 1939 to 60% by the end of the war, under dire wartime conditions, surely something had been wrong with policy before that?

One might ask: why did it take a war crisis to engender policy change? But it did. In food, the commitment was enshrined in the 1947 Agriculture Act, under Labour's Tom Williams MP. It reversed the former imperial power's reliance on its colonies; the Empire was haemorrhaging anyway. But the Act was informed by a moral duty to increase output and to ensure adequacy of supplies for public health. At the international level, similar motives spawned the creation of the United Nations' new Food and Agriculture Organization in the 1940s, headed by Sir John (later Lord) Boyd Orr.

Productionist food policy placed faith in a combination of science, capital and skills to defeat the old food enemies of want, unmet potential and social justice.[87] Productionism gave priority to technical advance but was informed by a social and health vision.[100] The assumption was that if farming could be induced to produce more, on more rational scientific advice, its output would increase and public goods and human welfare would follow. The public health message was: support agricultural output, which will increase supply, lower costs and make previously unaffordable food affordable. The old order of local food supplies being the sole route to health from food was to be banished by a new globalism, championed by the watchful and omniscient United Nations. A collective safety net could be built up by an international system of reserves.[101]

By the 1960s, optimists argued that the ambitious efforts that productionist food policies unleashed were proving effective. The combination of science, capital, state support and human endeavour was surely resolving the food problem. Wartime emergency systems were being made obsolete by new investment and state–farmer partnerships at global and national levels.[102, 103] Traditionalism was being transformed.[104] And output rose, food prices dropped, compared to previous era. Investment went into machinery, drainage, building. Hygiene accompanied efforts to improve distribution. To these ends, programmes were initiated throughout the world, turning unproductive land into production, sharing agronomic experience. In the Cold War era, east and west differed in who owned the land and how *dirigiste* and centralized their agricultural systems were, but they shared a vision of progress, albeit interpreted differently.[105] All states created funding schemes to support food production and distribution. Different regimes emerged.

The European Common Agricultural Policy (CAP) was created in 1957 by a new alliance of six countries previously fissured by war, Belgium, France, Germany, Italy, Luxembourg and Netherlands, now 27 countries of the European Union (EU).[106] The UK stayed out of this alliance, preferring its post-imperial links with its Commonwealth. In North America, then, as today, a powerhouse on world markets, the USA set out on a long sequence of subsidies (now in the Farm Bills) to fund particular food programmes, all designed on the one hand to suit national interests and on the other to deliver food security. Building on the New Deal (1929–54) and its 1933 Agricultural Adjustment Act, commodity price supports were introduced to attempt to provide confidence for farmers and to induce raised output. Farmers got paid for quantity; 'farm receipts were coupled to price and production'.[107] One view is that '[…] US farm policy has been described as a "cheap food" policy—in the broadest sense meaning the results of actions taken by the federal government to affect agriculture include lower retail food prices for consumers'.[108] If subsidizing farmers to raise output meant cheaper food for urban consumers, so be it. In the 1970s, this US price-support system evolved into income support for farming. The differences between US and European farm regimes need not detain us here; what matters is that this phase of food policy was altered by two shocks, bringing the first optimistic phase of postwar food policy to an end.

1970s: food policy for markets or development?

The shocks came in two forms.

Firstly, in 1971–74, public imagination was captured by two dreadful famines, in Sudan and Bangladesh, the latter sparking George Harrison of *The Beatles* to organize the first global rock concert in aid of development.[109] The famines questioned how effective and shared productionist policies were actually being, and whether food safety nets worked (see Chapters 7 and 8). Once more they raised the Malthusian spectre: could output keep up with population? A pessimistic prognosis had already been made by a US demographer Paul Ehrlich in a 1968 best-selling book.[110]

Secondly, Middle Eastern oil states raised oil prices, leading to escalating fuel and food prices. This exposed how oil-dependent Western societies had become in general and how food systems were particularly at risk. Analysts showed how oil had been the basis of much agricultural advance: tractors replacing animal power, agrichemicals, distribution systems. The over threefold rise of US maize (corn) yields in 1945–85, for instance, was due to a quadrupling of energy input.[111, 112] Oil was now shown to have underpinned much advance. The oil shock not only exposed farming but the powerful food processors and emerging food retailers, let alone Western car-owners. Whereas previously, Western Governments had relied either on imperial and military tentacles to secure oil supplies, by the 1970s they were locked into different options, needing Arab oil but constrained by Cold War politics.

These shocks—oil and famine—led to a flurry of policy action and analysis, suggesting that far from succeeding, the first phase of productionism had substituted one set of problems and failings for others. Neo-liberal economists seized their intellectual chance, arguing that the food system was heavily dependent on subsidies and that statist agri-economics were warped and irrational. Profesor D Gale Johnson, of Chicago University, for example, wrote that whether the European Community grew in numbers or not—as it was then poised to do—mattered less than that its agricultural support system distorted free markets and drained state funds.[113] Market liberalization, not state-funded support, would resolve the new difficulties. Agricultural support should be reduced to let markets drive food supply dynamics. The optimism and moral appeal of the Boyd Orr, Grondona, Astor and Rowntree generation's food policies was 'old'; they required a dose of market reality. The first step should be to reduce subsidies and the general goal should be to allow free markets to operate. Commerce had been held back for too long; it needed to be given free rein to be responsive to consumer needs rather than the depth of the public purse. Distortions only led to market failure.[114]

Giant commercial groups had already begun long-term futures research, which reinforced such thinking. The Club of Rome produced its influential *Limits to growth* report arguing the symbiosis of consumerism, oil use and threats to the environment and food security.[115] The FAO and UN system began the laborious process of bringing governments together to discuss policy implications of the crisis, culminating in the 1974 World Food Conference.[116] Academic researchers argued that the 30-year pursuit of food growth through investment in production needed more emphasis on social, not just technical, development.[117] New research bodies were created. In 1971, the Consultative Group on International Agricultural Research (CGIAR) was formed, a global network of agricultural research institutes investing in 'green revolution' plant breeding (funded by the Ford and Rockefeller Foundations, one with wealth from motor cars, the other from oil).[118] In 1975, the International Food Policy Research Institute (IFPRI) was created to bring a policy focus to the then four (now 15) institute membership CGIAR, injecting a food-policy dimension to what hitherto had been an agronomic, technical approach.[119]

Through this period, tapping into vibrant student and political awareness about development not necessarily being the Western route—arguments about individual versus collective wealth, societal versus individual progress—was threaded a burgeoning civil society presence. Organizations sprang up to lobby at the World Food Conference, heralding the first of now routine civil society or 'alternative' conferences. Worldwide, new non-governmental organizations (NGOs) sprang up in response to worries about food supply and starvation. This partly reflected the new planetary consciousness, and partly the counter-culture, the view that formal politics was not serving the public interest.[120] In the USA, the Institute for Food and Development Policy, now called Food First, was set up on earnings from Frances Moore Lappé's best-selling book *Diet for a small planet*.[121] In 1974, the Worldwatch Institute—publisher since 1981 of the annual State of the World reports—was founded by Lester Brown who, in the same year, wrote an early environmental analysis of food.[122] In the mid-1970s, too, the British Society for Social Responsibility in Science formed the Agri-capital and Politics of Health Groups.[123] Throughout Latin America, Africa and the Far East, solidarity organizations emerged to support liberation movements, many taking food as a key focus in their pitch for development. Development and environmental NGOs from Greenpeace and Friends of the Earth to Oxfam and church-based charities tapped and shaped public concern. The journal *Food Policy* was founded in 1975 with Geoff Tansey its first editor; its vision, according to Tansey, was broad: to bring together and make coherent the disparate perspectives and problems; to try to weave some order from the disparate inputs. Food policy was to be a rational exercise merging knowledge systems.

This, then, was the era that Maxwell and Slater characterized as the old food-policy. It was not in fact 'old' but itself a reaction to the perceived failings of the previous era, in turn a response to war and 1930s economic malaise. The 1970s was but another phase, not the founding phase, of modern food-policy. The confusion about historical starting points is, however, common in the literature.

John Tarrant's book *Food policies* published in 1980 was an early book attempting to apply academic rigour to the analysis of then current food policy, standing back from the policy-making process yet clearly engaged with the problems of development and environment.[124] Tarrant, surprisingly, barely defined food policy. The meaning is left implicit. The function of food policy is pure 1970s: to feed more people, equitably and soundly, with a focus on development. His use of the plural tense—policies not policy—in the title underlines that he was clear that food is something fought over by competing interests. He is equally clear about what over-arches and defines food policy:

> Two closely related spectres haunt the future world: a shortage of food and a shortage of energy. In both cases the trend in world consumption appears to be outstripping our capability to produce.

For Tarrant, food policy is about enlightened government intervention. The starting position for all government interventions is the need to bolster or otherwise shape agriculture. Agriculture is still the core issue for global food policy: '[f]ood policies and agricultural policies are two overlapping subsets of overall economic policy'. The goal is to achieve output within emerging energy constraints, an energy focus supported both by big industrialists and environmental scientists.[125]

A year earlier, the Centre for Agricultural Strategy at Reading University had published another view, a return to the public health theme of the 1940s. Christopher Robbins' *National food policy in the UK* was an important early recognition of the need to connect agriculture with the findings from public health nutrition, already troubled by epidemiological evidence about the impact of excess fat consumption on ill-health in rich countries.[126] Robbins' report, from an influential academic centre, delivered a salvo against the dominant model within UK and European agricultural policy, still confirmed in its belief that ensuring ample output would deliver health, welfare and progress. Robbins argued that health gain could no longer be guaranteed merely by farm output. He argued the need to analyse:

> [...] the relationships between the supply of foods, their distribution, and their role in health and welfare. These relationships are neither self-evident nor at present major considerations in providing the UK food supply.

This new nutrition focus stemmed from internationally shared research about the health impact in rich countries of excessive and inappropriate diets.[127] Developing countries meanwhile still faced burdens associated with deficiency. This bifurcated nutrition perspective—under-nutrition and over-/mal-nutrition—within food policy, still present in the early 21st century, first emerges in the late-1970s. But the malnutrition strand was pre-eminent. Only the US and UK alone had openly embraced the market-oriented approach, as had international finance bodies. The approach to food policy in the developing world was still statist and 'top-down'. Centrally-led initiatives aimed for sufficiency; consumerism was the preserve of affluent countries only. At this time, Dwyer and Mayer argued that food policy for the developing world must primarily take a nutrition-led approach, adapting to political processes:[128]

> Governmental nutrition policy, given appropriate conditions for the feasibility of its development, is determined by the body politic. Inasmuch as nutrition is usually recognized to be, at least in part, a technical area, scientists (health specialists, nutritionists and economists) are generally called upon to advise legislators, cabinet ministers, and planners in the formulation and implementation of policy.

In the 1970s and 1980s, we also begin to see a recognition that modern food-policy is only partly about *whether* and *how* food production can be raised; the other half is about *what* is produced and consumed and how equitably.[46] Robbins implicitly asked: if more fatty, sugary foods are produced and consumed, how is that a success? What is needed is a food system that delivers a health-inducing diet, not just quantity. He showed, for the UK, how dietary change was creating problems even for a rich country. UK standards of living had fallen in 1970–77, a time of inflation, with expenditure on food declining as a proportion of household disposable income, yet with rising food prices, 'suggesting that the composition of food purchases must also have changed'. He was correct. Diets had changed due to a revolution in food production and cultural change due to an explosion of new products, changed modes of consuming and marketing. Rising prosperity had led to changed lifestyles, such as foreign travel and shopping at supermarkets. This transition occurred first in the USA then throughout the West,[129] and is now rolling through the developing world.[130–133]

In the 1970s, the UK, for example, still had self-sufficiency as a formal goal for agriculture. Originally laid down in the 1940s, this altered its mode of delivery shifting from a system of deficiency payments (introducing canteens to enable workers to stay at work during breaks rather than return home) when the UK joined the Common Agricultural Policy in 1975.[134] The CAP, too, equated food policy with agriculture.[135] Robbins saw food policy's necessary adoption of the modern nutrition challenge through food planning, with the state in charge:

> In the light of current problems facing both the agricultural and food industries a national food policy would be a useful extension to the existing planning and policy machinery. Such a policy is both necessary and possible in the UK.

This emphasis on planning echoed the war-time experience, a high point of rational food policy. It was certainly the high point of food control. Lord Woolton, the Minister of Food in World War II, had been understandably proud of his Department's record. He was a practical man and saw food policy as a practical issue: 'The outstanding problem in feeding the nation became that of finding the necessary shipping space'.[33] In the section of his memoirs headed 'Food Policy', his focus was actually on planning and managing the planning process. His attention was on having a clear overall objective of feeding all the people; doing this equitably and to adequate nutritional standards defined scientifically; minimizing waste, rationalizng shipping and logistics space (for instance, requiring overseas suppliers to de-bone meat to save shipping space and weight); contributing to the war effort by helping labour be more efficient (introducing canteens to enable workers to stay at home in breaks rather than return home), thus building the eating-out market; and initiating new welfare food services to meet unfilled need, such as by the dependent elderly, and ensuring pregnant women received their requisite nutrition in dire times. For Woolton, food policy had been a practical task, harnessing state power. His approach, also catalogued by Hammond in the official history, provides the archetype of 'top-down' food policy.[32] It was not without reason that Sir William Beveridge titled his history of World War I experience *Food control*.[89] He was that World War I's lead civil servant in the experimental Ministry of Food, (reluctantly) set up in 1916, closed hastily in 1919 but deemed to have been so effective that its experience was the basis for the next war's ministerial control system.

To return to the second post-war phase, we find this statist top-down approach to food policy began to fragment. One emerging strand was development-oriented, the other more on mal-consumption. For both strands, the core solution still lay with agriculture. It is agriculture that Tarrant, Robbins and many others in the early 1980s wanted to reform, whether for health or welfare.[136] The key actor appealed to was the state; it is governments who can shape the direction and refine policy instruments using planning and co-ordination. As Robbins stated, the 'approach to food supply policy and national food policy outlined here is essentially a planning process which would seek to rationalise conflicting and coincident interests'.[126] The assumption was that food policy could be controlled; the implicit made explicit; the public good shaped by public action. There was conflict—such as health versus production interests—but this could be managed by a beneficent state.[137]

This appeal to a rational state may have been an honourable call to listen to evidence, but the confidence was misplaced. It coincided with the triumph of free-marketers over social democracy and Fabianism. Hayek, Friedman and Chicago economics replaced Keynesianism.[114] Markets replaced planning. Company-consumer dynamics replaced state policy and planning. Agricultural and food subsidies went from being conceived of as positive to being a drag on spending power. At the same time, market power and control began to move from food processors—who had mainly benefited from the plentiful and subsidized food commodities produced by supported farming— to the rapidly concentrating food retail chains who acted as gate-keepers to the new consuming classes.[138] The tectonic plates of food power were in the process of shifting, leaving food policy focused on a sector that had declining power. We return to this dynamic in Chapter 5.

One of the only attempts to set out a workable systematic definition of what is meant by food policy was made by the Organization for Economic

Cooperation and Development (OECD). In a report from its Agricultural Working Party in 1981, the OECD defined food policy as those policies affecting food—its supply and impact—that reflect 'the dominant priorities and objectives of governments…'.[139] Food policies are those that govern the food economy, defined as 'the set of activities and relationships that interact to determine what, how much, by what method and for whom food is produced'. Creating public policy on food is a 'dynamic [process] in which there is continual interaction and reaction'. As an inter-governmental research and advice body for rich countries—such as those who had suffered intellectual shock from the 1970s oil rises—the OECD had asked its Agricultural Working Party to provide a better and more up-to-date approach to food policy. It was aware that agriculture was increasingly subject to other demands from the supply chain. Processors wanted different products (frozen peas, uniform carrots, more potatoes for chips and snacks). Retailers were beginning to exert power on growers by setting tighter specifications. The OECD Working Party, therefore, adopted a 'systems' approach, reducing the focus on agriculture but instead taking an overview of all the constituent parts of the food system. Its systems approach carried assumptions. The key policy actor was still the state. Food policy is:

> … a balanced government strategy regarding the food economy, which takes account of the interrelationships within the food sector and between it and the rest of the national and international economy.

Food policy here is still what governments do; other actors are down-played. Consensus and identity of interest are also assumed; the system is rational and open to order. The task of food policy is to put policy in command of the dynamic nature of the food system, a position restated two years later by World Bank development economists, still agriculture-oriented:[15]

> Food policy encompasses the collective efforts of governments to influence the decision-making environment of food producers, food consumers, and food marketing agents in order to further social objectives.

For Tarrant, by contrast, '[f]ood policies and agricultural policies are two overlapping subsets of overall economic policy…'.[124]

1980s–2000s: the slow emergence of ecological crisis and market failure

From the mid-1970s, international bodies such as the FAO redoubled efforts to help build output. The engine on which they delivered this policy was in fact already underway, even before the early 1970s policy crisis had unfolded. A new 'green revolution' was already emerging from plant breeders in the late-1960s. This agronomic revolution combined F1 hybrid seed breeding, high use of agrichemicals (fertilizers and pesticides) and irrigation.[140] The technology was high input/high output and was developed under the auspices of the CGIAR research institutes for rice and wheat, particularly, and it won Norman Borlaug, known as the father of the Green Revolution, the Nobel Peace Prize in 1970 for his work sponsoring the new plant technologies in the developing world. The Green Revolution has been much debated. It raised output considerably but restructured peasant agriculture and favoured intensive monocultural systems. Within the developing world, its higher cost favoured peasants with larger, rather than small, holdings; it hitched development to commercial agri-business companies and made small-holders dependent on seed companies to buy new seed each year, rather than retained (free) their own seed for next year's planting. Supporters argue that Borlaug and colleagues saved hundreds of millions of lives, which otherwise would have faced Malthusian conditions. Critics argue that this tied agriculture to an intensive, unsustainable model.[141] It broke with traditional farming methods, which can be more environmentally benign and sustainable.[142] It was linked with rising evidence of health and environmental impacts, such as from pesticide use for farm labour, residues for consumers and run-off from fertilizers.[143–146]

Thus fed by the anxieties and crisis thinking at the 1974 World Food Conference in Rome, pressures to increase output continued; productivity was the measure for success. With important modifications, government-led productionism continued to be the dominant policy framework, but a social agenda was also strongly championed by pro-development NGOs such as Oxfam, arguing that human development required social justice not just technological fixes. A new tension in food policy came into the open, replacing the previous consensus (phase 1) and uneasy truce (phase 2). The tension was not just between agriculture and the land on the one hand and post-farm food forces on the other, but between technical and social means. Would food gain be better achieved by science and technology or by community empowerment? Hi-tech or low-tech? People-centred or expert-centred?

But even as this policy dilemma was being fought over by political processes—neo-liberal market approaches versus liberation movements, developing versus developed worlds, open versus closed political systems, etc.—evidence was mounting about four cross-cutting crises, all noisily championed by a new generation of public interest NGOs in the West; present but not articulated in the same way in the communist states. The first, as we have already suggested, concerned nutrition, specifically problems associated with mal-consumption. The second concerned community development.

The third was environmental. The fourth was food safety. In the 1970s–1990s, these all came to a head, with rising urgency partly due to the failure or reluctance of policy adequately to address them.

The first three issues have already been raised and are amplified in subsequent chapters (see Chapters 4, 5, 6 and 8), so here we will sketch the importance of food safety. Ironically, it was safety rather than the others that first seriously dented Western and then international food policies in the late-1980s. As with nutrition, a deep fissure between developed and developing worlds existed. Whereas poor hygiene has long troubled developing country food supplies, due to lack of investment, resources and harsh circumstances, rich countries prided themselves on having resolved the late-19th century problems of adulteration and safety. Municipal authorities had been given powers to inspect and control food quality at the local level from the late-19th century. Safety issues could be addressed by public health inspection and monitoring.[30, 147] Mid-20th century food-borne infections occurred, of course, but were deemed to be more of a problem where public health infrastructure was weak. Events such as the 1964 Aberdeen typhoid outbreak were judged rarities, albeit reinforcing the need for vigilance, particularly with public relations and internationally.[148] Western food policy-makers generally considered safety to be under control. Food monitoring systems and high scientific professional standards protected the public from unfit food.

This state of affairs was shattered in a few years, 1987–92, in Europe, largely due to a series of food scandals in the UK. After some years in which issues such as additive and pesticide safety had been championed as consumer and worker concerns by NGOs worldwide,[145, 149] a sequence of food safety crises erupted that exposed governments and politicians as complacent, food laws as inadequate and food production systems as lacking in requisite controls. Food-poisoning cases were rising on both sides of the Atlantic. New phage types of infection emerged, mostly with meat; salmonella incidents were becoming more prevalent due to mass catering. Countries had their scandals, Sweden with a 1950s outbreakthat killed 100 people; the UK in the early 1980s with salmonella in eggs and poultry.[150] Political sensitivities rocketed, most infamously and significantly, with an outbreak of bovine spongiform encephalopathy (BSE or 'mad cow disease') in the UK in the late-1980s. The aetiology and mishandling of this episode has been comprehensively documented.[48, 151] There are still competing interpretations of what happened but it is likely, either that consumption by UK cattle of rendered remains of sheep with scrapie, a related disease, or that a spontaneous mutation occurred. Either way, UK cattle were infected by an horrendous new neurological wasting disease, for which controls were only very slowly put in place.

The disease was identified in 1986 but tough controls did not begin to be put in place till 1988, and not before humans had been exposed through consumption of contaminated meat and meat products. Again, the precise aetiology cannot be confirmed, but 10 human cases of variant Creutzfeld Jakobs Disease (vCJD) were confirmed in 1996. As the official inquiry headed by Lord Phillips, a High Court judge, succinctly stated:[152]

> For ten years, the government told the people: there is no evidence that BSE can be transmitted to humans; it is most unlikely that BSE poses any risk to humans; and it is safe to eat beef.

All these statements were wrong, complacent and showed a presumption of risk that favoured industry before public health. The result was international fury, a crisis over food safety that spread worldwide, changes in laws, and even the resignation of the entire Commission of the European Commission. It spawned a new wave of food safety institutions—the European Food Safety Authority, the UK's Food Standards Agency, etc.—all set up at arms-length from day-to-day control by politicians. In the UK, it led to the abolition of the Ministry of Agriculture, Fisheries and Food. One of the first nations to create a Department of State dedicated to agriculture (in 1875) was one of the first to abolish it (in 2001), subsuming its residue into a more environmentally-focused department, the Department for Environment, Food and Rural Affairs (Defra). Food safety can truly be said to have heralded the demise of policy focus on agriculture.[77, 153]

We see this policy transition reflected in academic definitions. Mennell and colleagues, in 1992, gave a definition of food policy almost inconceivable before this period:[65]

> Food policies [are] intended to be coherent bodies of measures. There are two main goals: first, to prevent illness and to further public health by informing people about the importance of a 'prudent diet'. (...) Second, a food policy purports to guarantee the safety of food products, which means issuing and enforcing rules and regulations for food producing, food processing and food distributing companies.

Tansey and Worsley's 1995 *The food system* confirmed the arrival of food safety thus: '[w]e see the challenge of food policy as being to produce a safe, secure, sufficient, sustainable and nutritious diet for all, equitably.'[1] Acknowledging this transition—not just safety but cultural, environmental and health challenges—led Maxwell and Slater in 2003 to write:[76]

> ...the 'new food policy' cannot be ignored, even by the poorest countries. The world food system... is no longer the chrysalis it once was. The pace of change is accelerating. The challenges are daunting. They are immediate. And they need to be on the agenda of policy-makers throughout the developing world. A preoccupation with food security is no longer sufficient. It is necessary to rediscover food policy.

Food policy was thus cast as the bridge between competing perspectives: developing and developed; safety and nutrition; farm and consumer.

The emerging third phase agenda was complex and multi-dimensional. Arguably in the 1980s, food policy entered a confused period. In one direction, it was being pulled towards the language of markets. In another, new evidence about the environment, health, international divisions and consumer behaviour called for a renewed public protection agenda. Marketization was dominant with its language of consumers, choice and cheapness. The state's role in food should be minimal; nanny states should not be a barrier between consumers and their right to buy and eat what they want. Economically, farming had to be weaned off subsidies. But the food safety crises, which emerged around the world in the 1980s and 1990s, brought this ideological position into some disrepute. Surely urban consumers could not possibly know what was in their food, and deserved to be able to shop free from fear. Pressure to improve safety standards sent shockwaves down global sourcing supply routes, fanned by global media and consumer bodies calling for tougher controls.

Food safety thus began to erode the then dominant policy thinking known as the Washington Consensus, a term given by John Williamson, a World Bank economist, in 1989 to describe a policy package designed to wean the developing world—and any developed country that gets into fiscal crisis—from dependency on state funding.[154] The Washington Consensus suggested that policy should deliver ten features. Fiscal discipline should be defined in neoliberal terms. Economic growth is the route to public goods. Subsidies are frowned on. Trade should be liberalized. Exchange rates should be realistic and not artificially propped up by the state. Barriers to foreign direct investment (FDI) should be dismantled to allow big (usually Western) companies to enter markets easily, and free flow of capital across borders. State bodies should be, where possible, privatized; or, if not, deregulated. Property rights should be enshrined. These ten principles, championed by the world's economic powerhouses and their financial bodies, the World Bank and International Monetary Fund, over-arched any food policy initiatives, which were necessarily subservient. This led to considerable tension within bodies such as the FAO, which was heavily criticized for accepting fiscal rectitude above food justice. While the Western world continued to experience rising living standards and enough developing countries boomed to keep the economic paradigm in place, the distress from the losers could be kept at bay, although it was increasingly documented and acknowledged by the World Bank itself and the UN system in various annual reports.[155-158] Interviewed in May 2008, in the middle of the food crisis of that year,

Williamson himself remained convinced of the correctness of the Washington Consensus. 'My own view is that all those things are good for countries,' he said. 'But I'm not terribly sympathetic with the World Bank going in and laying down a list of things countries have to do.'[159] This, however, is what it tended to do.

The third phase of post-war food policy may thus be characterized as a period of fragmentation. It returned—with a vengeance—as a health issue in the developed world, while remaining a sore in the developing world, increasingly articulately championed by well-organized NGOs.[160–162] Mounting evidence about supposedly efficient food systems' social, environmental and health costs put the intensification model under strain. Environmentalists were particularly quick to document externalized costs,[163] but food and health policy analysts learned to do so too.[164] By the 2000s, official UK Government audits contained calculations of the high cost of 'cheap' food policies due to obesity and its on-costs alone.[165, 166]

In the wider economic sphere, the Washington Consensus and dominant policy-thinking came under pressure almost as soon as the Cold War ended with the Soviet Union's collapse from 1989. Far from the end of ideology,[167] the period saw the rise of China as an industrial power servicing the West, political realignments in Latin America and rising concern about energy, ecological and climate change threats.

The legacy of the first three phases of modern food policy development lies in the institutions and policies created. Table 2.1 illustrates some of these initiatives, globally, regionally, nationally, and locally.

21st century: rising to the challenge of ecological public health?

A new phase in food policy is unfolding. Evidence that the current food system was unsustainable had mounted throughout the last quarter of the 20th century, documented on a variety of fronts. They include the following:

- volatile world food prices in 2006–2008; reminded policy-makers that ever cheaper food cannot be assumed;[168]
- variable but peaking productivity growth;[169]
- a drop in world grain stocks and per capita grain availability;[170]
- fish stocks under strain and near or actual collapse in some areas;[171–173]
- concerns about the impact of meat consumption and the nutrition transition;[174–176]
- serious consequences of climate change;[177]

Table 2.1 Some examples of food-policy initiatives: global, regional, national and local

Policy level	Date	Body	Policy Occasion / Declaration
Global			
	1948	UN	Universal Declaration of Human Rights
	1974	FAO	World Food Conference
	1975	CGIAR	Creation of International Food Policy Research Institute to provide policy support to end world hunger and malnutrition
	1981	OECD	Agriculture Working Group 'Food Policy' statement
	1992	UN	Rio Declaration of the UN Conference on Environment & Development
	1996	UN	World Food Summit
	2000	UN	Millennium Development Goals
	2004	FAO/WHO	Global Strategy on Diet, Physical Activity and Health
Regional			
	1957	Europe	Common Agricultural Policy created at the Stresa Conference
	1988	WHO Europe	Healthy Nutrition strategy proposed
	2000	European Union	EU White Paper on Food Safety
	2000	WHO Europe	European Food and Nutrition Policy (51 countries sign on)
	2006	WHO Europe	Istanbul Charter on Counteracting Obesity
National			
UK	1947	Gov't	Agriculture Act
	1976	Gov't	Food from our own resources White Paper
	2000	Gov't	Food Standards Act
	2002	Gov't	Policy Commission on the Future of Food and Farming (Curry Commission)
	2005	Gov't	Defra Sustainable Food and Farming Strategy
USA	2008	Gov't	Farm Bill (settles subsidies for set period)
Local			
Canada	1991	City Council	Toronto Food Policy Council created to promote local food security
Scotland	1996	Scottish Executive	Scottish Diet Action Plan

Continued

Table 2.1 (continued) Some examples of food-policy initiatives: global, regional, national and local

Policy level	Date	Body	Policy Occasion / Declaration
Local			
England	1984	Greater London Council	London Food Commission created to be a 'food policy council' for Londoners on food health and education
	2006	FSA + NGC	Food Standards Agency & National Governors' Council agreed strategic policy framework on 'Food Policy in Schools'

+ rise of water stress and shortages hitting agriculture, as well as direct human drinking use;[178]

+ rapid rise in oil prices; these hit $140 a barrel in mid-2008 from $40 a barrel in 2006, exposing (again) the reliance of food systems on oil;[179]

+ realization that world markets could not be relied upon to feed people if their own financial strength is weakened;[180]

+ a recognition that agriculture is still a primary industry, the world's largest employer and key to human development;[156]

+ continued food insecurity in many low income countries;[158]

+ urbanization bringing new food dependencies for the remaining rural populations;[181, 182]

+ the impact and cost of changed dietary behaviour and the nutrition transition partly due to rising affluence but also due to marketing;[131]

+ the considerable footprint of animals' use of land, grain and water and the implications of rising meat and dairy consumption;[175]

+ deep ecological crisis threatening food capacity, biodiversity and soil.[6]

+ old as well as new forms of waste due to spoilage, packaging, inappropriate consumption.[183]

These new fundamentals suggest how marketized food policy has lost direction and that its benefits now need to be set against serious faults. Often 'solutions' offered for one problem create a knock-on effect elsewhere. A new vision for food will have to aim for improvement on all fronts. Scale, breadth and integration of response will be key words for 21st century food-policy.

Awareness of evidence about the new fundamentals contributed to a developing global food crisis in 2005–08, leading to high-level meetings at national and global levels throughout 2008.[184] Favourite formulae were much repeated by different interests: trade liberalization; the unfairness of trade rules; the need for GM foods and other technical solutions; the case for small-scale farming; the case for and against biofuels; the role of speculation; and more.[185] Government food policy-makers could no longer avoid the weight and range of evidence that the current policy paradigm was not delivering adequately and that new directions were appropriate and desired, even by large commercial enterprises.[186] A fourth phase of modern food-policy has begun, with decisions now being made that will shape the 21st century.[187] Much depends on whether this process is fully grasped or is fumbled. Optimists argue that this phase is but the slow march towards sustainable development, a re-alignment of economic, social and environmental policy, long heralded by the Brundtland Commission in 1987, the UN Conference on Trade and Development in 1992, and the World Food Summit in 1996. Others argue that, despite the need for change, paradigm shift has not occurred and that strong forces still favour a return to business as usual. Uncertainties could be identified; mapped in different scenarios.[169, 188]

For each of the new fundamentals of 21st century food-policy outlined above, there are competing solutions. As ever, in food policy, there is no single way; there are always options. The issue of water could be addressed, for instance, by more technology. The huge amount of water used in irrigation could be reduced and better targeted by droplet technology, releasing minute amounts of water slowly rather than in a rush (like a storm) into the soil or by building up soil structure to retain water, notably recycling plant, human and animal waste (which also builds fertility). Fertilizer prices could be addressed by genetically modifying plants to have leguminous nodules on their roots, thus helping them 'fix' nitrogen from the air rather than it being applied by farmers out of a bag; this has the advantage of giving quick results. Or the decision could be taken to build soil fertility by organic agriculture. There is a myriad of such options: intensive or organic? Functional foods or dietary change? Biofuels or food? In food matters, the mode of policy response to a problem is wide; rarely either static or fixed. Our point here is that there is wide agreement about the new fundamentals that food policy has to address. Unlike in the 1971–74 crisis, when the 'problem' was defined in terms mainly of energy and mal-distribution, today there are many: climate change, water, soil, land, biodiversity, urbanization, population, the nutrition transition, healthcare costs, as well as energy and social inequalities.

How could food policy-makers and institutions address this awesome array of problems? It will require considerable change, intelligence and effort.

Turning the fundamentals of ecological public health into goals for food policy

We see new cross-cutting food policy goals emerging as essential to address ecological public health. Six goals are outlined here and explored throughout the rest of this book. Each has a long record of being problematic for food policy; their emergence is not sudden, although the form and language they take may be.

Goal 1: achieving sufficiency of production on ecological terms

Food security is a term often used to indicate the perennial concern about hunger and famine at population level.[189] The goal of security of supply has been a persistent theme in many national and international food policies but the means for achieving, or claiming to achieve, sufficiency have varied, as have the geographical boundaries by which, and within which, this is deemed feasible.[117] The FAO encouraged governments in the aftermath of World War II to rebuild their national food systems by investing in food production to maximize output. Hence, the trauma of the early 1970s, outlined above, when the spectre of insufficiency of supply re-emerged. Was this because the policy recipe was wrong or badly implemented? Was it due, as some environmental demographers argued, to population growth reaching agricultural, if not planetary, limits?[190, 191] Or to failures of social justice?[192]

In fact, the evidence is that production kept ahead of the population curve. At least until the end of the 20th century, there was sufficiency of supply.[193] But the continued existence of malnutrition, famines and premature death due to insufficiency suggests that producing enough is not the same policy objective as distributing it equitably. Today, facing nine billion people by 2050, according to the UN,[182] the arguments for limits are being rehearsed. Under the Washington Consensus, until the 2000s, the dominant policy recipe for how to resolve hunger and food insecurity was international trade, a shift from the post-war focus on national supply systems and production. There is widespread agreement on the need to ensure a balancing of supply to demand, but the problems are about *how* to do so, within *which* political boundaries and with *what* incentives. Despite scientific and technical advances, 'efficient' food systems are hugely wasteful. It has been calculated that the UK, for instance, has a food system that operates as though it has three to five planets on which to draw—in land and sea, space and energy.[194] Although this food system has given unprecedented choice—30,000 items in hypermarkets— between one-third and a quarter of all sold as edible was thrown away each year, according to UK Government. Around 6.7 million tonnes (mt) of food waste is generated in UK homes each year, equivalent to a third of food bought. At least 50% of this could have been eaten and it generated the equivalent to 15 mt of CO_2. In financial terms, too, this was wasteful. A typical household in 2008 threw away between £250—£400 of food that could have been eaten.[195]

How can this wasteful food system be changed into one that feeds existing, let alone future, larger populations on sustainable grounds? This is no longer the Malthusian problem, but a problem of sustainable development, how to integrate nutrition with ecology and social justice.[6, 196, 197]

Goal 2: preventing diet-related ill-health (within a sustainable food supply)

Nutrition, microbiological safety and contamination have been troublesome for policy. They cast the state in the role of arbiter, if not always honest broker, of risks. Modern thinking about risk has put emphasis on consumer information but, ultimately, laws place the onus on food to be fit to eat before a consumer purchases it. This ideological element was a constant theme for late-20th century food policy-makers who were wary of being blamed for putting undue risks on public health, yet also keen not to be criticized for being the 'nanny state'. This theme had been voiced, too, in the 19th century as Western industrial societies debated what to do about health. Reformers won the argument then that prevention was preferable, less costly and more efficient than expecting families to protect themselves, which they patently could not. Hence, the classical period of public health. Engineering provided health solutions in the form of drains, clean water, better housing, work conditions... and food standards.[28, 29, 198, 199] And social reformers highlighted the ill-health of the industrial city poor, stressing how inequality of opportunity at society's base led to lost talent, a pool of dissatisfaction and a persistent reminder of market failure. Tackling hunger was not just humane but added to the greater good of all.[200] The poor and the unhealthy have needs, express them, yet they were badly fed, could not afford to eat healthily and thus suffered premature death and under-performance (see Chapter 7).

But can—if so how—that 19th and 20th century experience be translated for the 21st century? Technical solutions include altering food composition, fixing 'good' attributes into foods and lowering fat, for example. Since the mapping of the genome, nutri-genomics tantalizes policy-makers with the possibility of tailoring individualized solutions to dietary problems.[201, 202] Arguments about obesity policy have been a key site for such policy debates.[203] Now, however, food's health impact has to be dove-tailed with sustainability. After a century or more in which the goal has been to raise output to fill stomachs, is the agenda changing to one in which human physiological need is to be met sustainably? Rather than health being an outcome of food systems, the new vision is that health and ecology should be at their heart.[204]

Goal 3: harnessing all sciences to address the nature of production

Charting a course for food policy that is multi-functional, in that it meets various goals simultaneously, requires good information and exchange with a wide range of sciences and information sources. Part of the case explored in this book is that governance is partial, both in the sense that political processes filter what happens and in that policy is based on limited perspectives, blinkered by circumstance and ideology. Power inevitably filters knowledge. For centuries in regions with long settlement—China, India, Europe— private land-owners and rulers experimented with new techniques, plants and animals, designed to raise output (not necessarily to feed people but for profit). Land enclosure was central to power and gave wealth to fund improvements in techniques such as drainage, motive power and buildings. From the 18th century, this process of knowledge accumulation accelerated, fuelled by emerging scientific knowledge, particularly chemistry, biology and husbandry. With the industrial revolution, the process took off; output improvement and efficiency were the goals. But alongside these roles, the new sciences could be used to unmask adulterations and fraud.[29] In the 20th century, another bout of scientific advance helped to raise production together with changes in food processing; again science generated reactions to what was perceived as—and sometimes was—de-naturing and neo-adulteration of food.[150, 205, 206]

In the late-20th century, technical change was accused of out-stripping public knowledge and confidence. Questions emerged from radical science about whether increasingly private domination of research and technical development meant that the public interest was not always met; partially, yes, in that goods sold but not fully in that problems were left out of the efficiency equation. Such questions emerged about GM, irradiation and, more widely, about intellectual property rights (IPRs).[207, 208] New budgets, social institutions (food agencies) and research programmes had to be put in place to institute monitoring and enable appropriate controls.[48] In the 21st century, a new coalition of disciplines is required for food policy to address the complex challenges already manifest. In the case of fish eating, for instance, nutritionists advise routine consumption, whereas environmental scientists recommend drastic curtailment or restriction only to eating plentiful species; but they would suffer catastrophic fall in numbers if the entire world ate them. This illustrates the need for cross-sectoral, better co-ordinated evidence gathering within policy. What should an ecologically minded but health-desiring consumer do: eat or not eat fish? Similar problems arise with regard to mainstays of diet: does it matter whether we eat just lots of fruit and vegetables or only ones that have been grown in a sustainable manner? Given the huge environmental impact of meat and dairy production, should everyone keep their consumption to a minimum, if at all; or only those who inhabit lands that could grow other food sources? What would a bio-regionally ecologically appropriate, health-enhancing diet look like? And could it be produced?

Goal 4: lowering food's impact on the environment

Ever since FH King's classic study of Chinese agriculture suggested that a good production system was one that built and protected its soil, fertility and diversity,[209] it has been clear that a societally benign food system should have a beneficial ecological impact. King argued that keeping soil fertile, returning all waste, would keep its productivity in 'tune' with climate, terrain and use; yields would be enhanced; and the system would retain what, in modern terminology, is called sustainability. King's appeal, and that of other writers in similar vein,[210] was lost in the rise of the industrial model of production and scientific farming. But today, the need for closed systems or waste-minimizing and sustainable ones has resurfaced (see Chapter 6).

In the 1960s, evidence surfaced from ecologists, zoologists and environmental scientists that the armoury of modern farming and food production had a downside. Famously, Rachel Carson summarized the case in her 1962 book *Silent spring*, on pesticides in particular.[211] Such arguments were derided initially by the dominant policy-makers but by the 1980s and 1990s, after numerous scandals about food quality, the question of production's reliance on the environment once more became a legitimate policy concern. But by then, policy was locked in to a particular mode. A conundrum—quantity versus quality, food output versus its environmental impact—runs throughout modern food policy. But this is not a new problem. From Cobbett and Thoreau in the 19th century to Balfour and King or McCarrison in the 20th, concerns have been voiced about the cost of 'civilization' and intensifying food production on the natural world.[209, 212, 213]

From the 1980s, international policy began to build a perspective on environmental protection. Conferences, declarations and positions, often featuring food and particularly agriculture, called for, or outlined, new directions, beginning with the report of the Commission on Environment and Development,[16] consolidated at the UN Conference on Environment and Development,[214] and confirmed as the seventh goal of the Millennium Development Goals.[215] At a national level, admirable commitments have been made. In 2005, the UK Government, for instance, set one of its five cross-government principles to be 'living within environmental limits'.[216] Many countries pay lip service to the need for their people to live within environmental limits, but results have not been delivered. More movement has been exhibited on 'soft' policy measures; giant companies have begun carbon labelling of foods, showing the embedded carbon in a packet of crisps and other processed products.[217] Such measures help to improve awareness of carbon and greenhouse gas emissions (GHGs) but are not a fast track to lowering the entire diet's or food system's GHGs. The challenge today is to engender change across a variety of measures: water, energy/climate change (GHGs), land use, health, ethics and social justice. We return to this in Chapter 5 in relation to how supply chains might address complex standards.

Goal 5: achieving international development and social justice

One of the arguments for the productionist goals of the 1940s and 1950s was that only they offered the chance of raising production sufficiently to feed Asia, then the epitome of unmet needs. In World War II, Boyd Orr appealed for massive post-war effort to feed India. Today Africa is often depicted as the new India but it would be misleading to paint the global food picture in over-simple terms. For decades, analysts and international bodies have documented the gross inequalities within, as well as between, states—in their wealth, the disposable income for food, their food output, the gap between their needs and their consumption. The 2007/08 UN Human Development Report showed how inequalities underpin even climate change, with the poorest peoples and economies most at risk from temperature change, soil loss, water and food shortages.[218]

The challenge for 21st century food-policy is how to address inequalities within, as well as between, countries. One expression is the fair trade movement, which seeks to raise the funding that gets back to the primary producer from end-consumers. Fair trade is a riposte to the sometimes harsh realities of 'free' trade and the exploitation of the labour process.[161, 219, 220] Buying individual items is helpful but, like carbon labelling, is indicative but not sufficient for system change. That is why supporters of fair trade have articulated the need to alter trade rules and international flows. But they have looked less at fair-traded products through the lens of nutrition or carbon reduction. The food-miles debate has been a rare example of a policy issue that has sparked cross-cutting debate; does it matter if food is sourced locally or from far away? A tomato grown outdoors and seasonally, embodies less carbon than one grown in a heated greenhouse locally but a-seasonally.[221] Water is likely to be another confounding cross-cutting issue for food standards, too. If a single stem of a Kenyan green bean embodies four litres of potable water—from a water-stressed country—are trade-earnings taking priority over sustainability? Such issues are immensely complex and we are not arguing for or against such trade, only that ecological public health criteria require important considerations to be considered simultaneously not in policy 'silos'. This requires helping consumers to drive and eat within a new ethical food culture, where ethics and morality blend with social justice. Again, this requires cross-disciplinary input, with social as well as bio-physical indicators.

Goal 6: food democracy

We see food democracy—a term to indicate the process of holding food systems accountable from the 'bottom up'[30, 222, 223]—as a challenge for ecological public health. The reflex of public health practice tends to be expert-led and top-down. Its greatest Western moments are often cited as the classical interventions, such as drainage and pure water in the 19th century or smoking restrictions in the 21st. Restructuring the entire food system, however, is unlikely to be achieved by such *dirigisme*. Indeed, even those 'great moments' were only achieved due to sustained engagement with the mass of populations or the neutralization of opponents to restructuring. Either way, we propose that food policy-making needs to take full account of *how* to achieve the new market-consumption nexus in a framework of ecological public health and sustainable development.[224–225]

Food democracy is a term referring to the long process of striving for improvements in food for all, not the few, incorporating the principle of food citizenship with the rights and responsibilities this brings.[226] Its core idea is that food is a locus of the democratic process: the interest of the mass, the 'bottom-up' over 'top down', the building of social movements to embed rights into culture and expectations.[87] It may be a human right for all to have access to affordable, decent, health-enhancing food but this often has to be struggled for. By contrast, 'food control' is the use of food as a vehicle of control. One example is US Public Law 480 which used US food surpluses as food aid given on favourable terms, as part of US foreign policy.[46] An earlier example was the story of sugar, slavery and the British industrial working class diet.[228] The long tussle between food control and democracy has been manifest in campaigns as well as daily resistances, and in the slow march for decent food,[29, 30, 229] for living wages,[230] and for just welfare benefits for women and children sufficient to eat adequately.[231, 232] Without such pressures—of which many countries have their equivalent—the 'top-down' debate about food policy would have been different.

Governments today tend to talk of partnerships with industry when seeking change, but this down-plays the potential for democratic engagement.

Large food companies, by contrast, routinely use a formidable armoury of consumer research methods, from focus groups to analysing checkout till receipts, as indications of consumer preferences by demographic location (see Chapter 5 on the rise of supply chain power). From a democratic perspective, such methods are about the moulding of food consciousness, while playing to the language of choice. Companies in fact choice-edit products before the consumer sees them on shelves. Predilections to eat particular foods are also shaped by class, culture, tradition and income. This is why some food marketers see the checkout till as replacing the polling booth. Every time one buys a food, it is a 'vote' for that product. The more consumed, the higher the vote. Ecological public health perspectives, on the other hand, have to engage with the limits of choice that are also exposed.

In the 21st century, we inherit complex systems of accountability and governance (see Chapter 3). In distantly sourced, cleverly marketed and packaged food, consumers may not know what happens to their food before they see it. Somehow culture, as well as the supply chain, has to become more accountable for sustainability. Even in the 19th century, when policy-making was archetypically 'top-down', generating laws and regulations, popular pressure was an important factor in shaping supply. In the transition from a rural to an urban capitalist society, the UK witnessed a re-negotiation of social relations over food. The 'entitlement' that medievalism gave the villager was replaced by urban relations of market reliance and survival.[233] In the 20th century, reactions to the powerful food industry and retail interests, with their use of company regulations, contracts and specifications in lieu of law, has not gone unremarked or uncontested.[234, 235] If consumers feel constrained by market power, they voice it. In harsh or less democratic circumstances, the ultimate sanction is the food riot. The last UK food riots were in the 18th century; in 2008, 37 countries rioted over rapidly escalating global commodity food prices shaping what they could buy locally. Food democracy is expressed in different forms.

The emerging agenda

This chapter has introduced our understanding of what food policy is and is claimed to be. Our analysis is that food policy, like other policy spheres, has its own traditions, arguments and institutions. These are not hermetically sealed, the property solely of food policy. Nonetheless we can define food policy as shaped by those concerns. Table 2.2 provides an overview of how the fundamental problems outlined in this chapter might be conceptualized as being shaped by actions of actors and institutions in the food system, and how the

Table 2.2 New goals for food policy in an era of ecological public health

A new direction of travel is emerging shaped by...	...evidence on problems in issues such as these...	...requiring action by institutions covering these supply chain sectors...	...using policy levers ('soft' to 'hard')....	...to alter behaviour by food system actors....	...using managerial measures to reshape....	...in line with new ecological public health goals to deliver
ISSUES	◆ Water ◆ Energy ◆ Climate change ◆ Land use ◆ Human health ◆ Social justice ◆ Labour process ◆ Demographics ◆ Food availability & stocks	◆ Agriculture & rural affairs ◆ Environment ◆ Health ◆ Social welfare ◆ Trade ◆ International development ◆ Foreign affairs ◆ Industry ◆ Finance	◆ Labelling ◆ Education ◆ Public information ◆ Endorsements ◆ Welfare support ◆ Product standards ◆ Licensing ◆ Subsidies ◆ Competition rules ◆ Taxes & fiscal measures ◆ Bans ◆ Rationing	◆ Input industries ◆ Agriculture ◆ Transport & infrastructure ◆ Processing ◆ Distribution and logistics ◆ Retail ◆ Catering & foodservice ◆ Traders	◆ Standards ◆ Labour process & skills ◆ Markets & products ◆ Production and processing ◆ Distribution ◆ Full cost pricing ◆ Life cycle analysis ◆ Culture: from niche to mainstream ◆ Targets/metrics	◆ Sustainability (environmental economic) ◆ Energy efficiency, waste-minimisation and closed loop systems ◆ Capacity building (for nature, people & economy) ◆ Resilience to shock ◆ Eco-dietary advice ◆ Fairness and equitable access ◆ Confidence & trust ◆ Accountability (political & financial) ◆ Evidence-building for policy
COMMENTS	*Interdisciplinary thinking is required to face complex and sometimes competing evidence*	*The challenge is to improve co-ordination across these interests with all actors in the food system: Companies, Governments & NGOs*	*Policy has suffered a 'lock-in' which favours 'soft' interventions and focuses on consumers rather than upstream prevention*	*Globally, retailers and traders tend to hold power but the situation varies by country and sector*	*These are managerial foci*	*These are the new directions of travel for the food system; but subject to constant feedback loop and scrutiny....*

DIRECTION OF TRAVEL WITH FEEDBACK LOOP →

new goals outlined previously can be translated into managerial goals and measures with behavourial change to deliver ecological public health. It presages more detailed discussion in later chapters.

References

1. Tansey G, Worsley T. *The food system: a guide*. London: Earthscan, 1995.
2. Timmer CP. Food policy in the era of supermarkets: what's different? *Electronic Journal of Agricultural and Development Economics (eJADE)* 2004;**1**(2):50–67.
3. Knowles T, Moody R, McEachern MG. European food scares and their impact on EU food policy *British Food Journal* 2007;**109**(1):43–67.
4. Strategy Unit of the Cabinet Office. *Food: an analysis of the issues*. http://www.cabinetoffice.gov.uk/strategy/work_areas/food_policy.aspx. London: The Strategy Unit of the Cabinet Office, 2008:113.
5. Stapledon SG. *The land: now and tomorrow*. London: Faber & Faber, 1935.
6. IAASTD. *Global report and synthesis report*. London: International Assessment of Agricultural Science and Technology, 2008.
7. Lévi-Strauss C. *The raw and the cooked: introduction to a science of mythology: 1*. Harmondsworth: Penguin, 1966.
8. Evans-Pritchard EE. *The Nuer, a description of the modes of livelihood and political institutions of a Nilotic people*. Oxford: Clarendon Press, 1940.
9. Douglas M. Deciphering a meal. In: Douglas M, (ed.) *Implicit meanings: essays in anthropology*. London: Routledge, 1975:179–192.
10. Goody J. *Cooking, cuisine and class: a study in comparative sociology*. Cambridge: Cambridge University Press, 1982.
11. Goody J. *Food and love*. London: Verso, 1998.
12. MacClancy J. *Consuming culture*. London: Chapman, 1992.
13. Miller D. *A theory of shopping*. Cambridge: Polity, 1998.
14. Smith A. *The wealth of the nations*. Harmondsworth: Penguin, 1970 [1776].
15. Timmer CP, Falcon WP, Pearson SR. *Food policy analysis*. Baltimore, Maryland: Johns Hopkins University Press & World Bank, 1983.
16. Brundtland GH. *Our common future: report of the World Commission on Environment and Development (WCED)*. Chaired by Gro Harlem Brundtland. Oxford: Oxford University Press, 1987.
17. Intergovernmental Panel on Climate Change. *Climate change 2001: synthesis report and summary for policymakers*. Approved at the IPCC Plenary XVIII (Wembley, United Kingdom, 24–29 September 2001). Geneva: IPCC Secretariat c/o World Meteorological organization, 2001.
18. Intergovernmental Panel on Climate Change. *Climate change 2007: the physical science basis. Summary for policymakers*. Approved at the 10th Session of Working Group I of the IPCC, Paris, February 2007. Geneva: IPCC, 2007:18.
19. WHO. Diet, Nutrition and the Prevention of Chronic Diseases. Technical Report Series 797. Geneva: World Health Organisation, 1990
20. WCRF / AICR. Food, Nutrition, Physical Activity and the Prevention of Cancer: a Global Perspective. Washington DC / London: World Cancer Research Fund / American Institute for Cancer Research, 2007.

21. Marsden T, Flynn A, Harrison M. *Consuming interest: the social provision of foods.* London: UCL Press, 2000.

22. Atkins PJ, Bowler IR. *Food in society: economy, culture, geography.* London: Arnold, 2001.

23. Pritchard W, Burch D. *Agri-food globalisation in perspective: restructuring in the global tomato processing industry.* Aldershot, Hants: Ashgate Publishing, 2003.

24. Wilson B. *Swindled: from poison sweets to counterfeit coffee—the dark history of the food cheats.* London: John Murray, 2008.

25. Paulus I. *The search for pure food.* Oxford: Martin Robertson, 1974.

26. Lang T. Food, the law and public health: Three models of the relationship. *Public Health,* 2006;**120**:30–41.

27. Pyke M. *Industrial nutrition.* London: MacDonald and Evans, 1950.

28. Hammond RJ. *Food: the growth of policy.* London: H M S O/Longmans, Green and Co., 1951.

29. Woolton TE. *The Memoirs of the Rt Hon. The Earl of Woolton.* London: Cassell, 1959.

30. Humble N. *Culinary pleasures: cookbooks and the transformation of British food.* London: Faber and Faber, 2005.

31. Caraher M, Reynolds J. Lessons for home economics pedagogy and practice. *Journal of the Home Economics Institute of Australia* 2005;**12**(2):2–15.

32. Short F. *Kitchen secrets: the meaning of cooking in everyday life.* Oxford: Berg, 2006.

33. Pollan M. *The Omnivore's Dilemma: a Natural History of Four Meals.* New York: Penguin, 2006.

34. Pollan M. *In Defence of Food: The Myth of Nutrition and the Pleasures of Eating* London: Allen Lane, 2008.

35. Lawrence F. *Not on the Label.* London: Penguin, 2004.

36. Lawrence F. *Eat your heart out: Why the Food Business is Bad for the Planet and your Health.* London: Penguin, 2008.

37. Sinclair U. *The jungle.* Harmondsworth: Penguin, 1906/1985.

38. Accum FC. *A treatise on adulterations of food and culinary poisons.* London: Longman,, 1820.

39. Cruikshank EWH. *Food and physical fitness (Foreword by Sir John Boyd Orr).* Edinburgh: E and S Livingston, 1938.

40. Garrow JS, James WPT, Ralph A. *Human nutrition and dietetics,* 9th edn. Edinburgh: Churchill Livingstone (Elsevier Health Sciences), 2000.

41. Mayer J, Dwyer JT, with, Dowd K, Mayer L (ed.) *Food and nutrition policy in a changing world.* New York: Oxford University Press, 1979.

42. Cannon G. *The politics of food.* London: Century, 1987.

43. Kaput J, Rodriguez RL. Nutritional genomics: the next frontier in the postgenomic era. *Physiology & Genomics* 2004;**16**:166–177.

44. Shell ER. *The hungry gene.* New York: Atlantic Monthly Press, 2002.

45. Dowler E, Turner SA, Dobson B, Child Poverty Action Group (Great Britain). *Poverty bites: food, health and poor families.* London: Child Poverty Action Group, 2001.

46. George S. *How the other half dies: the real reasons for world hunger.* Harmondsworth: Penguin, 1976.

47. Ansell C, Vogel D (ed.) *What's the beef? The contested governance of European food safety.* Cambridge MASS: MIT Press, 2006.

48. van Zwanenberg P, Millstone E. *BSE: risk, science, and governance*. Oxford: Oxford University Press, 2005.

49. Curtin DW, Heldke LM (ed.) *Cooking, eating, thinking: transformative philosophies of food*. Bloomington & Indianapolis: Indiana University Press, 1992.

50. Korthals M. *Before dinner: philosophy and ethics of food*. Dordrecht NL: Springer, 2004.

51. Clarke PAB, Linzey A. *Political theory and animal rights*. London: Pluto, 1990.

52. Linzey A, Clarke PAB. *Animal rights: a historical anthology*. New York: Columbia University Press, 2004.

53. Singer P. *Animal liberation: a new ethics for our treatment of animals*. New York: Random House, 1975.

54. Singer P, Mason J. *Eating*. London: Arrow, 2006.

55. Chadwick R. Nutrigenomics, individualism and public health. *Proceedings of the Nutrition Society* 2004;**63**(1):161–6.

56. Conner M, Armitage CJ. *The social psychology of food*. Buckingham: Open University Press, 2002.

57. Shepherd R, Raats MM (ed.) *The psychology of food choice*. Wallingford (Oxon): CABI Publishing, 2006.

58. Tye L. *The father of spin: Edward L. Bernays and the birth of public relations*. New York: Crown Publishers Inc., 1998.

59. British Medical Association. Nutrition and the Public Health: Proceedings of a national conference on the wider aspects of nutrition, April 27-28-29, 1939. London: British Medical Association, 1939.

60. Surgeon General U. A Call to Action to prevent and decrease overweight and obesity 2001. Rockville, MD: US Department of Health and Human Services, Public Health Service, Office of the Surgeon General, 2001.

61. Donaldson L. Annual Report of the Chief Medical Officer for England 2002. London: Department of Health, 2003.

62. Newby H. *The deferential worker: a study of farm workers in east anglia*. London: Allen Lane, 1977.

63. Thomas WI, Znaniecki F. *The Polish peasant in Europe and America: monograph of an immigrant group*. Boston: G. Badger, 1918.

64. Murcott A. *The sociology of food and eating: essays on the sociological significance of food*. Aldershot: Gower, 1983.

65. Mennell S, Murcott A, Otterloo AHv, International Sociological Association. *The sociology of food: eating, diet and culture*. London: Sage, 1992.

66. Baudrillard J. Consumer society. In: Poster M (ed.) *Jean Baudrillard: selected writings*. Cambridge: Polity Press, 1970/1988.

67. Bourdieu P. *Distinction: a social critique of the judgement of taste*. London: Routledge, 1984.

68. Gabriel Y, Lang T. The unmanageable consumer: contemporary consumption and its fragmentation. London: Sage, 1995.

69. Taylor D, Field S (ed.) *Sociology of health & health care*. Oxford: Blackwell, 2003.

70. Lupton D. *Food, the body and the self*. London: Sage, 1996.

71. Kjaernes U, Harvey M, Warde A. *Trust in food: an institutional and comparative analysis*. Basingstoke: Macmillan/Palgrave, 2007.

72. Sustainable Development Commission. *Green, healthy and fair: a review of government's role in supporting sustainable supermarket food.* London: Sustainable Development Commission, 2008.

73. Cannon G. The rise and fall of dietetics and of nutrition science, 4000 BCE–2000 CE. *Public Health Nutrition* 2005;**8**(6a):701–705.

74. Lang T, Rayner G. Overcoming policy cacophony on obesity: an ecological public health framework for policymakers. *Obesity Reviews* 2007;**8**(Suppl.):165–181.

75. Maxwell S, Slater R. Food policy old and new. In: Maxwell S, Slater R (ed.) *Food policy old and new.* Oxford: Basil Blackwell, 2004:1–20.

76. Maxwell S, Slater R. Food policy old and new. *Development Policy Review* 2003;**21**(5–6):531–553.

77. Lang T, Millstone E, Raven H, Rayner M. Modernising UK food policy: the case for reforming the Ministry of Agriculture, Fisheries and Food. *Discussion Paper 1.* London: Centre for Food Policy, Thames Valley University, 1996:43.

78. Lang T, Robertson A, Nishida C, Caraher M, Clutterbuck C. *Intersectoral food and nutrition policy development: a manual for decision-makers.* Copenhagen: World Health organization, 2001.

79. Barling D, Lang T, Caraher M. Joined-up food policy? The trials of governance, public policy and the food system. *Social Policy & Administration* 2002;**36**(6):556–574.

80. Lang T, Barling D, Caraher M. 'Food, social policy and the environment: towards a new model'. *Social Policy and Administration* 2001;**35**(5):538–558.

81. Steinbeck J. *The grapes of wrath.* London: Penguin, 2000 [1939].

82. Boyd Orr J. *Food, health and income: report on adequacy of diet in relation to income.* London: Macmillan and Co, 1936.

83. Grondona LSC. *Commonwealth stocktaking.* London: Butterworths Publications Ltd, 1953.

84. Bateson FW. *Towards a socialist agriculture: study by a group of Fabians.* London: Victor Gollancz, 1946.

85. Blundell FN. *A new policy for agriculture.* London: Philip Allan, 1931.

86. Smith DF (ed.) *Nutrition in Britain: science, scientists and politics in the twentieth century.* London: Routledge, 1997.

87. Lang T, Heasman M. *Food wars: the global battle for mouths, minds and markets.* London: Earthscan, 2004.

88. Roll E. *The combined food board: a study in wartime international planning.* Stanford CA: Stanford University Press, 1956.

89. Beveridge SW. *Foodcontrol.* Oxford: Oxford University Press, 1928.

90. Malthus TR. *An essay on the principle of population, as it affects the future improvement of society with remarks on the speculations of Mr. Godwin, M. Condorcet and other writers.* London: Printed for J. Johnson, 1798.

91. Inter-departmental Committee on Physical Deterioration. *Report of the Inter-Departmental Committee on Physical Deterioration:* vol 1. Cd.2175 (chaired by Sir Almeric W. Fitzroy). London: H.M.S.O., 1904:v + 137.

92. Calder A. *The people's war: Britain 1939–45.* London: Cape, 1969.

93. Beveridge SW. *Social insurance and allied services,* Cmd 6404. London: HMSO, 1942.

94. Ostry AS. *Nutrition policy in Canada, 1870–1939.* Vancouver: UBC Press, 2006.

95. Mackintosh JM. *The nation's health*. London: The Pilot Press, 1944.

96. Boyd Orr SJ. *Food and the people. target for tomorrow no 3*. London: Pilot Press, 1943.

97. Astor WA, Rowntree BS. *The agricultural dilemma: a report of an enquiry organised by Viscount Astor and Mr. B. Seebohm Rowntree*. London: P. S. King, 1935.

98. Astor WA, Rowntree BS. *British agriculture: the principles of future policy*. London, New York: Longmans Green, 1938.

99. Robinson DH. *The new farming*. London: Thomas Nelson & Sons, 1938.

100. le Gros Clarke F. *Feeding the human family: science plans for the world larder*. London: Sigma Books, 1947.

101. Grondona LSC. *Utilizing world abundance*. London: George Allen & Unwin, 1958.

102. Fenelon K. *Britain's food supplies*. London: Methuen and Co., 1952.

103. Self PS, Storing HJ. *The state and the farmer*. London: George Allen & Unwin, 1971.

104. Schultz TW. *Transforming traditional agriculture*. New Haven: Yale University Press, 1964.

105. Dunman J. *Agriculture: capitalist and socialist*. London: Lawrence & Wishart, 1975.

106. Tracy M. *Agriculture in Western Europe: challenge and response, 1880–1980*, 2nd edn. London; New York: Granada, 1982.

107. Knutson RD, Penn JB, Flinchbaugh BL, Outlaw JL. *Agricultural and food policy*. 6th edn. London: Prentice Hall, 2007.

108. Miller JC, Coble KH. Cheap food policy: Fact or rhetoric? *Food Policy* 2007;**32**:98–111.

109. Harrison (and Friends) G. *The concert for Bangla Desh*. London: Apple Records, 1971.

110. Ehrlich PR. *The population bomb*. New York: Ballantine Books, 1968.

111. Pimentel D, Pimentel M. *Food, energy, and society*. London: Edward Arnold, 1979.

112. Heilig GK. Food, lifestyles, and energy. In: van der Heij DG (ed.) *Food and nutrition policy. Proceedings of the second European conference on food and nutrition policy*. The Hague, Netherlands, 21–24 April 1992. Wageningen: Pydoc, 1993:60–86

113. Johnson DG. *World agriculture in disarray*. London: Fontana/Trade Policy Research Centre, 1973.

114. Cockett R. *Thinking the unthinkable: think-tanks and the economic counter-revolution, 1931–1983*. London: HarperCollins, 1994.

115. Meadows DH, Club of Rome. *The Limits to growth; a report for the Club of Rome's project on the predicament of mankind*. New York: Universe Books, 1972.

116. FAO. *Report of the World Food Conference*, Rome, 5–16 November 1974. Rome: Food and Agriculture organization/United Nations Publication Sales No. E.75.II.A.3, 1974.

117. Barraclough S. *An end to hunger? The social origins of food strategies*. London: Zed Books & UN Research Institute for Social Development and the South Commission, 1991.

118. CGIAR. *Who we are: history of the CGIAR*. http://www.cgiar.org/who/index.html Consultative Group on International Agricultural Research, 2008.

119. von Braun J, Pandya-Lorch R (ed.) *Food policy for the poor: expanding the research frontiers—highlights from 30 years of IFPRI research*. Washington DC: Internationial Food Policy Research Institute, 2005.

120. Roszak T. *The making of a counter culture: reflections on the technocratic society and its youthful opposition*. London: Faber and Faber, 1970.

121. Lappé FM. *Diet for a small planet*. New York: Ballantine Books, 1971.

122. Brown LR, Finsterbusch GW. *Man and his environment: food*. New York: Harper and Row, 1972.

123. Lang T. Going public: food campaigns during the 1980s and 1990s. In: Smith D (ed.) *Nutrition scientists and nutrition policy in the 20th century*. London: Routledge, 1997:238–260.

124. Tarrant JR. *Food policies*. Chichester, UK; New York: J. Wiley & Sons, 1980.

125. Leach G. *Energy and food production*. Guildford: IPC Science and Technology Press for the International Institute for Environment and Development, 1976.

126. Robbins CJ. *National food policy in the UK*. Reading: University of Reading Centre for Agricultural Strategy, 1979.

127. Keys Ae. Coronary heart disease in seven countries. *Circulation* 1970;**41**(Supple.1):1–211.

128. Dwyer J, Mayer J. Beyond economics and nutrition: the complex basis of food policy. In: Mayer J, Dwyer J, with, Dowd K, Mayer L (ed.) *Food and nutrition policy in a changing world*. New York: Oxford University Press, 1979:3–16.

129. Lang T, Barling D. The environmental impact of supermarkets: mapping the terrain and the policy problems in the UK. In: Burch D, Lawrence G (ed.) *Supermarkets and agri-food supply chains*. Cheltenham: Edward Elgar, 2007:192–219.

130. Popkin BM. The nutrition transition and its health implications in lower income countries. *Public Health Nutrition* 1998;**1**(1):5–21.

131. Popkin BM. The nutrition transition in the developing world. *Development Policy Review* 2003;**21**:581–597.

132. Reardon T, Swinnen JFM. Agrifood sector liberalization and the rise of supermarkets in former state-controlled economies: comparison with other developing countries. *Development Policy Review* 2004;**22**(5):515–523.

133. Reardon T, Timmer PC, Berdegué JA. Supermarket expansion in Latin America and Asia Implications for food marketing systems. In: Regmi A, Gehlhar M (ed.) *New directions in global food markets*. Washington, DC: Economic Research Service/USDA, 2005.

134. Ministry of Agriculture FaF. *Food from our own resources*. White Paper. Cmnd. 6020. London: HMSO, 1975.

135. Laing H. Common Food policy for Europe. *Food Policy* 1978;**3**:223–225.

136. Clutterbuck C, Lang T. *More than we can chew: the crazy world of food and farming*. London: Pluto Press, 1982.

137. Walker C, Cannon G. *The food scandal*. London: Century, 1983.

138. Burch D, Lawrence G (ed.) *Supermarkets and agri-food supply chains*. Cheltenham: Edward Elgar, 2007.

139. OECD. *Food policy*. Paris: organization for Economic Co-operation and Development, 1981.

140. Conway G, Pretty JN. *Unwelcome harvest: agriculture and pollution*. London: Earthscan, 1991.

141. Shiva V, Third World Network. *Monocultures of the mind: perspectives on biodiversity and biotechnology*. London; Penang, Malaysia: Zed Books; Third World Network, 1993.

142. Pretty J, Hine R. *Reducing food poverty with sustainable agriculture: a summary of new evidence*. Colchester: Centre for Environment and Society, University of Essex, 2001:http://www.essex.ac.uk/ces/esu/occasionalpapers/SAFErepSUBHEADS.shtm.

143. Lang T, Clutterbuck C. *P is for pesticides*. London: Ebury, 1991.

144. Dinham B. *The pesticide hazard: a global health and environmental audit*. London; Atlantic Highlands, NJ: Zed Books, 1993.

145. Bull D. *A growing problem: pesticides and the Third World poor*. Oxford: Oxfam, 1982.

146. WHO. *Public health impact of pesticides used in agriculture*. Geneva: World Health organization, 1990.

147. Penningon TH. *When food kills*. Oxford: Oxford University Press, 2003.

148. Smith DF, Diack HL, with, Pennington TH, Russell EM. *Food poisoning, policy and politics: typhoid and corned beef in the 1960s*. London: Boydell Press, 2005.

149. Millstone E. *Food additives*. Harmondsworth: Penguin, 1986.

150. London Food Commission. *Food adulteration and how to beat it*. London: Unwin Hyman, 1987.

151. Phillips (Lord Phillips of Worth Matravers), Bridgeman J, Ferguson-Smith M. *The BSE inquiry report: evidence and supporting papers of the inquiry into the emergence and identification of Bovine Spongiform Encephalopathy (BSE) and variant Creutzfeldt-Jakob Disease (vCJD) and the action taken in response to it up to 20 March 1996*. London: The Stationery Office, 2000:16 volumes.

152. Phillips (Lord), Bridgeman J, Ferguson-Smith M. *The BSE inquiry report: evidence and supporting papers of the inquiry into the emergence and identification of Bovine Spongiform Encephalopathy (BSE) and variant Creutzfeldt-Jakob Disease (vCJD) and the action taken in response to it up to 20 March 1996*. London: The Stationery Office, 2000:16 volumes.

153. Lang T, Millstone E, Rayner M, Thames Valley University. Centre for Food Policy. *Food standards and the state: a fresh start*. London: Thames Valley University Centre for Food Policy, 1997.

154. Williamson J. What Washington means by policy reform. In: Williamson J (ed.) *Latin American readjustment: how much has happened*. Washington DC: Institute for International Economics, 1989.

155. World Bank. *Health, nutrition, population sector strategy paper*. Washington DC: World Bank Health, Nutrition and Population Division., 1999.

156. World Bank. *World development report 2008: agriculture for development*. New York: World Bank, 2007.

157. UNDP. *Human development report 2006: beyond scarcity: power, poverty and the global water crisis*. Washington DC: United Nations' Development Programme, 2006.

158. FAO. *The state of food insecurity in the world 2006: eradicating world hunger—taking stock ten years after the World Food Summit*. Rome: Food and Agriculture organization, 2006.

159. Fitzgerald A, Gale J, Murphy H. World Bank 'Destroyed Basic Grains' in Honduras. *Bloomberg News Service* 2008 May 5 2008 (1618 h).

160. Watkins K. *Rigged rules, double standards*. Oxford: Oxfam Publications, 2001.

161. Madeley J. *Hungry for trade: how the poor pay for free trade*. London: Zed Books, 2000.

162. Madeley J. *Food for all: the need for a new agriculture*. London: Zed Books, 2002.

163. Pretty JN, Brett C, Gee D, Hine R, Mason CF, Morison JIL *et al*. An assessment of the total external costs of UK agriculture. *Agricultural Systems* 2000;**65**(2):113–136.

164. Rayner G, Rayner M. Fat is an economic issue: combatting chronic diseases in Europe. *Eurohealth* 2003;**9**(1, Spring):17–20.

165. National Audit Office. *Health of the nation: a progress report.* HC 458 1995/96. London: Report by the Comptroller and Auditor General, 1996.

166. National Audit Office. *Tackling obesity in England.* London: Stationery Office, 2001.

167. Fukuyama F. *The end of history and the last man.* New York: Free Press, 1992.

168. FAO. *Food price index* (May 2008 report). http://www.fao.org/worldfoodsituation/ FoodPricesIndex. Rome: Food and Agriculture organization, 2008.

169. OECD, FAO. *Agricultural outlook 2008–2017.* Rome & Paris: organization for Economic Co-operation & Development and Food & Agriculture Organization, 2008.

170. FAO. *Food outlook: global market analysis.* Rome: Food and Agriculture Organization, 2007.

171. FAO. *The state of world fisheries and aquaculture 2006.* Rome: Food and Agriculture Organization, 2007.

172. Pew Oceans Commission. *America's living oceans: charting a course for sea change.* Washington DC: Pew Charitable Trusts, 2003.

173. Royal Commission on Environmental Pollution. *Turning the tide: addressing the impact of fishing on the marine environment,* 25th report. London: Royal Commission on Environmental Pollution, 2004.

174. WHO. *World Health Report 2002: reducing risks, promoting healthy life.* Geneva: World Health organization, 2002.

175. FAO. *Livestock's long shadow—environmental issues and options.* Rome: Food and Agriculture organization., 2006.

176. WCRF/AICR. *Food, nutrition, physical activity and the prevention of cancer: a global perspective.* Washington DC/London: World Cancer Research Fund/American Institute for Cancer Research, 2007.

177. Intergovernmental Panel on Climate Change. *Climate change 2007*: the IPCC Fourth Assessment Report (AR4)—the Synthesis Report. November 17. Geneva: IPCC, 2007.

178. Brown L. *Outgrowing the earth: the food security challenge in an age of falling water tables and rising temperatures.* New York: WW Norton, 2004.

179. Sustainable Development Commission. *$100 a barrel of oil: impacts on the sustainability of food supply in the UK.* A report by ADAS, commissioned by the SDC. London: Sustainable Development Commission, 2007:112.

180. Committee On Commodity Problems. *Food security in the context of economic and trade policy reforms: insights from country experiences*; 2005 11–13 April 2005. Food and Agriculture organization.

181. FAO. *Globalization of food systems in developing countries: impact on food security and nutrition.* Rome: Food and Agriculture organization, 2004.

182. UNFPA. *State of world population 2007: demographic, social and economic indicators.* http://www.unfpa.org/swp/2007/english/notes/indicators.html. Washington DC: UN Population Fund, 2007.

183. UNEP. Agri-food facts and figures. *UNEP Industry and Environment* 1999:1–6.

184. FAO. *World food security summit.* June 3–5 2008. Rome: Food & Agriculture organization, 2008.

185. Evans A. Rising food prices: drivers and implications for development. *Food Supply Project Briefings*. London: Chatham House, 2008:11.

186. Cabinet Office Strategy Unit. *Recipe for success: towards a food strategy for the 21st century*. London: Cabinet Office, 2008.

187. von Braun J. *Agriculture for sustainable economic development: a global R&D initiative to avoid a deep and complex crisis*. Charles Valentine Riley memorial lecture. Capitol Hill Forum, Washington D.C., February 28, 2008. Washington DC: International Food Policy Research Institute, 2008.

188. Chatham House. *UK food supply: storm clouds on the horizon?* Preliminary findings of the Food Supply in the 21st Century Project. London: Royal Institute of International Affairs, 2008.

189. Shaw DJ. *World food security: a history since 1945*. London: Palgrave Macmillan, 2007.

190. Commoner B. *The closing circle: confronting the environmental crisis*. London: Cape, 1972.

191. Harrison P. *The third revolution: environment, population and a sustainable world*. London: I.B.Taurus & Co (with World Wide Fund for Nature), 1992.

192. Dumont R, Rosier B. *The hungry future*. London: Deutsch, 1969.

193. Dyson J. *Population and food: global trends and future prospects*. London: Routledge, 1996.

194. Birch R, Ravetz J, Wiedmann T. *Footprint north west: a preliminary ecological footprint of the north west region*. Manchester and York: Stockholm Environment Institute (York), Centre for Urban and Regional Ecology, Action for Sustainability (North West Regional Assembly) 2005.

195. WRAP. *Love food hate waste: UK Household food waste campaign facts*. Banbury (Oxon): Waste Resources Action Programme (WRAP) http://www.wrap.org.uk/, 2008.

196. McMichael AJ. Integrating nutrition with ecology: balancing the health of humans and biosphere. *Public Health Nutrition* 2003;**8**(6A):706–715.

197. Lang T. *Retailing & sustainable development*. First Lecture to the Sustainable Consumption Institute, University of Manchester. http://www.sci.manchester.ac.uk/news/. Manchester: Susainable Consumption Institute University of Manchester, 2008.

198. Porter D. *Health, civilisation and the state. a history of public health from ancient to modern times*. London: Routledge, 1998.

199. Fee E, Brown TM. The Public Health Act of 1848. *Bulletin of the World Health Organization* 2005;**83**(11):866–867.

200. Vernon J. *Hunger: a modern history*. Cambridge: Harvard University Press, 2007.

201. Food Ethics Council. *Getting personal: shifting responsibilities for dietary health*. Brighton Food Ethics Council, 2005.

202. Lang T. Functional Foods. *British Medical Journal* 2007;**334**:1015–1016.

203. Foresight. *Tackling obesities: future choices*. London: Government Office of Science, 2007.

204. Lang T, Rayner G. *Why health is the key to farming and food*. Report to the Commission on the Future of Farming and Food chaired by Sir Don Curry. London: UK Public Health Association, Chartered Institute of Environmental Health, Faculty of Public Health Medicine, National Heart Forum and Health Development Agency, 2002.

205. Huxley EJG. *Brave new victuals: an inquiry into modern food production*. London: Chatto & Windus, 1965.

206. Cooper D. *The bad food guide*. London: Routledge & Kegan Paul, 1967.

207. Tansey G. Patenting Our Food Future: Intellectual Property Rights and the Global Food System *Social Policy and Administration* 2002;**36**(6):575–592.

208. Tansey G, Rajotte T (ed.) *The future control of food: a guide to international negotiations and rules on intellectual property, biodiversity and food security*. London & Ottawa: Earthscan & IDRC, 2008.

209. King FH. *Farmers of forty centuries, or permanent agriculture in China, Korea and Japan*. Emmaus, pennsyhania Rodale press, 1911.

210. Balfour LEB. *The Living Soil: evidence of the importance to human health of soil vitality, with special reference to post-war planning*. London: Faber, 1943.

211. Carson R. *Silent spring*. Boston/Cambridge, Mass.: Houghton Mifflin/Riverside Press, 1962.

212. Cobbett W. *Rural rides*. London: J.M.Dent & Sons, 1932 (1853).

213. Thoreau HD. *Walden or life in the woods*. Oxford: Oxford University Press, 1999 [1854].

214. UNCED. *Rio Declaration*. Made at the UNCED meeting at Rio de Janeiro from 3 to 14 June 1992. Rio de Janeiro: United Nations Conference on Environment and Development, 1992.

215. United Nations Development Programme. *Millennium development goals*. http://www.undp.org/mdg/basics.shtml. New York: United Nations, 2000.

216. HM Government. *Securing the future: delivering UK sustainable development strategy*, Cm 6467. London: H.M.Government, 2005.

217. Carbon Trust. *Tesco and Carbon Trust join forces to put carbon label on 20 products*: http://www.carbontrust.co.uk/News/presscentre/29_04_08_Carbon_Label_Launch. htm [June 3 2008]. London: Carbon Trust, 2008.

218. UNDP. *Human Development Report 2007/2008—Fighting climate change: Human solidarity in a divided world*. New York: UN Development Programme, 2007.

219. Coote B. *The trade trap: poverty and the global commodity markets*. Oxford: Oxfam, 1992.

220. Lamb H. *Fighting the banana wars and other Fairtrade battles*. London: Rider/Ebury, 2008.

221. Smith A, Watkiss P, Tweddle G, McKinnon PA, Browne PM, Hunt A *et al. The validity of food miles as an indicator of sustainable development*. Report to DEFRA by AEA Technology. London: Department for the Environment, Food and Rural Affairs, 2005.

222. Lang T. Towards a food democracy. In: Griffiths S, Wallace J (ed.) *Consuming passions: food in the age of anxiety*. Manchester: Manchester University Press, 1998.

223. Lang T. Food control or food democracy: Re-engaging nutrition to civil society, the state and the food supply chain. *Public Health Nutrition* 2005;**8**(6A):730–737.

224. Barling D, Lang T, Caraher M. Joined-up food policy? The trials of governance, public policy and the food system? In: Dowler E, Jones Finer C (ed.) *The welfare of food: rights and responsibilities in a changing world*. London: Blackwell, 2003:1–19.

225. Barling D, Lang T. Trading on health: Cross-continental production and consumption tensions and the governance of international food standards. In: Fold N, Pritchard B (ed.) *Cross-continental food chains: cross-continental food chains*. London: Routledge, 2005:39–51.

226. Barling D, Lang T, Sharpe R. *The re-governance of food supply for the UK: policy routes to integrating sustainability with national food security*. Paper to Food Security and Environmental Change Conference, Oxford University, 2-4 April 2008. http://www.gecafs.org/documents/PS10Barling.pdf. London: Centre for Food Policy, City University, 2008.

227. Lang T. Food policy for the 21st century. In: Koc M, MacRae R, Mougeot LJA, Welsh J (ed.) *For hunger-proof cities: sustainable urban food systems*. Ottawa: International Development Research Centre/IDRC Books, 1999:216–224.

228. Mintz SW. *Sweetness and power: the place of sugar in modern history*. Harmondsworth: Penguin Books, 1985.

229. Accum FC. *A treatise on adulterations of food and culinary poisons*. London: Longman, 1820.

230. Hannington W. *Unemployed struggles 1919–1936*. London: Lawrence & Wishart, 1977 (1936).

231. Rathbone E. *The disinherited family: a plea for the endowment of the family*. London: Edward Arnold, 1924.

232. Spring Rice M. *Working class wives: their health and conditions*. Harmondsworth: Penguin, 1939.

233. Thompson EP. The moral economy of the English crowd in the eighteenth century. In: Thompson EP (ed.) *Customs in common*. Harmondsworth: Penguin, 1993 [1971]:185–258.

234. Vorley B. *Food Inc.: corporate concentration from farm to consumer*. London: UK Food Group, 2004.

235 . Simms A. *Tescopoly: how one shop came out on top and why it matters*. London: Constable & Robinson, 2007.

Chapter 3

Public policy and governance

Food supply is mediated and regulated by interventions from both state and international institutions and bodies. These range from production supports to safety and quality standards, and from health guidelines to environmental standards. Public policy on food is generally depicted as emanating primarily from governments and from the apparatus of the state, but the success of public policy on food depends upon successful engagement with the actors across the food system from food producers to consumers and those who figure in-between. Food is fundamental to human survival, and the adoption of agriculture played a key role in human settlement and to the development of a settled civil society. This historical development underpinned the need for more complex systems of public policy and rule over civil society. In short, food, civil society and public policy are inextricably linked.

The first part of this chapter draws on academic studies of the public policy process to identify some key concepts that have been deployed to aid understanding of the making and implementation of public policy, and the factors that might contribute to its final form and features. The key concepts that are introduced to this modern conception of food policy are the notions of power relationships, historical institutionalism, governance, governmentality, policy networks and multi-level governance. The nature of the contemporary governance of food in relation to, and under, the 'rule' of public policy is then examined and explained. Within these explanations, a clearer picture is sought of some of the dynamics that will shape the future trajectories of food policy, and the consolidation of both environmental and health priorities raised in the last chapter and later in the book.

The evolving trajectories of food policy are being shaped by these public policy dynamics and by the transfer of ideas and ways of thinking about food and its value to health, society and the environment. The political institutions and public policy processes mediate the processing of these ideas, and of new bodies of evidence and new evaluations of the role and value of food in society. For example, now that obesity is identified as a major health problem, even in developing countries, how can and should public policy address it? How is it interpreted as a problem? Is it a problem that needs to be addressed on behalf of society and for the greater public good? If so, is it interpreted in terms of public education, industry formulation of food products and its marketing, or of individual consumer choice, or a combination of these and, if so, in which order? Where are the decisions being made and by whom? Which are the policy institutions and which stakeholders are around the table? Levels of government and governance, institutions, ideas, evidence, actors and groups all interact to shape public policy. In this chapter some of the key variables in policy-making and how we can understand them are presented in order to understand more clearly the dynamics of food governance and of the public policy of food.

Analysing public policy: some key definitions, concepts and relationships

Policy is simply defined as a plan or course of action. To this extent, each one of us may have a policy that we apply to a situation in terms of a plan of action that we are pursuing or an established plan of action that we apply to a given situation,or to areas or challenges in our life. Likewise organizations, such as corporations or universities, will have policies laid down that guide their actions in defined areas of activity. The primary focus for public policy is upon the 'public and its problems' and why and how governments pursue particular problems, and how and to what extent (if any) the institutions of government handle these problems.[1] This focus leads into the analysis of a series of questions and dimensions of public policy and the way that it is processed. Some examples of key questions that emerge from an analysis of public policy and public policy processes, presented as an indicative but far from exhaustive list, include:

- How do issues come on to the public policy agenda?
- What issues do not get on to the public policy agenda and why? Are there structural constraints that condition what becomes part of the public policy agenda and what does not?
- Who is involved in this policy processing, and on what terms and conditions are participants involved?
- How are issues are defined and by whom? What types and terms of policy discourse are deployed and what impact does this have on the policy-making process?
- How are such issues then processed? In what policy sectors are they processed, and by whom—which institutions, which stakeholders and through what mechanisms?
- How does policy change and how significant can this change be?

- To what extent can we observe who has influence over the decision-making processes on public policy? Can we identify who has power and how they exercise it?
- How successfully is policy carried out once it has been agreed? How is policy implemented in practice? What are the impacts of the implementation? How do we measure success?
- Does change in policy direction bring change in the lives of the targeted public or publics?
- Does the implementation process give rise to identification of new problems or a rethinking on how to address existing concerns?

The analysis of public policy throws up a range of important questions, but there are some common observations or themes that lie behind these questions and may help the quest for answers to these questions, and help to inform this chapter. Firstly, the questions point to a range of dynamics and relationships that shape public policy. Secondly, government and governing plays a central role in the policy process. This role may be more fully played out by agencies of the government in some policy areas, or agencies of the state (to give government and its various organizational appendages their more collective title). Thirdly, however, it is clear that governments and the state do not act alone as other actors and interests are present and these other actors may play a more central role in certain stages of the policy process, such as at initial formulation stage and the later implementation stag, where policy is carried out on a day to day basis. In addition, interests within the public may seek to reject and resist policy initiatives that emerge, and seek to force further change from the public policy-making process and public officials overseeing the implementation of such initiatives.

The dynamics and relationships that interact to shape public policy, its coverage and its form and content can be conceptualized, in turn, in three related ways that are: firstly, in terms of power relationships; secondly, the relationship between the state and the market economy; and, finally, in terms of the relationship between structure and agency. In the first instance, there are a series of power relationships that exist amongst and between governing institutions and actors, and these relationships may be very entrenched and/or may change over time. The political outcomes of these power relationships, and the conflicts and the degree of consensus reached, shape the form and scope of the resulting food policies. Secondly, adopting a more structuralist perspective, that is, a perspective that identifies key structural constraints upon the scope of agency, a dialectical relationship can be discerned between the state and the market economy. That is, the state and the market economy interact in an iterative way to shape and reshape each other. States regulate and so influence the workings of the market economy through public policy; for example, through international trading agreements or through minimum safety requirements of food products. Likewise, the market economy evolves and acts to constrain the ability of states to act autonomously in terms of policy initiatives. Not least, this is because the co-operation of key players in the market economy, in this instance in the food sectors of the economy, is needed to implement policies effectively (such as food safety standards or animal welfare or environmental safeguards). Only with widespread market acceptance and conformity with state policy can the rogue traders and law-breaking companies be targeted efficiently.

Contemporary food policy must engage with the market economy and key market place players, such as large food trading and processing corporations and large food manufacturers and grocery retailers, who are increasingly concentrated in terms of market share, at national and international levels. Also, consumers emerge as key players in food policy. In the past two decades or more, in some areas of food policy, the public and their interests have been defined not in terms of their rights as citizens but rather in terms of their rights as consumers. From the 1990s, the introduction of Food Safety and Standards' agencies in European States were depicted as institutional innovations designed to protect and account for the consumer interest. In other words, the dominant ideological discourses of the times interact with the structural realities of governing a market economy; as exhibited during the contemporary era of international trade liberalization. As we will see, the mechanisms of the market have become central to the debates over how to improve food policy, where using policy instruments that are designed to impact upon consumer choice are increasingly in vogue (such as labelling and certification of food products). However, questions arise as to whether the market mechanisms, with their emphasis upon consumer choice, are indeed adequate for a food policy that incorporates ecological public health. Ecological public health, as explained in the last chapter, challenges some key structural features of modern industrial states. For example, the environmental impacts of modern food production and the complexities of modern supply chains have had severe environmental impacts, and threaten the stability of the ecosystems within which food must be produced and harvested. Furthermore, the challenges to the *modus operandi* of the contemporary food supply are coming largely from civil society. Civil society organizations, environmental and other public interest groups, have aroused the attentive publics to the uncertainties in the safety and impacts of the food supply, and of the methods used in production and some of the industrial and technological inputs for pesticides to GMOs. Issues such as fair terms of trade for developing world producers selling on to developed worlds markets and animal welfare have originated from civil society organizations. These challenges are expressed through the market place but invoke some fundamental critiques of the operations of the food system.

Finally, there emerges from debates around the exercise of power a continuing relationship between structure and agency. That is, the relationship between the structural social, economic and political settings for public policy, and the way that such settings both serve to constrain and yet offer some scope for the actions of agents to have an impact to effect change. In turn, the actions of the agent, that is their agency, can modify and change the institutional and structural settings that act as their constraint in the first place. Hence we can view 'the relationship between structure and agency as dialectical; that is interactive and iterative... structures may constrain or facilitate agents, but agents interpret structures and, in acting, change them'.[2] To move food policy to an ecological health orientation involves the efforts of policy actors and groups, structural and institutional changes, and the promotion and acceptance of refreshed ideas and interpretations of the world.

Power relationships and public policy

Identifying the exercise of power and power relationships is important for interpreting the question of how public policies are shaped and so take the forms that they do. John Scott has identified two broad streams to the study of power.[3] The main strand of analysis has been based around exploring the location and exercise of sovereign power, i.e. who exercises it and where, in the policy process. A secondary strand has been around discursive power, which has focused on how power is acted out or performed throughout society, drawing particularly on post-structuralist thinking.

The sovereign power approach or dominant stream of power studies has sought to identify who has the power in policy-making and who exercises their influence upon the final shape and content of public policy. Power as a concept is seen as relational in that power can only exist and be exercised over someone else and so with a degree of consent from the recipients. Scott explains power in terms of a principal agent and subaltern agent relationship, where the existence of the subaltern is necessary for the principal to be able to have influence.[3] As a result, the subaltern may seek concessions as part of the interaction of the relationship. Alternatively, the subaltern may accept the exercise of power without ever questioning it or, indeed, without ever having realized that power was being exercised.

Public policy analysis as it emerged in the 1950s, primarily in the USA, adopted a technocratic and rationalist approach based on the belief that you could improve policy by adopting the rational and scientific management techniques that were influencing public discourse at this time. This approach was ideologically rooted in its faith in human reason to provide objective and successful solutions. The scientific management approach was supported by functionalist models, which looked at the policy process and saw it in terms of a system with inputs and outputs and feedback loops in the style depicted in Fig. 1.2 (see Chapter 1).[4] These models adopted a view of public policy as a process of different stages, such as: policy formulation and policy-making, policy legislation, and, in turn policy implementation and administration. Shortcomings in policy identified in the final stage of the process would be identified and feed back into the front end of the process, leading to fresh policy formulation and so on. In this manner a rational and ever improving public policy would evolve. However, faith in the application of this rational technocratic approach broke down with the experience of large-scale policy interventions and their implementation in the 1960s, notably where the interventions sought to shape social outcomes. The classic account of this was Pressman and Wildavsky's work on *Policy implementation* or as it was more graphically subtitled: *How great expectations in Washington are dashed in Oakland; or, why it's amazing that federal programs work at all.*[5] In short, they found the more stages that exist in the implementation process (such as from federal or national level, through state level down to local municipal level) the more latitude there was for change in direction by actors at different levels and stages of implementation, and so for the original intent of the policy to be distorted.

Equally, it was clear that policy-making involved a range of actors and institutions, and their interaction—and this was political in nature and not always rational or straightforward. Indeed, political and social scientists had begun to investigate empirically how different interests were able to influence policy decisions from the 1950s, including studies of decision-making at local government and municipal level in the USA, the so-called community power studies. At a national level, the concept of an interlocking economic and social elite had been identified (the 'power elite'), drawing on a longer tradition of elitist interpretation of political and social organization.[6, 7] The power elite were in the commanding positions of political, economic and social organizations, and so power was interpreted as following structural position. Conversely, pluralist thinkers saw society as more fragmented, with a range of different (and sometimes overlapping) groups who organized to promote and defend these interests. Rather than subscribing to the elitists' view that there inevitably exists a situation of oligarchy (rule by a few), the pluralists identified a polyarchy (rule divided by many different interests).[8] In a study of decision-making at the local government level, in the city of New Haven,

Robert Dahl[9] found that different interests had influence in different policy areas. There was no common presence across different policy areas. However, Dahl looked only at observable decisions. Critics asked what about decisions that never made it on to the political agenda? Matthew Crenson,[10] in a comparative study of city governments' policy on air pollution, found that in one city, Gary, Indiana, where the steel industry was a major employer, air pollution was not a policy issue and was not on the agenda. This was identified as a politics of non-decision-making. Bachrach and Baratz had termed this non-decision-making as being the second and hidden (or non observable) face of power.[11] For public policy analysts, the politics of agenda control, identifying which issues failed to make it on to the public agenda and why, became a further focus for study.[12] For food policy this remains an important dimension, as to which issues remain off the agenda and why, and, subsequently, how they may emerge on to the agenda and in what form they are defined and presented, and through whose efforts. Put another way, how has dietary health emerged as an issue for food policy, or how has diet emerged within health policy, and how and where has it appeared on the public policy agendas, and what issues have not appeared or have been effectively sidelined within debates around dietary links to health? Why and how have they been kept off the agenda and by whom (see Chapter 4)?

The critique of the behavioural approach to observing power, as explored by Dahl, continued with Steven Lukes who identified a third face of power.[13] For Lukes, the third face of power exists when actors do not realize what is in their interests, and accept the parameters within which policy is set due to the controlling ideas and interests inherent within the public policy system. This interpretation of power points to an ideological control exerting a false consciousness upon actors who do not realize what is in their own best interests. It suggests that there may be a radical agenda that is latent but not addressed by public policy, as the actors who should be concerned with advocating such an agenda do not recognize it. Presumably, this agenda is so radical that it involves an overthrowing or displacement of the contemporary economic, social and political orders.[14] This more radical interpretation can be matched to some of the deeper green environmental critiques and their prescriptions for change to the current food system, and human society's use and abuse of natural resources and the global ecosystem (see Chapter 6).

The bias that may exist around how public policy is formulated and determined led pluralists like Dahl to adopt a more critical take on their views of pluralist democracy, identifying continuing inequalities and bias within the policy process, evolving what has been termed a neo-pluralist analysis.[15] Charles Lindblom identified that policy makers within the state are necessarily receptive to economic interests, such as business corporations and trade associations, as they govern a market economy.[16] Governments' political progress benefits from an economic management record of prosperity and growth, and so those interests that occupy a more structural position in the economy gain advantage in terms of policy access and degree of influence on policy makers. The neo-pluralists further acknowledgement of structural advantage for some economic interests, and so bias in the policy process, points to the dialectical nature of the relationship between the state and the market economy.

The emphasis of structural constraints that inhibit the scope or freedom of policy makers to change existing policy and its direction is most closely identified with Marxist analyses of the policy process and the role of the state, where the state is pictured as the instrument of the ruling class who dominate society and the economy. Modern Marxist-based analyses of policy processes have diverged along different lines, but the structuralist approaches embedded in these lines of interpretation have in their revisions allowed for a greater range of roles for political actors, not least within the agencies and apparatus of the state.[17, 18] These more recent structuralist analyses are not static, nor do they necessarily see the dominant interests in political systems as monolithic.[18] The interests of economic actors, such as corporations and trade associations, can diverge as examination of the relationships along food-supply chains clearly demonstrates. Similarly, the agencies of the state can have different policy priorities and act as competing agents in the policy process. Structuralist approaches to public policy offer, at the very least, some fixed points of departure in analytical terms, such as the symbiotic relationships between the state and the market economy.

The existence of structural factors and bias points investigations of sovereign power to the importance of institutions and the role that institutions and policy processes play role in processing issues. Historical institutionalism is an approach to understanding public policy that covers, not just the institutions themselves but also, the norms and values that underpin their operating procedures and their interrelationships.[19] Hence, a public policy process will be conditioned by the historical direction of past policy and the agreed norms and operating rules of the processes and institutions involved. The implication is that past policy decisions can create paths of dependency that are subsequently hard to change significantly. For food policy, this can make it hard to integrate policy initiatives and lift them from the policy sector silos that have dominated in the past. Any institutional change that does occur needs careful analysis as to the rationales, discourses and expediencies incorporated into such institutional change and what informs the new operating procedures created, as with the wave of new food safety agencies created throughout Europe in the 2000s. For social interests, there will be established modes of governance, incorporating rules and norms that are accepted by the participants. For new participants into such policy arenas, acceptance of these rules may be a condition of entry.

The structural factors that shape policy institutions, and the relationship of the state and policy processes to the market economy and its workings, do not preclude the role of agency. Individuals, political parties, interest groups and social movements, all can influence the shape of public policy. Ideas play an important role in shaping actions to policy challenges. The contemporary era (phase 3 in Chapter 2) has seen the re-emergence and dominance of neo-liberal thinking and its implementation through a range of policy approaches from increased international trade liberalization, to welfare reform, to agricultural subsidy reform. The extent and transfer of these ideas through to policy action has varied across national states and across policy sectors. Here, actors through their agency actualize and realize both the transfer of ideas into policy direction and content and, also, their resistance and compromise. The transfer of ideas takes place in a policy environment where structural biases are found both in the greater influence of some actors and in the institutional processing of ideas into policy. However, such bias is not free from challenge and resistance, or to the pushing of alternative prescription. One enduring refrain of this book is that food policy is contested space—even if the contest has a structured bias. The connection between structure and agency can be depicted as a relational one of interaction and adaptation over time. The relationship of the policy process and, central to that process, the state to the market, has a similar dialectical energy—each part influencing the other. In the food-supply chain there are structural advantages that when strategically asserted let one set of players exercise greater power over others. The questions are to what extent do the dominant players in the market, or the food-supply chain, operate their influence in relation to the state and so in the policy process, and how and when does this influence take place, and to what ends and with what consequences? Also, is the state addressing the consequences of the contemporary supply chain relationships adequately? Chapter 5 on the food-supply chain addresses some of these questions.

The second theoretical approach to power stems from the work of Foucault and deliberately by-passes the focus on sovereign power and such attempts to judge who has influence upon policy decisions.[3, 20] The focus is no longer on government and governing. Instead, the second stream focuses on how power is operated and deployed throughout society, notably through the terms and language of the policy discourse that act as discursive structures that shape how society thinks and acts.[3] These may well be a contested set of processes but the approach sees power as a method of disciplining society to conform. The policy discourse approach is informed by the post-structuralist premise that knowledge is shaped by the terms of discourse used to frame and present it. There is no single or true rationality, but only differing interpretations of reality, all interpretations are socially constructed. The questions are which one(s) are dominant and how is that dominance performed? The Foucaultian approach does not see power as being measurable in terms of a quantity that some groups can have at the expense of others. Rather, it is a totality of relationships and structures brought to bear by some on the actions of others. As Nikolas Rose suggests, visible government is only part of the picture and more important are the social relationships that underpin government.[21] Governing is about making people governable subjects and the 'discursive formations' that socialize people to conform to accept social discipline. The outcome is similar to Lukes' third face of power, although for Lukes such power was structural and embedded in class controls in society. As a result of these discursive formations and calculative practices, people accept ways of conforming as detailed by a range of agencies and actors such as: teachers, social workers, doctors, planners and so on. This range of calculative practices and tools make up what are termed contemporary governmentalities and so the focus is on the ways and forms that 'seek to shape conduct so as to achieve certain ends'.[21] Rose emphasizes that: 'To analyze political power through the analysis of governmentality ... is to start by asking what authorities of various types wanted to happen, in relation to problems defined how, in pursuit of what objectives, through what strategies and techniques'.[21]

Within the second strand of work into power relations, the studies on governmentality see themselves as theoretically distinct from public policy studies that focus on sovereign power and government and its agencies.[21] However, the contention supported in this chapter is that there are complementarities that can be drawn from both streams of work that can help to inform our understandings of food policy. In this account of the relationship between food and public policy, the point of analytical departure remains that of the state. The more institutional and governing focus of sovereign power is complemented by the policy discourse focus upon the role of expertise and how it is utilized and deployed in the policy process and through wider governance arrangements. The importance of expertise and the challenges to expertise are central to our understanding of the application of technology to food, and the critiques of expertise emerging from policy conflicts around areas such as pesticide use, GM crops and functional foods (see Chapter 6). In addition, the move from more confined processes of governing to wider, more fluid forms of governance is dependent upon networks of agents interacting around discernible policy sectors or indeed subsectors—such as say health policy and in turn nutrition policy, or agricultural policy and say animal welfare policy. The forms of discourse that these networks take may frame the scope of policy action—in terms of definitions of problems and methodologies referenced and chosen and decisions made, and therefore the impacts of policy. In other words, structures and processes interact with ideas and policy discourse to effectively direct policy along certain paths.

Also, the deployment of the consciousness industries to shaping food choice and their interactions with culture at national levels, and the interaction of fast foods and food service and so called fast foods are dimensions that come to the fore in looking at the interactions of culture and food policy (see Chapter 7). The industrialization of food and the globalization of brands and tastes are mediated at national levels, but they reinforce the important role that the market economy with its globalizing or internationalizing trends, and so the powerful actors in the market, play in shaping and editing both food choice and food policy (see also Chapter 6 for a discussion of choice-editing).

The state, governance and policy networks

The concept of governing depicts a command and control approach to law making and enforcement from the national state, which in modern times has been underpinned by the state's successful claim to political legitimacy. In the past three decades, at least in the countries of Western Europe and other advanced (or post-) industrial democracies, the state has lessened its control and command over economic sectors on the one hand, while on the other, it has sought to extend its regulatory and strategic reach, partly achieved through new governance forms.[22, 23] In this context, governance implies more indirect and softer forms of direction from the state than command and control, and reflects collaborative outcomes, involving a wide range of actors often from the private sector as well as from government bureaucracy, as much as deliberate interventions by the state.

The relationship of the state to such governance forms, as opposed to governing, is a very useful departure point for understanding the unfolding dynamics of policy-making in the contemporary agri-food sector and the extent to which policy is conducted away from the more immediate environment of the state or is emerging beyond the state. It also allows us to look at how the state may be seeking to enrol other actors, and to delegate to them the task of realizing desired policy and social outcomes. In this fashion, governing is extended to include a variety of groups from within and outside government, leading to this use of term governance—suggesting a veiling of the boundaries between public and private sectors for policy delivery. This may reflect, in part, the spread of the new public management credo of government and public administration, focusing more effort on steering rather than rowing the ship of state and public policy; in turn, diversifying the range of service providers and the criteria for efficient public services. The state increasingly relies on a range of mechanisms, professions and actors to shape order in society. In addition, the state may be taking the opportunity to further its regulatory reach, relying more on regulation rather than distributive or redistributive policies. Distributive policies allocate resources to actors or groups in society, such as subsidies for farmers; redistributive policies take resources away form some sectors and re-allocate them to others, such as with taxation and social welfare.[24] Regulatory policies, unlike the other types, potentially transfer the bulk of the economic costs to the regulated, while extending and enhancing the reach and influence of the state and its officials.[25, 26] Governance becomes a strategic approach by the state to enable desired outcomes—it is the 'enabling' state in action.

These trends involve embracing a range of non-state actors in service or policy delivery. The regulated can become the deliverers. This is not an entirely new phenomenon, of course. Traditionally, the state has had to look outside for expertise in framing its laws and in ensuring their effective implementa- tion, making for functional representation. Hence, representative bodies for specific economic interests and economic or social groups can become incorporated by the state (or pan-national bodies such as the European Commission) into the policy process. The corporatist state was the most for- mal and extreme model of incorporation, involving key peak interest groups from the economy and society, and was a feature of fascist states in the 1930s in Europe. In more pluralistic polities and times, interest groups may gain insider status; for example, in the case of the National Farmers Union in UK agricultural policy from the late-1930s until the 1980s and 1990s.[27]

A dominant theme of the research into how governing has given way to looser governance arrangements has focused on the role of networks. Central government authority is more dispersed and dependent upon a multiplicity of actors located in a variety of arenas to reach policy solutions. The actors provide necessary resources for these solutions and engage in bargaining and compromise within institutional norms and rules that, in turn, can shape the outcomes.[28, 29] Resource dependency is a feature of policy networks identified in modern governance arrangements in the UK, leading to governance through networks, some of which are depicted as virtually self-sustaining and separated from government in implementing and administering public policy.[30, 31] In the USA, the metaphor of policy communities was put forward initially to suggest a stable configuration of participants, government department(s) and/or agency(ies) and selected interest groups. The concept of issue networks was developed to suggest a more fluid and open set of arrangements, where participants could vary depending on the issues within the policy area—and so the configuration was less stable. In the case of food policy, we might see agricultural policy as being a relatively stable policy community, which has fragmented into a variety of issue networks;[32] for example, around food safety or commodity based concerns, such as dairy, grain crops and so on.[33] Conversely, it can prove difficult to demarcate a clear distinction between a policy and issue. For example, food standards may be an issue in agricultural policy, but can be a policy area in its own right, containing a range of issues such as: authenticity, nutritional content, safety from pathogens and so on. In the European public policy literature there has been a preference for the more generic metaphor of policy network as a means for mapping the players and their presence and actions across the range of issues that make up policy sectors.[34]

Network analysis has been developed as a separate methodology to map, with the aid of mathematical modelling, the presence of different interests (private as well as public) within and across different policy sectors (agriculture, health, energy and labour) in the USA's national policy process.[35] The studies sought to determine the extent that there was a centre of dense and close network relationships in each policy area. What they found was that there was no central core of influence or presence in any area, rather there was a 'hollow core' in each, giving a picture of complexity and diffusion.[35, 36] The actual operating arrangements for the networks differed from policy sector to policy sector, and different coalitions appeared and re-appeared as well, reinforcing other studies' findings that there are different modes of operation in different policy sectors. Across the policy sectors that fall within our remit of food policy, well-positioned groups may gain access across a range of sectors and a range of issue networks—such as food industry trade associations or peak associations from farming, manufacturing or retail. In the UK, prominent groups such as the National Farmers Union and peak associations for trade groups such as the Food and Drink Federation (food and drink manufacturers), the British Retail Consortium (retailers) and the British Hospitality Association (food service industry) are represented on a wide range of food policy stakeholder and consultative committees in government agencies (such as the FSA) and departments (such as Defra).

Food governance

Governance in the food sector can occur in the absence of direct state involvement when private and societal interests seek to exert forms of control within the market economy. However, the shadow of the state does loom over these arrangements, usually providing some enabling or operating context for this governance. Examples include: standards setting and grading of produce, process- and product-based food assurance schemes, contractual specifications from food manufacturers and retailers to growers, or from retailers to manufacturers through own-brand labelled foods.[37–40] Private governance forms throw up new power relationships along supply chains, particularly through the extraction of economic value. Academic concepts such as global commodity chain analysis and global value chains have focused on the governance strategies and forms that are deployed along international food-supply chains.[41] Corporate retailers are at the forefront of what are now characterized as buyer-driven food-supply chains. The positions of control gained by supermarkets, as the buyers with a dominant market position and acting as gatekeepers to the consumer, have altered relationships and changed who adds value and appropriates profits along the supply chain. Product and process specifications are set out by individual retailers or consortia of different retailers. In short, the setting of standards entails forms of private sector governance of supply chains. This governance can impact upon both the social and environmental standards of contracted suppliers and their livelihoods. These relationships and their impacts are looked at in more detail in the Chapter 5 on the food-supply chain.

New and alternative modes of ordering may emerge from civil society as 'alternative food networks' arise to challenge the dominant supply chains, setting new criteria as in the case of fair trade foods.[42] The growth of the fair-trade movement provides a good example of how the governance of agri-food standards can originate from civil society organizations, as has been the case with animal welfare standards, such as the Freedom Foods classification developed by an animal welfare NGO in the UK. NGOs and corporations can combine to produce their own criteria, traceability and labelling systems for food produce, as with the example of the Marine Stewardship Council set up as a result of collaboration instigated by Unilever with WWF, the NGO, in 1997 to certify produce from sustainable fisheries.

The development of private-sector forms of governance are subject to redirection and intervention from the state and inter-governmental organizations and polities (such as the EU) to address specific public policy goals around food. In the case of food safety reform, EU public policy makers have sought to utilize the private governance arrangements to achieve their goals of safe and audited handling and processing of food—pushing responsibility on to the food retail point initially but ultimately requiring responsibility for audited safety procedures back along the food-supply chain and on to the farm.

Responsibility was allocated through the requirement of due diligence from all food handlers up to the point of sale to the public. Due diligence was enshrined in the UK 1990 Food Safety Act and the EU's Food Hygiene Directive in 1993. The extension of due diligence, all the way back to the farm itself, arrived with the EU's reform of the general food principles of food law in 2002.

A first example of this private–public governance interaction and symbiosis was through the adoption of Hazard Analysis and Critical Control Points (HACCP) procedures. HACCP is a process-based system aimed at good hygiene practice and inspection in food businesses, which focuses on the points where contamination of food is most likely to occur at each stage of the food-supply chain. HACCP, as a process for identifying risk points, was developed from the mid-1980s in the agri-food sector, although its origins lay with the NASA space programme in earlier decades. Codex also developed HACCP-based standards at the international level for countries to use. HACCP is a regulatory process that relies upon the voluntary compliance by industry, and government (approved) inspection of the processes (usually paperwork records) is the main form of state enforcement. In the UK, the Home Authority Principle was introduced, which allowed the large corporate retailers with multiple branches across the country to designate one branch, usually near the company headquarters, that would serve as the token and lead branch for food hygiene inspections. The inspections would be conducted by that local government (or home) authority, which would cover the inspection standards for all of the other branches for that retailer across the country.[43]

The widespread adoption of food assurance schemes in EU states provides another related illustration of the private–public governance and auditing interface. In the case of the UK, the introduction of due diligence stimulated industry collaboration along commodity supply chains in animal meat products and combinable crops in the form of assurance schemes. The schemes were designed to ensure that the farming and food and related industries (such as transportation) could exhibit the existence of systems of due diligence (including HACCP protocols). The schemes also had the advantage of offering reassurance to the consuming public that high standards were being met by British producers. The dominant corporate retailers also had some of their own assurance schemes, which, in many ways, were an extension of the contractual-based standards required by retailers of their food suppliers. As these schemes developed in the UK, the NFU developed a common system and a label, for farmer-producer led assurance schemes, which the UK Government endorsed. As this scheme evolved into the Assured Food Standards (AFS) and incorporated a wider range of stakeholder organizations from along the food-supply chain, it came to embrace over 78,000 farmers under its little red tractor scheme. Further recognition from the state for the AFS came from the Food Standards Agency, who conferred further legitimacy under the implementation arrangements of the EU General Hygiene Regulations in 2007. Under the agreed terms of implementation only 2% of farms would be audited by local government inspectors as against 25% of non-scheme farms, a process of 'earned recognition'.[44] In effect the AFS is providing a private-based form of co-regulation for the state. Michael Power,[45] in his examination of the audit society, observed that this has become a widespread trend of governance: 'Instead of regulation seeking to penetrate organizational culture from the outside, the image proffered is more that of a form of self control embodied in quality control systems'.[45] For Power, the delegation of regulatory control helps solve legitimacy problems for the state and enhances compliance 'but the state remains an important sponsor of private interest regulation'.[45] In this way, there is a bridging, or indeed a virtual, dissolution of the public–private governance divide. The state is able to devolve responsibility and the bulk of the work of governance to industry, or other non-governmental actors, including much of the auditing task.

The execution of policy is often mediated by private interests that are business interests from along the food-supply chain in this governance model. Private-interest government is a concept that has been deployed to understand the close relationships between industry and government in policy-making; for example, in the dairy sector and in food retailing.[43, 46, 47] It was a clear basis for policy development in many agricultural sectors in the UK from the late-1940s until the late-1980s. However, from the 1990s the concerns of civil society around food production have resulted in both institutional reforms and policy changes at UK and EU levels. Government's concerns with food policy have broadened out once again from production supports to regulating the damaging outcomes of intensive production, such as food safety and environmental harm, and a greater focus upon consumption (see Chapter 2). Nonetheless, the key industry players in the food sector remain firmly in the policy networks around food and agriculture policy. For example, in response to the crisis in farming with plunging farm-gate prices from the late-1990s, the Ministry for Agriculture Fisheries and Food (MAFF), the predecessor to Defra, set up a food-chain group to look at how to improve the efficiency of food production. Subsequently, after the reports of the Curry Commission and Defra's subsequent farming and food strategy, the government sponsored the creation of the Food Chain Centre (FCC) in 2002, which was located within the IGD, formerly called the Institute for Grocery Distribution, a research think-tank sponsored by the grocery retailers.[48] The FCC's role was to improve the efficiency of UK farming through more efficient co-ordination of supply chains from British produced foods. The FCC employed the lean production paradigm model from car manufacturing pioneered by Toyota, which sought to integrate their suppliers into the manufacturing process.[49] By 2006 it had carried out 33 value chain analyses, seeking efficiency improvements along a range of food product lines and disseminating improved benchmarking criteria for each product line back to farmers as food producers.[50] The broader aim for the government was to create leaner and more competitive food producers and supply chains for the international market-place. The original board representation included the key trade associations along the UK food-supply chain: the British Retail Consortium (BRC), the Food and Drink Federation (FDF), the National Farmers Union (NFU), as well as IGD and MAFF. Similar governance approaches have been used by the UK State to improve the environmental performance of food-supply chains, with the creation of enabling bodies, such as the Waste Resources Programme (WRAP) and Envirowise and the Carbon Trust, to work in partnership with industry (see Chapter 6 for a more detailed explanation). Another example was in the area of public procurement, with the setting up of the School Food Trust in 2005 to take forward the setting of nutritional standards for school meals in the state-school sector in England.

This interaction of private and public forms of rule and governance presents us with a clearer understanding of what we can term food governance. This is an interactive process of state and public laws and policy with private interests and actors. The private sector governance may be corporate led or originate from civil society, as depicted in Fig. 3.1. These different sectors interact and each can play a shaping role upon the actions of the other. Policy networks tend to portray a consensual process of negotiation and co-operation amongst participants, but the interaction of these sectors may be one of relative conflict and tension as well. The results can still have a policy impact in terms of shaping corporate practice. The watchdog role of civil society based NGOs, and the potential for (negative) publicity, can act as a pressure on corporate actions with attendant market-place effect, from ensuring dolphin-free tuna to preventing the use of child labour by contract suppliers. The rise of corporate social responsibility (CSR) has gone hand in hand with both civil society scrutiny and state regulation. In the UK, there has been a rush of CSR initiatives by the corporate food retailers.[51] This follows growing civil society scrutiny of aspects of their product-choice and supply-chain instructions to farmers and growers; including exercises that score the supermarkets according to environmental and other criteria, such as the health-supporting nature of their products.[52, 53] In the case of pesticide residues, the UK Government's regulators had made public the results of governmental inspections of residue levels found on fresh produce on the shelves of the multiple retailers from 1998. Friends of the Earth then tabulated the results to compare the environmental and health performance of the retailers.[52] Two of the smaller high street supermarkets, which specialize in own-brands, responded to these pressures by raising their standards. Marks and Spencer, which has a strong high-value-added food profile, phased out 79 pesticides, some of which remained state approved.[54] The company's stated goal of selling residue-free produce would have a significant impact on its 47 fresh-produce suppliers, who in turn work with 1,000 farmers worldwide. The Co-operative Group, a retailer with a lower socio-economic customer-base but a strong ethical tradition and with around 4 per cent UK market share, unilaterally banned 24 pesticides for which there are alternative growing options; six of them were approved by the UK regulatory system.[55]

The picture here reflects an interaction between: state inspection and data collection, civil society organization, in the form of Friends of the Earth's use of this data to create a new set of standards or rankings, and the retailers' private governance response in the form of raising their own standards to ban certain pesticides from their supply chains. Food governance can involve actors from each of these sectors, the state, corporate sector and civil society, as well as the professions who may be based within the state (environmental health officials) or be independent of the state (food scientists) or sit in both (nutritionists and doctors). The UK State has opened up and reformed its institutional structures around food to incorporate the consumer interest with the creation of the Food Standards Agency (FSA).[56] The state can use these other spheres of governance to implement policy or to help achieve public policy goals, such as rolling out community food projects (in Chapter 8) or strategies to reduce food waste, audit carbon on the food-supply chain, or to audit water-use (see Chapter 6). Equally the initiatives of private governance can lead the policy, as in animal welfare standards or ethical trade. For these initiatives, the state may play a more back-seat role, monitoring and approving developments when deemed necessary; or it may be left behind by the actions of civil society and the corporate sector, and be required to catch up with the shifting agenda. A graphic presentation of this account of the governance flows that operate through food policy in the UK, through the interaction of the public and private sectors (divided into the corporate sector and civil society) is given in Fig. 3.1. This represents what can be termed as the scope of food governance in UK.

Multi-level governance of food policy

While the focus of public policy is at the level of the national state—much important food policy takes place at levels within and below the national

Legislation and regulation: EU and national (and international regime commitments) → **state framing of policy initiatives** → **governance flows via:**

State agencies and bodies implement and/or direct policy
- Directing policy from central government – e.g. Defra and Department Health
- Devolved assembly administrations (Scotland, Wales and N. Ireland) with separate jurisdiction and decision-making, e.g.:
  - Agriculture and Environmental Health
- Directing policy at arm's length from the central government – e.g:
  - Food Standards Agency: powers at arm's length from central government
  - Local authority trading standards officers (LACORS); environmental health officers
- Arm's length via "new governance" bodies - e.g.:
  - School Food Trust
  - Food Chain Centre
  - Assured Food Standards (AFS)

And/or
Private forms of governance:
Implementation of regulations or introducing new initiatives, standards and criteria
- Corporate sector origins: e.g. new audit and certification schemes e.g.
  - Air Miles labels from retailers
- Civil Society sector origins: audit and certification e.g.
  - RSPCA – Freedom Foods; Fair Trade schemes
- Corporate and civil society origins: e.g.
  - Marine Stewardship Council - Unilever & WWF
- State & corporate sector implementation: e.g.
  - Home Authority Principle
  - "earned recognition" for members of AFS schemes less inspection

KEY: Governance flows

Fig. 3.1 Food Governance: UK policy and governance flows.

and, increasingly, above and beyond it. Sub-national levels of public policy activity vary in their degree of autonomy and impact, conditioned by the legal-constitutional order in which they exist and degree of delegated law-making and power available to local state and local policy-making. In food policy, local government levels have played an important role in attempting to address food access and poverty issues, such as with the Toronto Food Policy

Council (see Chapter 8). In the UK, some key parameters of food policy have moved to regional administrative levels and to elected devolved government assemblies (in Scotland, Wales and Northern Ireland) as a result of constitutional and administrative reforms since the late 1990s.[57]

The increased role of international trading regimes, such as NAFTA and Mercosur and especially the more mature EU, which can be viewed as having many of the features of a self-standing political process or polity, have impacted upon the role of the state in making public policy. At a global level, the WTO agreements, with their binding rules on food standards and food production supports, are another level of impact upon national policies. As Bob Jessop points out 'there is a complex trend towards the internationalisation of policy regimes. The international context of domestic state action has extended to include a widening range of extra-territorial or transnational factors and processes; and it has also become more significant strategically for domestic policy'.[58] The combination of devolution of power and policy input downwards to local and regional governments and upwards to international regimes, with the state's withdrawal from some areas of activity such as ownership of industries and utilities, has been characterized as the 'hollowing out of the state'.[59] However, the state still remains a key player in these policy processes, but shares this governance with outside actors and other levels of political authority—leading to the development of the concept of multi-level governance to embrace these developments.

The concept of multi-level governance was developed first in the context of the EU and its member states and sub-national governments.[60] The determination of some key decisions by the EU and its member states has been explained within a framework of multi-level governance, in the form of two-level or multi-level strategic bargaining and decision-making.[29, 60, 61] Domestic considerations impact on international decisions, but international decisions also catalyse domestic considerations.[62] There may be a range of decisions taking place simultaneously according to different institutional rules and in slightly different domestic policy contexts, which are shaping each other to some extent.

Some recent academic work on food governance has extended the concept for the agri-food sector to include international-global level agreements and rules.[56, 63, 64] Notably, these include the impact upon national and local levels of decision-making of: the WTO's Agreement on Agriculture, the Sanitary and Phytosanitary (SPS) Agreement (based in part on Codex standards), the Technical Barriers to Trade (TBT) Agreement and the Trade-Related Intellectual Property Rights Agreement (TRIPS). In agriculture, the negotiation of the General Agreement on Tariffs and Trade (GATT) Uruguay Round agreements and the so-called McSharry reforms of the CAP (achieved in 1992) took place simultaneously. The negotiations involved: international, EU and national-level bargaining games (including the US, countries in the Cairns group of commodity exporting countries, developing countries and so on).[65, 66] The Agenda 2000 reforms of the CAP were shaped, at least in part, by the terms of the trade rules laid out in the AoA.[66] The agreement allowed for government supports for agriculture that have 'no, or at most minimal, trade distorting effects or effects on production' nor have 'the effect of providing price support to producers'. Such supports were seen as truly de-coupled from production and so were put into the so-called 'green box'. Direct payments to farmers, that seek to reduce production under Agenda 2000, such as arable area and livestock headage payments, were also allowed under the Agreement on Agriculture. However, such supports are supposed to be phased out over a period of time under the 'blue box' classification.

There were several ambiguities in the wording of the Agreement on Agriculture, reflecting the fraught diplomatic negotiations and compromises that produced it, and a review was built in from 2000, originally due to be completed in 2003. The Agriculture review was subsumed within the Doha or 'development' round of negotiations over revision of the WTO agreements that was agreed in 2002. This was termed the 'development' round, as it was agreed that the negotiations should seek outcomes designed to benefit the development of the agricultural producers of less developed countries under the trade rules. In part, the completion of the Agriculture review was seen as being contingent upon the outcomes of the mid-term review of the Agenda 2000 reform of the CAP subsidies. This EU-level reform of CAP was completed in 2003 with the agreement for a single-payment scheme of de-coupled payments. The European policy-makers saw this reform as being in compliance with the existing rules of the Agreement on Agriculture. Nonetheless, the CAP reform, along with the USA's desire to maintain its farm supports for food and feed commodity producers, were seen as insufficient by many developing nations negotiating over agricultural reform under the Doha round. As a result, the completion of this round of trade liberalization negotiations ground to a halt in July 2006. While negotiations continued within the WTO's permanent committee rooms, no satisfactory resolution had been found to move the talks back to the Ministerial level by the end of 2008.

The process of mutually contingent regime reviews is illustrative of the context within which multi-level governance leads to strategic policy choices, and multi-level bargaining and game playing, by states and other participants such as international organizations. In the case of the CAP Agenda 2000 mid-term review, the European Commission led a further shift from production subsidies, a process termed de-coupling, to more qualitative supports under the single farm-payment schemes. The EU has sought to frame these supports as green-box compliant and 'non- or minimally trade distorting' under the terms of the Agreement on Agriculture. The UK Government has supported the Commission's policy direction on CAP reform. The introduction of the Department for the Environment, Food and Rural Affairs (Defra) as a government department merging environment with agriculture and rural affairs, marked an institutional affirmation of this policy approach of wider agri-environment and rural development supports for British agriculture. Hence, an important factor in the UK's domestic approach to food policy reform was the calculation of the likely direction of trade-liberalization agreements and CAP reform, and was reflected in Defra's subsequent *Strategy for sustainable farming and food*.[48] Strategic decision-making, of course, is just that. It is highly contingent upon rational calculations of policy at other levels playing out in certain directions. Exactly what type of supports are indeed 'green-box' compliant is still open to interpretation, and has been challenged by the so-called 'G20' developing countries in WTO negotiations. At the same time, then, multi-level governance may not only lead to a process of gradual harmonization through compromise but also, witness political contest, conflict and stalemate.

Corporate, industrial and civil society organizations monitor and seek to influence the different policy arenas at these multi-levels. European and international levels of governance have seen a multiplication of new NGO alliances and trade associations and their sponsored organizations engaging, as what have been termed as, trans-national networks entering a trans-national policy space.[67] In addition, professional bodies and experts, notably in the form of epistemic communities, i.e. bodies of experts who claim authoritative knowledge and are recognized within international regimes, can be instrumental in both national and international policy formulation. International organizations themselves, such as the European Commission and the secretariats of the WTO, play important roles in prompting policy solutions by helping to frame the terms of the debate. The trans-national approaches emphasize the role of these multiple and non-state actors and the international settings of policy-making. Taken further the impacts of globalization have led to theories of global governance, where the lines of interpretation emphasize the diminished role of the state and of governments, and the dominance of hegemonic discourses over public policy.[68] However, once the focus of global or international policy-making alights on individual international regimes, it becomes clear that states play key roles as decision-makers and brokers of competing interests in such regimes. This is illustrated by studies of the WTO's agriculture and food safety regimes and the related decision-making in the Codex Alimentarius, which is the joint FAO and WHO food standards setting body, whose decisions inform the WTO rules.[39, 69] Multi-level governance allows for these state and international level interactions over public policy to be related and explained.

The state and market economy relationship informs the rise to prominence of international trade-based regimes in the contemporary governance of food. International sourcing of agricultural commodities as ingredients to final processed or manufactured foods, and of fresh fruits and vegetables, has increased with the globalizing trends in the economy. There has been the rise of global brands in food service, food manufacturing and drink and beverages along with multi-national grocery retailers. Corporate concentration is a clear feature of some segments of the food economy, as is explained in more detail in Chapter 5. Among the competing interests deployed across the international regimes and organizations ruling on food, agriculture, health and the environment, the presence of large corporations and trade associations looms large. The corporate interests and their trade organizations have the resources to guarantee a lobbying presence across a range of relevant international regimes and organizations—they are able to shift the debate across a range of policy-making arenas. The neo-pluralists' identification of structural bias at national policy level is reiterated at the international and global levels—although the regimes at the higher levels greet a larger size of market player through their portals. These realities point to a structural framing of policy discourse and the comparative influence of competing interests. The spread of a dominant neo-liberal policy discourse underpins the operation of these regimes, although this set of ideas is contested and the momentum of the neo-liberal consensus shows signs of faltering—not least in the breakdown of the Doha round of world trade negotiations.

The previous sections have introduced a range of actors that engage and seek to influence public policy outcomes around food. From dietetic and nutritional standards and healthy eating advice and food composition, to farm subsidies and supports, to food safety assurance processes. A summary of some of these key actors, institutions and actors are drawn from the discussion in this chapter and throughout the rest of the book, as presented in Table 3.1. The table utilizes a multi-level governance structure and classifies the actors according to their location in:

- the public sector;
- the food industry sector differentiated by stage of the supply chain: primary production, primary processing, manufacturing, retail and catering; and more briefly:
- other relevant industrial sectors (e.g. distribution);
- the consuming public.

Table 3.1 Policy actors, organizations and institutions at local, national, regional and international levels: some examples

Policy Actors, Organizations and Institutions	Local	National (UK)	European (Regional)	International/Global
Group 1— STATE & PUBLIC SECTOR	Food control/safety authorities, statutory responsibilities fulfilled by local authority employed officers (often professions' based). For example: Public health doctors and nutritionists (monitoring nutrition status of populations), veterinarians (e.g., food hygiene in abattoirs), trading standards officers (food regulations, labelling, food product safety); environmental health (food safety and hygiene of retailing and catering premises), local health services (e.g. school nurses, laboratories).	Government Ministries: Main food policy focus: agriculture, health, environment. Plus influential: economy, trade and competition, industry consumers, education, etc.	Regional economic areas and agreements: e.g. EU and broader European Free Trade Area (EFTA), NAFTA, Mercosur, ASEAN.	World Trade Organization Committees on Agriculture, SPS, etc.
		Government agencies: Food Safety Agencies Environment Agencies National Institutes of Public Health/Health Protection Agencies	EU regulators European Commission: e.g. DG Sanco (Health and Consumers), DG Agriculture, DG Environment, etc.	United Nations: Food and Agriculture Organization, World Health Organization, Joint FAO/WHO Codex Alimentarius (food standards). UN Conference on Trade and Development, United Nations Conference on Environment and Development,
		Legislatures: MPs—devolved assemblies.	European Parliament & MEPs.	World Food Programme.
		Government sponsored bodies across industry and civil society sectors: e.g. Schools Food Trust (England).	EU agencies: European Food Safety Agency, Food and Veterinary Office, European Environment Agency, etc.	Consultative Groups on International regimes. Framework Convention on Climate Change Biodiversity Convention.

PRIVATE & CORPORATE SECTOR 1: FOOD INDUSTRY	Local	National (UK)	European (Regional)	International/Global
Primary producers	Individual farms and farmers. Urban agriculture and horticulture; allotments associations.	National Farmers Unions. Producer product associations: e.g. National Beef Association. Large Landowners: e.g. Country Landowners and Businesses (UK) Marketing boards—produce sector focused, e.g. English Levy Boards. Farmer-grower co-operatives vertically integrate up supply chain: e.g. Danish Tulip become major policy influencers. Alternative agriculture: e.g. UK Soil Association—organic food and farming trade association. e.g. France—Confederation Paysanne: peasant farming movement.	EU trade associations and lobbying—notably on CAP. COPA/COGECA—farmers confederations—powerful in CAP. European Landowners Association.	Governed under trade rules of the WTO—notably Agreement on Agriculture and SPS agreements. Farmer-grower co-operatives move into processing, etc. e.g. Fronterra in Dairy—NZ farmers co-operative—multinational business. National trade associations can have strong international lobbying presence, e.g. American Soybean Association. Via Campesina—international peasant and small farmers movement (supported by European alternative and more radical farming organizations).

Continued

Table 3.1 (continued) Policy actors, organizations and institutions at local, national, regional and international levels: some examples

PRIVATE & CORPORATE SECTOR 1: FOOD INDUSTRY	Local	National (UK)	European (Regional)	International/Global
Agricultural input industries	Decline in local companies—increasingly agents of multi-national corporations from agricultural machinery to seed merchants to fertilizers.	Lobbying presence at national levels: e.g. pesticide companies mainly international but national lobbying and regulatory focus orientation. Trade Associations such as: Agricultural Industries Confederation (AIC)—pesticides, fertilisers, seeds and animal feed. British Society of Plant Breeders (BSPB).	Strong European lobbying presence as individual corporations and trade association: e.g. EuropaBio (life sciences and biotech companies).	Life science corporations: e.g. Bayer, Novartis, Aventis, Monsanto: multinational corporations with international political reach.
Primary food and feed processing and trading industries	Some local producers and craft processors; bakers; cheese makers, etc. Overall sector marked by large corporate concentration in main food and feed commodities.	National Trade Associations: e.g. flour millers NABIM—National Association of British and Irish Millers. Increasingly key policy actors are based in multinational corporations.	Euro-trade associations: e.g. animal feed; Fefana; EU Association of feed additives and pre-mixtures operators. e.g. European Dairy Industry (EDA).	Multinational corporations such as: Cargill, Bunge, ADM dominate trading in major food and feed commodities and the first stage processing in oils and flours & Fronterra (Dairy).

	Local	National	EU	Global
Food Manufacturing		UK National trade associations; e.g. Food and Drink Federation FDF (UK). Individual manufacturing sectors e.g. UK Federation of Bakers. Large scale Bread making.	CIAA: EU focused food manufacturers association.	Large multinational corporations: e.g. Unilever, Danone, Nestlé, and Kraft have extensive international lobbying reach. International Life Sciences Institute (ILSI)—is an manufacturing industry based network of food scientists and technologists at the forefront of promoting functional foods, etc.
Food retailing	Small local retailers associations give some critical mass, e.g. in UK Farma—Farm Shops, corner shops and farmers' markets. Local regional: Booths (NW England).	Corporate multiple retailers (supermarkets) strong individual lobbying presence, e.g. top four: Tesco, Asda Wal-Mart, Sainsbury, Morrisons. British Retail Consortium Trade Association. IGD—grocery retailers think tank policy research organization.	EuroCommerce: European Retail industry trade Association.	Supermarket chains with global reach: e.g. Wal-Mart (USA), Ahold (Nether-lands), Carrefour (Fr), Tesco (UK).
Catering	Small private restaurants and canteens.	Mass caters; national presence in work and private and public canteens (Compass; Sodexho). British Hospitality Association: trade association—weaker of the UK Trade associations.	Agreements between neighbouring countries on a regional basis—franchise between different restaurant chains.	McDonald's, Pizza Hut, Kentucky Fried Chicken—global reach and presence with strong lobbying presence at national levels.

Continued

Table 3.1 (continued) Policy actors, organizations and institutions at local, national, regional and international levels: some examples

PRIVATE & CORPORATE SECTOR 2: other relevant industries to food policy	Local	National (UK)	European (Regional)	International/Global
Financial services	Banks and micro-credit organizations.	National banks, lending facilities, insurance companies.	Agreements between neighbouring countries on a regional basis: e.g. for governing the euro, stockmarkets and share-holdings. EU regulatory and banking bodies. European Central Bank. European Bank for Reconstruction and Development.	World Bank, International Monetary Fund—public sector institutions direct large scale funds to impact upon structures of national economies and in the case of developing countries' their agricultural and food sectors.
Marketing/ Advertising industries	Newspapers, local media, through hospitals and health facilities.	Newspapers, women's magazines, TV, internet, etc. Trade association: Advertising Association—federation of 30 plus trade groups across marketing, advertising, media.	European market regulation focus of Marketing and advertising industries lobbying. European federations of trade associations, e.g. European Association of Communication Agencies and more specialized lobbying organizations, e.g. European Advertising Standards Alliance.	Multinational advertising companies like WPP (world's largest advertising company) and international public relations corporations like Burston Marsteller. International Chamber of Commerce (ICC).

	Local	National (UK)	European/Regional	Global
Distribution	Local haulage companies and farmers set up protest groups, e.g. in UK Farmers for Action (base for fuel protest movements in UK).	National Road Haulage Association.	European Roundtable of Industrialists (ERT)—lobby and promote EU road transport infrastructure projects. Very influential pressure group in EU. Airline companies (air freight of food).	Airline companies (air freight of food).
Group 3—CIVIL SOCIETY				
Public Interest NGOs	Food poverty action groups.	Consumer associations. National Heart Forum. Sustain (food NGO alliance). Friends of the Earth. RSPB.	Pesticides Action Network (Europe/Asia Pacific/Americas, etc.). European Heart Forum. Birdlife International. Friends of the Earth Europe. EuroCoop.	Consumers International, IACFO—International Association of Consumers Organizations, Greenpeace International, La Leche League International.
Government sponsored NGOs	Community food projects.	National Consumer Council (UK).	BEUC, the European consumers organization; European Environmental Bureau.	

Continued

Table 3.1 (continued) Policy actors, organizations and institutions at local, national, regional and international levels: some examples

Group 3—CIVIL SOCIETY	Local	National (UK)	European/Regional	Global
Professions	Professions are recognized and organized primarily on a national basis, with regional and international associations of national bodies. Cross both private and public sectors or more common in either public or private sectors.	Mainly public sector in the UK: Doctors. Nutritionists. Dieticians. Environmental Health and Trading Standards. Officers. Scientists in food and agriculture research Institutes. Mainly private sector: food scientists, pharmaceutical chemists. Royal Society Professional Unions (e.g. Chemistry, Agriculture, etc.).	European Scientific Associations/ Unions range across life sciences, food science and technology, nutrition, etc. European Science Foundation— sponsored by national governments via national scientific unions—influential on lobbying on science and technology.	International Scientific Associations. Scientific advisory experts to international organizations, e.g. Codex Alimentarius. Epistemic communities prevalent in international regimes.
Group 4—THE CONSUMING PUBLIC	The public is organized at a local level (individuals) or at a national level via mechanisms in all democratic countries. Also the public are organized through civil society based organizations (public interest NGOs), campaigns (fair trade) and social movements.			

Food policy change

An established picture of public policy change depicts change as incremental, minor adjustments taking place over a period of time.[70] Peter Hall has identified the need to differentiate between different degrees of policy change, drawing from a study of change in economic policy-making.[71] First-order change is incremental; second-order change will involve the development of new policy instruments; and, third-order change may see a change in the prevailing policy paradigm—i.e. a change in the pattern of ideas that are accepted by the actors and within the main policy institutions. Third-order change will see a challenge to an established policy paradigm, from a wider array of participants mobilizing new ideas and solutions.[71] These participants may include political parties competing for elected office and governmental control, but also the ascendancy of different expertise and interpretations advocating different policy solutions—often in the form of advocacy coalitions more widely drawn from different sections of society, which may include different professional bodies informed by differing disciplinary or epistemic views.[72] The more persuasive models attempting to explain the conditions for policy change include a mix of challenges to both the prevailing policy ideas and discourse, and to the hierarchy of accepted expertise, that are voiced in wider society-based debates. These debates may draw on existing evidence or solutions and generate the search for new evidence or new ways of gathering and assessing evidence, such as economic costs of the externalities of diet-related ill heath or environmental and natural resource degradation (see Chapters 4 and 6 for examples). In addition, institutional change or adaptation and changes in policy instruments and solutions feature.[73, 74]

In the case of food safety reforms in the 1990s onwards, new ways of defining control of food and its safety, with a more consumer focus, were put forward and accepted, leading to institutional change and a wider incorporation of interests into policy deliberation under the new FSA, in the case of the UK.[56] However, the significance of such change needs to be judged over a longer term horizon. Any underlying bias of interests of the policy sector may not have been fundamentally challenged, and key established interests may be able to move with the changes and take the reins over new initiatives, such as with the previously cited example of food assurance schemes and the NFU. New policy initiatives, designed to alter existing practices and outcomes and address different areas of need, may well end up retreating to a position of policy confinement, where the established interests re-enter as key actors in the policy execution.[57] Changes may occur within established policy networks allowing in new ideas or paradigms, accepting them and seeking to share in moulding their transfer into policy in ways that meet their own perceived interests; not necessitating any significant change in policy institutions.[33]

Policy change is shaped by a mix of ideas, evidence, actors and institutions and their interaction. The trajectories of contemporary governing have more consciously incorporated wider ranges of actors, from not only the professions, but also from civil society and of course the corporate sector. The result is forms of governance that allow for more diversity in achieving public policy goals, with the state and governments seeking to achieve their goals through a mix of regulatory frameworks, economic and market incentives and wider stakeholder and participant action. For food policy, there are episodes of policy change that are occurring, which signal the growing awareness of the ecological public health prerogatives, as the chapters on the environment and nutrition illustrate. However, these processes of change in food policy are complex and still have a long way to go.

References

1. Parsons W. *Public policy*. Chelthenham: Edward Elgar, 1995.
2. Lister M, Marsh D. Conclusion. In: Hay C, Lister M and Marsh D (ed.) *The state: theories and issues*. Basingstoke: Macmillan, 2006:248—261.
3. Scott J. *Power*. Cambridge: Polity, 2001.
4. Easton D. *A systems analysis of political life*. New York: John Wiley, 1965.
5. Pressman J, Wildavsky A. *Policy implementation: how great expectations in Washington are dashed in Oakland; or, why it's amazing that federal programs work at all*. Berkeley: University of California Press, 1973.
6. Mills CW. *The power elite*. New York: Oxford University Press, 1956.
7. Hunter F. *Community power structure*. Chapel Hill: University of North Carolina Press, 1953.
8. Dahl RA. *Polyarchy: participation and opposition*. New Haven: Yale University Press, 1971.
9. Dahl RA. *Who governs?* New Haven: Yale University Press, 1961.
10. Crenson M. *The un- politics of air pollution*. Baltimore: The Johns Hopkins University Press, 1971.
11. Bachrach P, Baratz M. Two faces of power. *American Political Science Review* 1962;**56**:947–952.
12. Cobb R, Elder C. *Participation in American politics*. Boston: Allyn and Bacon, 1972.
13. Lukes S. *Power: a radical view*. London: Macmillan, 1974.
14. Wilson GK. *Interest groups in the United States*. Oxford: Oxford University Press, 1981.
15. Dahl RA. *Dilemmas of pluralist democracy*. New Haven: Yale University Press, 1982.
16. Lindblom C. *Politics and markets*. New York: Basic Books, 1977.
17. Dunleavy P, O'Leary D. *Theories of the state the politics of liberal democracy*. Basingstoke: Macmillan, 1987.
18. Jessop B. *The future of the capitalist state*. Cambridge: Polity Press, 2002.

19. Evans PB, Rueschemeyer D, Skocpol T (ed.) *Bringing the state back in*. Cambridge: Cambridge University Press, 1985.

20. Foucault M, Gordon CE. *Power/knowledge: selected interviews and other writings, 1972–1977, by Michel Foucault*. New York: Pantheon Books, 1980.

21. Rose N. *Powers of freedom: reframing political thought*. Cambridge: Cambridge University Press, 1999.

22. Pierre J. *Governance, politics and the state*. Basingstoke: Palgrave, 2000.

23. Pierre J, Peters BG (ed.) *Debating governance*. Oxford: Oxford University Press, 2000.

24. Lowi T. Four systems of policy, politics and choice. *Public Administration Review* 1972;**32**:298–310.

25. Majone G. *Regulating Europe*. London: Routledge, 1996.

26. Moran M. *The British regulatory state: high modernism and hyper innovation*. Oxford: Oxford University Press, 2003.

27. Smith MJ. *The politics of agricultural support in Britain*. Aldershot: Dartmouth, 1990.

28. Kooiman J. *Governing as governance*. London: Sage, 1993.

29. Scharpf F. Introduction: the problem-solving capacity of multi-level governance. *Journal of European Public Policy* 1997;**4**(4):520–38.

30. Rhodes R. The new governance: governing without government. *Political Studies* 1996;**XLIV**:652–667.

31. Rhodes R. The governance narrative: key findings and lessons from the ESRC's Whitehall Programme. *Public Administration* 2000;**78**(2):345–363.

32. Smith MJ. From policy community to issue network: salmonella in eggs and the new politics of food. *Public Administration* 1991;**69**(2):235–255.

33. Coleman W, Skogstad G, Atkinson M. Paradigm Shifts and Policy Networks: Cumulative Change in Agriculture. *Journal of Public Policy* 1996;**16**(3):273–301.

34. Jordan G, Schubert J. Policy Networks: special issue. *European Journal of Political Research* 1992;**21**(1–2):1–205.

35. Heinz J, Laumann E, Salisbury R, Nelson R. Elite networks in national policy subsystems. *Journal of Politics* 1990;**52**:356 -90.

36. Laumann EO, Knoke D. *The organizational state*. Madison: University of Wisconsin Press, 1987.

37. Reardon T, Farina E. The rise of private food quality and safety standards: illustrations from Brazil. *International Food and Agribusiness Management Review* 2001;**4**(4):413–421.

38. Busch L. The moral economy of grades and standards. *Journal of Rural Studies* 2000;**16**:273–283.

39. Barling D, Lang T. Trading on Health: Cross-continental production and consumption tensions and the governance of international food standards. In: Fold N, Pritchard B (ed.) *Cross-continental food chains: cross-continental food chains*. London: Routledge, 2005:39–51.

40. Henson S, Reardon T. Private agri-food standards: implications for food policy and agri-food system. *Food Policy* 2005;**30**:241–253.

41. Ponte S, Gibbon P. Quality standards, conventions and governance of global value chains. *Economy and Society* 2005;**34**(1):1–31.

42. Whatmore S, Thorne L. Nourishing networks: alternative geographies of food. In: Goodman D, Watts MJ (ed.) *Globalising food. Agrarian questions and global restructuring.* London: Routledge, 1997:287–304.

43. Flynn A, Marsden T, Harrison M. The regulation of food in Britain in the 1990s. *Policy & Politics* 1999;**27**(4):435–446.

44. Kirk-Wilson R. *Review of uptake of FSA food assurance scheme guidance by UK scheme operators.* London: Food Standards Agency, 2008.

45. Power M. *The audit society: rituals of verification.* Oxford: Oxford University Press, 1997.

46. Streeck W, Schmitter P (ed.) *Private interest government: beyond market and state.* London: Sage, 1985.

47. Grant W (ed.) *Business interests, organizational development and private interest government: an international comparative study of the food processing industry.* Berlin: de Gruyter, 1987.

48. Defra. *Strategy for sustainable farming and food: facing the future.* London: Department for Environment Food and Rural Affairs, 2002.

49. Simons D, Zokaei AK. Application of lean paradigm in red meat processing. *British Food Journal* 2005;**107**(4):192–209.

50. Defra. *Review of food chain initiatives.* London: Department of Food and Rural Affairs, 2007.

51. Lang T, Barling D. The environmental impact of supermarkets: mapping the terrain and the policy problems in the UK. In: Burch D, Lawrence G (ed.) *Supermarkets and agri-food-supply chains.* Cheltenham: Edward Elgar, 2007:192–219.

52. Friends of the Earth. *Pesticides in supermarket food.* London: Friends of the Earth. http://www.foe.co.uk/resource/briefings/pesticide_supermarket_food.pdf [Accessed 9 June 2006], 2004.

53. Dibb SE. *Healthy competition: how supermarkets can affect your chances of a healthy diet.* London: National Consumer Council, 2005.

54. Buffin D. Food retailer aims to restrict pesticide use. *Pesticides News* 2001(54):3.

55. Buffin D. Retailer bans suspect pesticides. *Pesticides News* 2001(53): 3.

56. Barling D. Food Agencies as an institutional response to policy failure by the UK and the European Union. In: Harvey M, McMeekin A and Ward A (ed.) *The qualities of food.* Manchester: Manchester University Press, 2004:107–128.

57. Barling D, Lang T, Caraher M. Joined-up food policy? The trials of governance, public policy and the food system. *Social Policy & Administration* 2002;**36**(6):556–574.

58. Jessop B. *The state and the contradictions of the knowledge-driven economy.* Lancaster: Department of Sociology, Lancaster University, 2000.

59. Rhodes R. The hollowing out of the State. *Political Quarterly* 1994(**65**):138–151.

60. Marks G, Hooghe L, Blank K. European integration since the 1980s: state-centric verses multi-level governance. *Journal of Common Market Studies* 1996;**34**(3):341–378.

61. Moravcsik A. Preferences and power in the European Community. *Journal of Common Market Studies* 1993(**31**):473–524.

62. Putnam R. Diplomacy and domestic politics: the logic of two-level games. *International Organization* 1988;**42**(3):427–60.

63. Lang T, Barling D, Caraher M. Food, social policy and the environment: towards a new model. In: Cahill MAFT (ed.) *Environmental issues and social welfare*. Oxford: Blackwell, 2001:70–90.

64. Morgan K, Marsden T, Murdoch J. *Worlds of food: place, power and provenance in the food chain*. Oxford: Oxford University Press, 2006.

65. Paarlberg R. Agricultural policy reform and the Uruguay Round: synergistic linkage in a two-level game? *International Organization* 1997;**51**(3):413–444.

66. Moyer W, Josling T. *Agricultural policy reform: politics and process in the EU and US in the 1990s*. Aldershot: Ashgate, 2002.

67. Coleman WD, Grant W, Josling T. *Agriculture in the new global economy*. Cheltenham: Edward Elgar, 2004.

68. Roseneau J. Governance in the 21st century. *Global Governance* 1995;**1**(1):13–43.

69. Peine E, McMichael P. Globalization and global governance. In: Higgins V, Lawrence G (ed.) *Agricultural governance: globalization and the new politics of regulation*. London: Routledge, 2005:19–34.

70. Lindblom C. The science of 'muddling through. *Public Administration Review* 1960;**19**:79–88.

71. Hall P. Policy paradigms, social learning and the State. *Comparative Politics* 1993;**25**:275–296.

72. Sabatier P. An advocacy coalition framework of policy change and the role of policy oriented learning therein. *Policy Sciences* 1988(21):129–168.

73. Kingdon J. *Agendas, alternatives and public policies*. Boston: Little Brown, 1984.

74. Baumgartner F, Jones B (ed.) *Agendas and instability in American politics*. Chicago: University of Chicago Press, 1993.

Chapter 4

Nutrition

This chapter explores how and why nutrition has the long policy pedigree already noted. During over a century and a half of existence, nutritional science has provided advice in times of war, 'technical fixes' for health deficiencies, and helped shape agricultural policy and commercial product ranges. Its range of influence has been considerable, yet its impact has varied—more at some times than others—and the relationship between nutrition and policy-making is often problematic. Its findings sometimes imply, if not overtly call for, changes in supply. Its researchers have had a long track record of pointing to unmet health potential and evidence of inequality, all of which has been known to disconcert sectional interests, let alone policy-makers.[1] This is the case again today when there is ample evidence about diet's bad effect on public health.[2]

We suggest, too, in this chapter that nutrition has not one but three distinct traditions and foci, each of which has different messages for policy. One stresses the bio-chemical basis of nutrients and their implications for health. Another centres on how social factors shape dietary intake. The third, which we term ecological or environmental nutrition, explores how nutrition is a function of humanity's environmental infrastructure. The 21st century ecological public health challenge requires each nutrition tradition to address both environmental protection generally and how to eat sustainably in particular. It is highly likely that diets will be reshaped by the need to lower food's climate change and water impact, for example (see Chapter 6). These two considerations alone might well alter current dietary advice and which foods are produced and distributed. Over and above that policy requirement, all three nutrition traditions face a difficulty in the lag between their generation of evidence and policy engagement. Evidence of the need to tackle over-consumption has been strong for decades but the policy response has been patchy. This gap between evidence and policy suggests the need to consider whether the complex architecture of institutions, which emerged involving nutrition in the 20th century, is complete. Nutrition science now sends complex messages to policy-makers, and a doubt may be voiced as to whether this more complex and sophisticated understanding is an example of the problem of policy cacophony, where competing voices, each with good evidence, fail to deliver policy coherence. The challenge for nutrition is how to integrate its three traditions.

Why nutrition matters

Although nutrition has played a big part in food policy (see Chapter 2), its importance has been contested. One criticism is that neither the state nor any other powerful entity has the moral right to be involved in food choice; food intake is a private matter, an engagement between the eater and the market. This argument has been influential within the consumer movement and also championed by neo-liberals.[3] The right to choose was one of President John F Kennedy's four consumer rights in his 15 March 1962 speech, which are still enshrined in the now eight Consumer Rights of Consumers International (CI), the world consumer alliance.[4] It has led to nutrition policy stressing the 'right to know', a combination of two of CI's Consumer Rights (to information and to education), and to debates about whether nutrients should be labelled, and if so how.[5] The effectiveness of nutrient labelling in shaping consumer behaviour change depends on many other variables, such as knowledge, preparedness to act, price signals, culture, household role. Labelling can, however, encourage processors to reformulate product recipes. Its effectiveness, in short, resides in encouraging manufacturers to 'choice-edit' rather than leave it to 'choice' by consumers.

A second criticism voiced of nutrition is that it is riven by contradictory evidence and thus not able to give public policy advice and, more extremely, that its experts are wrong. These arguments have been addressed elsewhere.[6, 7] The rebuttal is that, like all areas of scientific inquiry, there are debates and uncertainties but that nutrition evidence is sufficiently consistent and strong to help shape policy; that overall disease profiles, at the population level, are seriously affected by food intake and quality; that the resulting ill-health is costly to individuals and society; that poor nutrition at the population level adds to healthcare budgets; and that it is in the interests of all to prevent their worsening. Health institutions, however, are sometimes nervous about being seen to be too didactic, a situation that can be exploited by interests who do not want nutrition taken seriously.[8] As a result, leadership and policy direction are not always clearly charted, a situation exacerbated by the different foci of interest from the three traditions (explored in more depth below).

Reflecting the general consumerist and non-interventionist policy frameworks of recent decades, the mainstream nutrition policy message has been couched in health education terms, relying on individual choice and consumer power. The counter view to this is that what is required is a whole population shift which requires change upstream in the food-supply chain. If fat is being produced in large quantities, for instance, it is likely to be consumed somewhere in some form or other, often 'hidden' in processed or catered food.[9] Between 1967–69 and 1997–99, the production of fat per capita in North America and the European Community rose by 26% and 31%, respectively, suggesting oversupply.[6] The onus on individual behaviour change is probably inadequate in such a situation.[10] The case for distinguishing between relying on individual behaviour change and trying to engender population change was articulated by epidemiologist Geoffrey Rose.[11] He was clear that a population focus allows for (and assumes) continued variation within populations. The need to address social determinants of health at that population level was the purpose of the WHO's Commission on the Social Determinants of Health.[12] Appealing to individual change can have the perverse effect of action by 'worried well' or those aware of need to change, rather than social groups most at risk. Good public health requires systemic change to help frame choices in a healthy direction. This raises the politically thorny issue of how 'soft' or 'hard' policy approaches can and should be. Soft ones include information, labelling and education, while harder more systemic ones include choice-editing (before consumers see products), bans and fiscal measures (see Chapter 7 for further discussion of choice). The range of policy approaches is hotly debated with regard to the big nutrition challenges such as obesity and reducing food's carbon load to prevent climate change. In such matters, structural and society-wide responses are recognized and required.[13]

A third criticism levelled at nutrition is that it is flawed by reductionism, confusing social and cultural meanings for scientific facts. Gyorgy Scrinis has termed this 'nutritionism',[14] a notion and position adopted by Michael Pollan in his critique of nutrition.[15] The argument proposes that nutrition's appeal to policy wrongly reduces 'food' into component bio-chemical parts, when it would be far better to see it primarily as a social function (see Chapter 7). Nutritional reductionism, the argument continues, encourages consumers and policy to pursue the unrealizable Holy Grail of an ideal combination of nutrients; it is a fantasy that breeds public neurosis, encourages food processors' to exploit health by adding or extolling nutrients, adding value and thus distorting culture. The nutritionism argument attempts to relocate eating as a cultural activity first and foremost, severing nutrition from the production and growing of food. Its message to policy-makers and public alike is that consumers ought to reassert their cultural power against scientism on the one hand and food processors on the other hand. It calls on policy-makers and consumers to follow simple or common-sensical dietary behaviour, rooted in culture and tradition. This requires no-one to be a nutritionist. 'Don't eat anything your great grandmother wouldn't recognize as food,' suggested Pollan.

While we sympathize with the argument that foods have been altered by changed production and processing, it would also be absurd to romanticize the past or rudimentary diets; not everyone had access to the Mediterranean diet. Too often diets were restricted, monotonous and lacking in range. Wealth raises access to a variety of foods, even if the quality of ingredients is de-natured. In the time of great grandmothers, nutrient deficiencies led to ill-health. This is too often still the case around the world today, as the WHO catalogues. Iodine deficiency, for instance, leads to cretinism and goiter.[16] Protein deficiencies lead to kwashiorkor, malnutrition or vitamin deficiencies.[17, 18] Scientific understanding of deficiencies has been a major contribution from nutrition science, not just to famine relief but the routine monitoring of whether food markets provide what they should. The standard nutrition policy response to proven deficiencies is to fortify foods, usually by adding the deficient nutrient(s) as ingredients in staple foods.

The message from nutrition for policy becomes more challenging if the direction of dietary change is moving in an inappropriate direction at the population level. More people globally now suffer overweight and obesity (1.1 bn) than hunger (c.900 million). Certainly, as populations get wealthier and are subject to powerful marketing and changed availability of foods, they do seem quickly to consume 'feast day' foods every day. When this happens, health profiles alter, a shift known as the epidemiological transition, itself affected by the nutrition transition, a term coined and a phenomenon studied by Barry Popkin.[19] A series of country profiles show this to be happening as many developing countries modernize, industrialize and become wealthier.[20–23] Their diets tend to shift from traditional staples to processed foods, which are fattier, saltier and sweeter, and from simple to sugary soft drinks, for instance.

The Nutrition Transition covers three changes in supply, culture and health.[9] The supply shift emerges due to investment and strategic choices, notably around agriculture and import/export of foods.[24] The arrival of foreign brands to a developing country can have a dramatic effect, not just in the presence of international food companies seeking new markets but in food expectations and culture. Access changes and choice widens as food becomes more abundant and the supply chain changes; in this process, marketing of 'new' foods opens up consumers to highly processed energy-dense foods. Some features of the nutrition transition improve, such as safety, while others have a more dubious legacy, for instance, the use of additives and colorants enabling longer shelf-life but cosmetic appeal.[25, 26] Overall Popkin and colleagues have documented how calorie intake rises with this shift in food processing and culture.[23] The disease pattern follows later.

Policy and institutional responses to this more complex nutrition picture are emerging, as we discuss below, but there has been less attention to the environment's impact on nutrition and whether nutritional advice needs to be refined by living within environmental limits. Western nutrition science tends to assume limitless sources of nutrients, a fragile assumption applicable to rich rather than poor countries, not least because of inequalities in the food-supply chain and within and between societies (see Chapter 7).

Big problems, low policy profile?

For such an established branch of science, nutrition still suffers from relatively low engagement with mainstream public policy, yet nutrition is in a perfect place to contribute to the food-environment policy debate now emerging. Food's nutritional impact on, within and between populations is shaped by the relationship between food supply, modes of production, environment and society. Like all animals, humans live or die by what they consume, what is in their food and how appropriate the range of foods consumed is. In classical times, the ancients never lacked advice about what to eat and where diet fitted within the cosmos. The literature from the past that has come down to us today is in a language of understanding that modern nutrition puts aside—the reference to the 'passions' and 'humours' lacks biological resonance—but the fact that food affects health, has medicinal properties and potential, was hard-wired into culture everywhere.[27, 28] Nutrition emerged as a modern body of knowledge, however, in the 19th century, building on the sciences as they evolved in the 18th century Age of the Enlightenment. Studying the role of food's constituent parts was integral to the pursuit of understanding the unified order of things. It was helped by work such as James Lind's investigation of scurvy.[29] His interest was aroused by reading of how scurvy killed many crew members of Admiral Anson's fleet circumnavigating the world; over half of one ship's crew died from it. Lind found that it could be prevented by consuming citrus fruit. The precise mechanism he identified was not known for nearly two centuries until Gowland Hopkins' discovery of vitamins in the 1920s. Lind is often credited with having achieved practical success by running real-life experimentation to see what abated the symptoms, but there is some debate about whether this narrative completely fits what happened.[30, 31]

By the early 20th century, there was a clear body of work available to policy-makers. They could improve the diet of both humans and farmed animals. Diet shaped how humans perform adequately, let alone optimally.[32–34] The lineage of modern, systematic, scientific understanding of what nutrients are, which foods have them and their impact on the body and health (or ill-health), can be traced to the work of people such as Lind and, in Germany, to Justus von Liebig. The latter worked from 1820 to the 1870s on the chemical and mineral basis of nutrients in human food and the natural environment. Today, when sciences tend to be specialized, the breadth of von Liebig's work is striking. He bridged science, agriculture and industry. In 1865, von Liebig created beef extract, arguably one of the first industrially-created nutritional 'technical fixes' and an early 'laboratory spin-off' for a nutritional deficiency. His beef extract was rebranded as 'Oxo' after his death, a brand that still exists. The only advertisement allowed to be displayed facing London's River Thames is the formation of the letters 'Oxo' built into the chimney above the Oxo Building just downstream from Parliament, now a restaurant! Von Liebig pioneered not just nutrition but chemistry itself, discovering the role of nitrogen in plant growth and developing nitrogen fertilizers.[35, 36] His work had an inspirational effect on agricultural research, not least the Rothamsted field trials on use of nitrogen fertilizers in the UK. This was arguably the beginning of scientific agriculture, a long collaboration between Sir John Bennett Lawes and the chemist John Gilbert who had worked with von Liebig. Between them, this generation clarified what affected plant and animal growth.

If one impact of early nutritional science was the development and refinement of products, another was its use in measuring behavioural performance, defining how much food a manual as opposed to a sedentary worker needed, for example. This had a powerful effect when the West learned the lessons of disruptions to food supply in the World Wars and the recession in-between. Another strand of work by the mid-20th century was into the impact of diet on non-communicable diseases (NCDs). Ancel Keys' Seven Nations study in the 1950s produced strong epidemiological evidence of diet's population-wide effect. Building on earlier work into nutritional deficiency, Keys and colleagues showed how the Japanese and Greek balance of nutrients explained their longevity and lower incidence of circulatory diseases compared to other richer countries.[37, 38] The people on the Greek island of Crete, whom Keys studied, were not the affluent Greeks or Cretans of today who suffer high levels of obesity. They lived frugal lives, literally consuming lots of fruit within what is now called the Mediterranean diet, honed by a close relationship to home production and environment, i.e. their diet had evolved in tune with local ecology; for example, combing the Mediterranean flora to maximum effect in the case of herbs rich in essential oils. They had a remarkably low incidence of heart disease. Keys' approach laid the foundations for a new era of population approach to food supply. He sent an alert warning to policy-makers on inappropriate consumption. Like another public health sore, tobacco and smoking, this has taken half a century to receive serious policy engagement.

At the same time as the American Keys' findings, Thomas McKeown, a British epidemiologist, proposed an association between greater wealth, consequent improvement in diet, and increased longevity or an absence of particular diseases. McKeown argued that much of the increase in life-expectancy in England and Wales from the 19th century was less due to improvements in medicine than to nutritional advances as the population improved its living standards and disposable income.[39–42] He proposed that there were five possible reasons to explain the decline of mortality. These were: medical intervention, such as immunization; public health measures, such as sanitation and food hygiene; changes in the nature of micro-organisms, such as by mutation; reduced contact with micro-organisms and a decline in contagion; and increased and improved nutrition—in short, a better diet. Subsequently McKeown has been criticized for having underplayed the role of medicine but what he was arguing was that its role was less important than had been portrayed generally. He proposed that other factors—notably improved living standards and greater expenditure on food—were more important.

McKeown's thesis attracted huge academic attention. Some have criticized his use of the data. (McKeown was able to do his analysis in the first place due to the long line of cohort data on England and Wales.) Others have criticized the baseline assumption that high mortality before the 19th century was due to lack of food. RW Fogel, the 1993 Nobel Laureate in Economics, has argued that McKeown confused or conflated diet and nutrition.[43–45] The historian Simon Szretzer has argued convincingly that the impact of medicine in eradicating big killers—cholera, typhoid and smallpox—cannot be under-estimated but nor can it be denied that the public health measures took some time to have effect.[46] The McKeown thesis, although propounding a social rather than medical account of nutrition's impact, has chimed with economists who have seen it as evidence that dietary problems are linked to general economic welfare. They depart from McKeown, however, in generally favouring the view that nutrition is a private choice, not a matter for population shift, which implies public intervention. Although the debate on McKeown continues, with most agreeing with Fogel that in the real world the factors interweave,[45] few economic historians now argue that nutrition is unimportant for population health.

An overview of the global nutritional picture

The global picture of nutrition is given annually in WHO and FAO reports. They portray a patchwork of over-, mal- and under-consumption. In the latter part of the 20th century, the numbers of under-nourished people fell, largely due—if we follow McKeown—to efforts with food production and rising wealth, but the rate of reduction has slowed, and mal-nourishment grew again from the early 2000s.[47, 48] At the same time, evidence of the 'new' issues associated with over-consumption emerged from the 1970s.[6, 49, 50] If under-nourishment symbolized the focus of food policy in the 1970s, over-consumption looked set to shape the 21st century's.[51] Policy conflicts and tempers rose over issues such as marketing and inappropriate food supply as a result. Evidence of rising child obesity and its association with soft drinks and confectionery was a case in point, leading to growing frustration among health analysts about the policy reliance on the language of choice, consumer information and health education.[10, 52-55]

A refrain emerged from nutrition science of inappropriate consumption determining major non-communicable diseases (NCDs) such as coronary heart disease, strokes, hypertension, diabetes, obesity and more. This analysis emerged, as we have seen with Keys decades ago; it was consolidated and officially accepted at national levels too.[7, 56] The connection between inappropriate and excessive consumption of fats, salt and sugars and the rise of NCDs is now accepted as fact.[6, 49, 57-60] Across the globe, health bodies have confirmed and subscribed to this overall position. There have been, and still are, furious debates among them about, for example, which fats matter in diets, what proportions, what the impact of physical activity is in 'burning off' excess calorific intake, or about the role of sugars, but that health advances are being curtailed by an inappropriate mix of food and exercise (i.e. the utilization of nutrients) is not in question. This consensus was summarized in a WHO report in 1990, and reviewed and confirmed by a joint report from the WHO and the FAO in 2003.[6, 49]

The WHO's 2002 World Health Report calculated the source of these preventable deaths. Figures 4.1–4.4 provide summary data on this conventional view of the global nutrition situation. Figure 4.1 gives the assessment of annual deaths worldwide associated with 15 major risk factors. Diet is implicated in all except unsafe sex, tobacco, indoor smoke, urban air pollution (unless that was stretched to include emissions from food transport). Figure 4.2 looks at how those risk factors have an impact in countries with different levels of economic development. Water hygiene, for example, disproportionately affects low income countries with worse water and sanitation infrastructure. Figure 4.3 aggregates those factors affecting both under-nutrition and other dietary and physical activity associated deaths; again these figures are given for different levels of development. Figure 4.4 presents some of the already cited key risk factors by the WHO's six regions (Africa, the Americas, Eastern Mediterranean, Europe, South East Asia and the Western Pacific). It shows

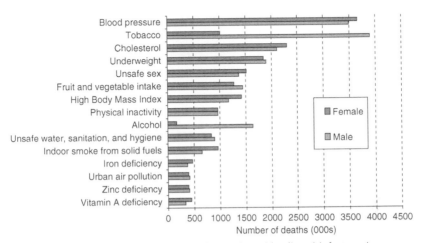

Fig. 4.1 World deaths in 2000 attributable to selected leading risk factors, by sex.

Source: World Health Organization (2002). World Health Report. Geneva: WHO

considerable variation across the regions but there is not the simple rich–poor divide between the regions one might expect. Even South East Asia and the Western Pacific regions exhibit high impact of risk factors associated with inappropriate or over-consumption rather than under-consumption. The picture, as so often for modern food policy, is one of social gradients within and between countries.[12]

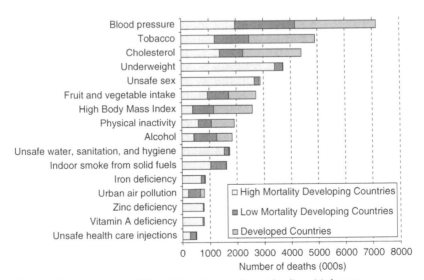

Fig. 4.2 World deaths in 2000 attributable to selected leading risk factors.

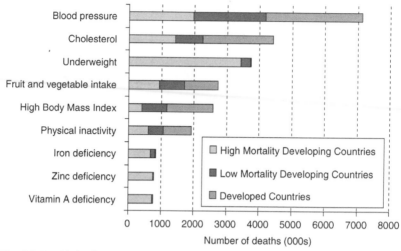

Fig. 4.3 World deaths in 2000 attributable to under-nutrition and diet-related risks and physical inactivity.

With such consistency in the big picture, one might ask why policy-makers have not taken action on nutrition as a result. They have, but this has overwhelmingly been in the 'soft' form of health education and information, rather than upstream prevention. The harder policy response is not yet forthcoming, but is being helped by real appreciation about the formidable healthcare implications of obesity, whose visibility is everywhere.[61] Cost calculations of the impact of dietary health sharpened policy-makers' attention.

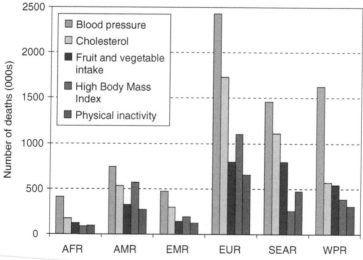

Fig. 4.4 WHO regions deaths in 2000 attributable to selected leading risk factors.

The World Bank and WHO have collaborated in developing methodologies, calculating how many disability-adjusted life-years (DALYs) result from different food and cost regimes. [62–64] This focus on economic costs, however, cannot deviate from the social costs of persistent diet-related ill-health. Developing countries, without the same health infrastructure as rich developed countries, are particularly affected by the double burden of under- and over-consumption.

The cost: obesity as a case study in policy failure?

Although overweight and obesity afflicts growing numbers, even in developing countries, most policy 'noise' has been expressed in developed countries. In the USA, for example, two-thirds of the population are overweight and one-third is clinically obese. An estimated one-fifth of US healthcare expenditures will have to be devoted to treating the consequences of obesity in the future, if current trends continue. [65] In the early 2000s, the US Surgeon General estimated obesity costs up to 6% of healthcare budgets, a figure exceeding $100 billion. [66] The Rand Corporation calculated the big implications for US healthcare costs, concluding that severely obese people are more than twice as likely as people of normal weight to be in fair or poor health and have about twice as many chronic medical conditions. US healthcare costs are 69% higher for overweight men and 60% higher for women compared with people of normal weight. [65, 67] In addition to direct costs, there is also the impact on decreased household incomes, earlier retirement and higher dependence on state benefits; these are likely to exceed the medical costs alone. [68] The weight problems of children and teenagers threatens to convert into lifetime disease, mental health and other social costs. [69] Similar calculations have been run in Europe. In France, obesity was estimated to account for 2% of total healthcare costs by 1995. [70] In England, the National Audit Office estimated in 2001 that obesity cost the NHS an annual £480 million (€720 million) and the wider economy a further £2.1 billion (€3.2 billion). [71] By 2004, that cost was estimated to have risen to £3.3–3.7 billion (€4.95–5.55 billion) for obesity alone and £6.6–7.4 billion (€9.9–11.1 billion) for obesity plus overweight. [72] In the Netherlands, a 2004 study estimated that the proportion of the country's total General Practitioner expenditure attributable to obesity and overweight was around 3–4%. [73]

With data such as these emerging from European member states, the European Commission (EC) Commissioner for Health and Consumer Affairs looked at US incidence as the warning for Europe. In 2003 he pronounced that '[i]t will take nothing short of a behavioural revolution to stop this epidemic in its tracks.' [74, 75] The process of initiating policies and bringing stakeholders together to try to address the problem began. [76]

Globally, the World Health Report 2002 estimated that more than 2.5 million deaths annually were weight-related, with 320,000 deaths directly related to overweight and obesity a year in Europe and more than 300,000 in the USA.[57] In some developing countries, the fear is that an already high incidence of overweight will add further burdens on health systems. In Egypt, for example, an estimated 70% of women and 48% of men are overweight or obese. In 2004, 40% of Moroccans were overweight and 12% of Kenyans.[77] This is in addition to health problems from underweight. With regard to that issue, in 2000 the UN Commission on the Nutrition Challenges of the 21st Century, reporting to the UN's co-ordination body (now the Standing Committee on Nutrition),* concluded that, although progress had been made in lowering the number of children who were underweight, the possibilities to lower that number drastically were still not being taken. 150 million children were being consigned to unnecessary, preventable ill-health.[60]

Diabetes type 2, a diet-related disease, kills approximately 3.8 million people a year worldwide. Not all is weight-related but the incidence of what is, is rising. In 2007, an estimated 246 million people worldwide had diabetes.[59] The incidence of very young people having diabetes type 2 is increasing, suggesting unnecessary premature death and/or many years of costly healthcare. Already, 46% of all those affected are in the 40–59 age group. With obesity and overweight rapidly rising worldwide, diabetes was estimated in 2007 as on course to affect over 380 million people by 2025. In the UK, the state public health observatories estimated that incidence would rise from 2.8 million to 4.2 million sufferers by 2025, out of a population of approximately 60 million, a 46% increase.[78] In many poorer countries in Asia, the Middle East, Oceania and the Caribbean, diabetes affects 12–20% of the population. In 2025, 80% of all cases of diabetes are set to be in low- and middle-income countries.

The UN-affiliated International Diabetes Federation (IDF), launching its 2006 Diabetes Atlas, acknowledged the 'complex interplay of genetic, social and environmental factors' driving the global explosion in type 2 diabetes. But it recognized the policy urgency too and that, as people get richer and supply chains alter, their aspirations to eat differently and their capacity to 'burn' energy alters too. The IDF summarized the global situation thus:[79]

> In low and middle-income countries, economic advancement can lead to alterations
> to the living environment that result in changes in diet and physical activity within a
> generation or two. Consequently, people can develop diabetes despite relatively low

---

* The SCN is the contemporary title of the committee that previously had one of the longest names in food policy institutional architecture: the Administrative Committee on Coordination, Sub-Committee on Nutrition (of the United Nations) (ACC/SCN).

gains in weight. In the developed world, diabetes is most common among the poorest communities. Either way, wherever poverty and lack of sanitation drive families to low cost-per-calorie foods and packaged drinks, type 2 diabetes thrives.

For decades, as the European Union (EU) grew in wealth and policy influence, there was a split between health policy, which was largely monitored by the WHO's European region, and economic policy, a EU responsibility. By 2006 the EU was 27 countries, all within the WHO's 52-member state European Region (WHO-E). In 1992, the demarcation began to blur, with the EU adopting slightly stronger health powers, first under the Amsterdam Treaty article 129 and then in stronger form under the 1996 Maastricht Treaty article 152. These powers gave small but useful budgets to work on human health, mainly through education and research programmes. But it meant closer liaison with the WHO-E, which, like all UN bodies, lacked powers other than mainly to provide advice to member states.

The WHO-E runs from the Atlantic to the Pacific and down to the Caspian sea, a region with rich countries, some not; some long urbanized, others not; some large countries with big populations, others not. The general picture from WHO-E supports the view that nutrition is an important factor shaping health. Using the World Bank/WHO notion of disability-adjusted life-years (DALYs) to measure how factors have an impact on health, poor nutrition was estimated to account for 4.6% of the total disease burden in 2002. There is no widespread acute malnutrition in rich Western Europe but food insecurity is documented in the poorer Eastern Europe. Based on 2002 World Health Report data, chronic malnutrition due to micro-nutrient deficiencies extensively affects vulnerable populations.[80] Malnutrition is reported among the elderly, chronically ill patients and disabled individuals 'to a variable extent throughout the European Region'. Across the region, obesity had 'now reached epidemic proportions', accounting for an additional 7–8 % of DALYs.[57] More than two-thirds of the population did not take enough physical activity, a failing that contributed a further 3.3% of DALYs. The rate of exclusive breast-feeding at 6 months was low everywhere, ranging from 1% to 46%, and one review concluded that some member states did not even comply with the policies agreed by all governments at the World Health Assembly in 2002, let alone the preceding UN Innocenti Declaration of 1990.[81] These policies were designed to give coherence and impetus to a massive increase in breast-feeding, the advantages for which there is ample evidence.[82, 83]

The long struggle to tackle hunger, famine and food insecurity

The possibility of inadequate sources of food has shaped human culture, provided religions with rules for daily life and determined the panorama of historical events. Hunger is rediscovered by each generation. There were an estimated 25 major famines in the period of the Roman Empire. And well before its imperial period, Britain experienced an estimated 95 famines before AD1500. Eastern Europe had an estimated 150 famines between 1500 and 1700. Russia experienced famines regularly both before and after the October 1917 revolution, not least that of Stalin's enforced collectivization in 1946–47.[84, 85] Between 1000 and the 19th century, France experienced 150 'serious famines', one every 6 years.[86]

No-one needed to inform early civilizations of the importance of food. Droughts, floods, plagues and poor harvests have been the nightmares of societies since settled agriculture emerged approximately 10,000 years ago. Dumont and Roisier, in their 1960s appeal for a more coherent agricultural and development policy, proposed that its moral goal should be to avoid two nutritional failures: under-nourishment ('nourishment inadequate in quantity') then affecting 300–500 million, and mal-nutrition ('nourishment which is defective in quality') then affecting about 1,600 millions.[86] The language and the demographics of their argument may have been new, shaped by the spectre of feeding rising populations and by the sophistication of nutritional science, but their core argument that politics and economic progress must be harnessed to avoid hunger is not new. A voluminous literature is testament to the political effort into how to avoid, manage and explain it.[45, 87–91] The simplest analyses—that famine is due to absence of food or inadequacies of availability of food or pestilences and disease[92]—has been shown not to be the full explanation. Of course, if foodstocks are contaminated by ergot (in rye) or blight (in potatoes) or rust (in wheat), yields and availability will be seriously curtailed; but whatever the myth, hunger cannot be reduced to crop failure. Vice versa, just to raise output does not mean that hunger is dissolved; it all depends on such issues as distribution, income inequalities and access.

The classic illustration of this is the Irish Famine of 1845–49. The common-sense narrative is that it was caused by the spread of potato blight, which meant that the potato crops on which the Irish poor depended were devastated, leading to famine. The blight certainly makes potatoes rot and shrivel and the devastation was nowhere harsher than in the parts of Ireland where families existed on tiny plots of lands and used the high-yielding and filling potato in repetitive mono-cropping, thereby increasing their crop's susceptibility to disease. On small holdings, potatoes were the only crop that might produce enough to fill the bellies of large families. To understand the Irish Famine one therefore needs to locate the problem within that social and economic context. Other factors shaped its path: landownership; unscrupulous landlords; high taxation; indifference to Ireland by the English; a strict localist system of welfare relief; religious identities; and trade relations. In the famine, the Quakers were a key Protestant group to protest and proclaim the need for relief. Throughout the famine, traders continued to export food.[93, 94] To reduce this one famine to the single issue of blight would be wrong. Famines are not 'acts of God' but, as one review of the blight pathogen has stated: '(t)he Irish had had, for two centuries, little or no control over their own affairs'.[92]

The necessity of putting hunger into its social context was the core message of the now classic study by Amartya Sen of the 1943 Bengal Famine, when India was still under British rule. Sen, subsequently the 1998 Nobel Prizewinner for Economics, showed that the 3 million excess deaths in the 1943 tragedy occurred, not so much due to absence of food as to social inequalities that shaped people's expectations and their notions of entitlement to food.[95] Rather than the stereotypical explanation of 'food availability decline' (FAD), Sen proposed that famines can occur—as in Bengal—when there is no substantial FAD; or to express it differently, the drop in food availability may be small, but the famine great. Sen's 'poverty and entitlements' study made the powerful distinction between whether enough food is in a market and whether the famine victim had access to it. In the 1943 famine, there was no collapse of food availability but the rural labourers, who were the most significant famine victims, did suffer what Sen called lack of 'trade entitlement', despite the general economy being in a boom state.[96] In the 1974 famine in Ethiopia's Harerghe province, by contrast, there was a food availability collapse, exacerbated by the general Ethiopian economic slump. In the 1974 Bangladesh famine, as in Bengal in 1943, there was no collapse of food availability, but rural labourers' entitlement was again absent or redefined and, unlike in 1943, the economy was in a mixed rather than a boom state. Sen's point, from these and other comparisons, is that availability is not the key determinant of famine. Money and a belief in one's right to food can find a way. Food may be—and usually is—available beyond the immediate geography of crop reduction (if there has been one). Entitlements and a sense of democracy, freedom and rights are fundamental;[97] their presence or absence is reflected in legal structures such as ownership rights, contractual obligations and legal exchanges.

The range of academic studies on hunger and under-nutrition is enormous.[98] Trying to understand how people starve has spawned a new literature and new concepts, such as food (in)security, food poverty, food entitlement, food rights, food availability, food access. The literature on hunger ranges from the micro-management of hunger relief[99] to studies of how changing food-supply chain dynamics have altered the form that modern mass hunger takes.[88, 100–102] Within the literature on food security alone, there has been a gradual shift in focus from the population level to the household 'micro' level, and to an emphasis on generations (young/old), gender and urban/rural differences. This has led to a shift in policy thinking from increasing food supply at the national level—still apparent at the 1974 World Food Conference—to a combination of promoting more liberalized trade plus 'micro' management of household and individual access to food.[103, 104]

Hunger is not just an issue for developing countries; there is also a strong body of work identifying relative hunger and food insecurity in richer country.[105, 106] The US Government, one of the wealthiest countries in the world, acknowledges it has a food insecurity problem. In 2002, for instance, the US Department of Agriculture estimated that 11% of American households were food insecure at least some time in that year, meaning that they did not have 'access, at all times, to enough food for an active, healthy life for all household members'. The prevalence of US measured food insecurity rose from 10.7% in 2001 to 11.1% in 2002, and the prevalence of food insecurity with hunger rose from 3.3% to 3.5%.[107, 108] This was despite the successes of the Women, Infants and Children welfare food programme (WIC). WIC provides central (federal) grants for supplementary foods, and funds nutrition education for 'low-income pregnant, breastfeeding, and non-breastfeeding postpartum women, and to infants and children up to age five who are found to be at nutritional risk'.

Three nutritions: life science, social, and ecological

How can policy make sense of this complex picture from nutrition? As ever, policy-makers hope for (rather than expect) unanimity from expert advice; they hope for it particularly within professions more than between disciplines. In fact there is, as we have stressed, an impressive consistency about the importance of diet's effect on health in general and of the existence of under-, mal- and over-consumption problems. But the foci within nutrition are somewhat different from three distinct traditions; there is no nutrition; there are nutritions.[109] Each tradition has a distinct approach, appeal and knowledge-base. Each has a way of couching the role, remit and task of nutrition. These vary, not just in focus and perspective but in influence, support and funding. Table 4.1 summarizes the differences.

The first tradition, which Lang and Heasman termed the 'life sciences' approach, locates nutrition as drawing on the life sciences, on the interface of biology and chemistry originally, but now also genetics, since the announcement of the double helix in the spring of 1953.[110–113] The completion in 2003 of mapping the human genome's 20–25000 genes in 3 billion chemical base pairs has unleashed another remarkable bout of scientific endeavour with

Table 4.1 A typology of the three main approaches to nutrition

Features	Life Science Nutrition	Social Nutrition	Eco-Nutrition
Approach to food science	A natural science.	A social science. Or a natural science working with and shaped by social goals.	Nutrition has to accept its environmental basis and implications.
Key contributing sciences	Old dominance of chemistry now giving way to biological sciences.	Social sciences such as sociology, demography and cultural anthropology.	Ecology and environmental sciences; energy and physics.
Core 'directions of travel'	'Mining' down the natural sciences. Unlocking their interactions.	Embedding nutrition within society, culture and living. Strong social justice emphasis.	Diet in an era of climate change. Juxtaposing two meanings of ecology: interactions and the wider environment. Ecological nutrition + nutritional ecology.
Core concept/ proposition for nutrition advance	Individuality. in 19th and 20th c., nutrition advances came through understanding and integrating biology and chemistry; in the 21st c., the linkage is thence to genetics.	Sociability. Nutrition is socially mediated. The shape of society and social relations determines who eats what, who well and who poorly.	Biodiversity. Up to the 18th c., focus was more on improving soil, plants and animals. Today, re-emerging as formulating new rules for ecological eating and ecological supply chains.
Current emphasis/ challenges	Clarifying the relationship between nutrients and biological pre-programming. The 'omics': genomics, nutrigenomics, metabolomics.	How to reshape culture and economy in an era of globalisation. Food as a right.	Carbon counting. How to juxtaposition of various 'single issues': from animal welfare.
Industrial appeal	Food manufacturers; pharmaceuticals; biotechnology; life science-based companies.	High interest among marketing and taste-changers from the consciousness and cultural industries.	Non-existent until recently. Now a source of niche products: 'green' foods.

Continued

Table 4.1 (continued) A typology of the three main approaches to nutrition

Features	Life Science Nutrition	Social Nutrition	Eco-Nutrition
State appeal	Competitive advantage from unlocking food as intersection point between the life sciences.	Currently poor. Seen as welfare-oriented.	Until recently generally low but rapidly changing.
Research (funding) appeal	Currently high; appeals as generator of new 'niche' products. Offers way out of saturated food markets.	High appeal to social movements but these tend to have low funds.	Likely to grow rapidly. Currently appeals to pursuit of niche markets but this is likely to be transient as more structural aspects emerge: energy, water, climate change.
Consumer appeal	Varies. Walks a narrow dividing line between being too 'hi-tech' and 'modern'.	Depends on ideological times. Can appeal to nationalism and individual rights. Ethical consumerism reconnects with 19th c. co-operative movement.	Potentially significant but carries dangers of association with choice restriction. Environment as 'choice editor'.
Scientist appeal	High. Reasserts nutrition scientist as expert. Reopens role as 'top-down' expert.	Unfashionable, but likely to re-emerge with societal problems from globalisation and geo-political uncertainties.	Largely untapped but likely to create new synergies across previously discrete research areas.
Core message	Better understanding of complex interactions between diet and physiology will enable diet to be tailored to individual requirements.	Consumers need to be more in control of the food supply chain. Food democracy must be asserted over food control.	We must eat within environmental limits and eat foods produced in a way which is sustainable. Simpler diets and variety are achievable.

immense implications for nutrition.[114] The core idea of Life Science Nutrition now is to unlock the dynamics and mechanisms of how nutrients interact with this increasingly well-understood but complex physiology. How might genetic pre-potential be activated by diet at particular times in the life cycle? How might particular food ingredients or nutrients or combinations affect health outcomes?

Of the three, Life Science Nutrition is currently dominant. Once Gowland Hopkins and others had unlocked the mechanism for vitamins in the 1910s and 1920s, this approach was set fair. The old certainties about the broad role of macro-nutrients and micro-nutrients have been shaken by the complexity and interactions of genomics and the multiple emergence of branches of '-omic' science. New policy routes are being championed, such as functional foods with added and tailored specific health attributes.[115] Life Science Nutrition's Holy Grail is to be able to design foods for a person's genetic pre-potential, thus personalizing health and allowing policy to seek at-risk groups with new accuracy. The analytic possibilities of nutri-genomics are, however, not yet yielding big breakthroughs in either dietary change or marketed products, although food industry interests, having resisted diet-health connections for decades, now see advantage there.[115-118]

The second approach, social nutrition, centres on how food fits into, or is shaped by, societal processes. Social nutrition sees food as a location for social interaction; nutrition conveys social forces and reflects its wider social context.[119] Social nutrition's political high point is undoubtedly its legacy in the global system of famine relief and in the watching brief on food prices within welfare safety nets. But its policy influence has ebbed in the developed world, paradoxically with the rise of those welfare systems. Institutionalized safety nets often contain embedded nutrition standards but there continue to be heated arguments about whether such welfare is adequate or was intended to be.[120-123] Boyd Orr and the 1930s' generation developed the notion that nutrition is held back by social inequality and is best promoted by the pursuit of more equitable access and affordable food, with welfare rates as the safety net for food security.[106, 124] Food policy, from this perspective, is about the social determinants of nutrient intake.

Social nutrition is an intellectual bridge from the natural to social sciences, whether it casts nutrition as a natural science with firm social goals or as a social science, which incorporates the natural sciences and biological pathways. If food is identity, as the anthropologists and sociologists propose,[125] then nutritionists must understand how those identities and social relations shape nutritional intake. Looking at nutrition through this societal lens, has been incorporated into marketing and advertising whose practitioners closely monitor the changing meanings of food and the effect of demographic shifts.[126] Food intake thus becomes a vignette of society. In the 19th and early 20th centuries, writers such as Engels, Booth and Rowntree recorded, and were shocked by, the dire state of food provision and culture among people on low incomes.[127-129] Despite huge growth in aggregate wealth, gross inequalities within industrial societies determined whether needs were met, a finding reinforced by European colonialism.[130, 131] Researchers and colonial administrators were both fascinated and troubled by the different mores and culinary traditions they encountered, arguing the need for medical science to help address the nutritional problems encountered.[132] The spread of Western researchers generated a rich understanding of how culture shaped food roles and routines and how societies created food cultural rules, related not just to domestic life but to economic roles and religious beliefs.[133]

The third approach to nutrition is environmental or ecological nutrition, which focuses on how nutrition is shaped by its environmental context. This locates diet with the wider eco-sphere. Like the other traditions, environmental nutrition, too, has long roots. Nutrition pioneers like von Liebig, Gibson and Lawes saw the quality of nutrition as shaped by what the environment could offer; the point of science was to alter that relationship. Their project was a resistance to Malthus; production could and would be raised to defeat the spectre of population. Today the environmental ethos is gentler or more respectful, seeing nutrition as needing to protect and reflect the environment. The terminology varies. Modern nutritionists at the University of Giessen, where von Liebig worked, have suggested using the term 'nutritional ecology' to emphasize how nutrition has to adjust to wider ecological principles.[134, 135] Leitzmann and colleagues see eco-nutrition as offering a narrower focus on 'the interactions of nutrition and environment', whereas they suggest nutrition should be located within wider sustainability. In this sense, they see nutrition returning to an older philosophical project, locating human physiological needs as one (albeit complex) 'unit' within a wider cosmos.[136]

However defined—ecological nutrition or nutritional ecology or environmental nutrition—this tradition is by far the junior partner within policy of the three nutritions described here, but its relevance for nutrition research is returning and will strengthen.[137] The need to link appropriate nutrition to diet's CO_2 emissions, level of embedded water and wasted output is pressing.[138, 139] It is not yet sufficiently clear what a sustainable diet is.[140]

Whichever term is used, this environmental approach locates nutrition within ecology in two senses. Haeckel first used the term 'ecology' in 1866 to refer to the relationship of organisms to their physical conditions of living.[141, 142] In the present context, it has two meanings. Firstly, nutritional adequacy has to fit environmental limits. Humans can only produce and eat what is possible within the capacities of soil, geography, climate, water availability and so on.[137, 143–145] Secondly, nutrition is ecological in that it is about the interactions across the sciences. Eco-nutrition is intrinsically inter-disciplinary; therein lies a difficulty for policy. Judging by the evidence of diet-related ill-health, there is a mismatch between physiological needs, the legacy of evolution over hundreds of thousands of years and what is delivered by the food system.[146, 147] The answer depends on the starting point. If the prime concern is the environmental impact of eating to suit human wants, as distinct from needs, the evidence suggests that Western diets, at least, may be exceeding planetary capacities. But as Cohen has argued globally, and as Fairlie has for the UK, how and what people eat has different impacts on use of land.[148] A study of the UK, for instance, showed considerable differences in ecological footprint according to whether the diet included meat and dairy products. An officially designated 'healthy' diet used 0.6 global hectares per person (gha/cap) to achieve that diet, whereas the actual UK diet had an average of over 0.8 gha/cap An assessment of Scotland's school lunches, before nutrition standards were introduced, compared with after, showed a drop of 42% in its ecological footprint. If a vegetarian diet lowers the footprint further, and a seasonal, organic, local, vegetarian and 'healthy' diet is the lowest of all measured by that study,[149] this suggests a potential 'win-win' for policy: healthier diets carry less environmental burdens.

But if the starting point is biological legacy rather than environmental limits, a different avenue of policy thinking emerges. One group of authors, for example, has argued that complex nutritional capacities developed in the Darwinian process of evolution, such that at least seven nutritional characteristics were shaped by 'ancestral hominin diets'. These were: glycaemic load; fatty acid composition; macro-nutrient composition; micro-nutrient density; acid–base balance; sodium–potassium ratio; and fibre content.[150] The future of nutrition, it follows, would be to shape diet to suit our biological givens. One illustration of where this restrictive line can end up is the so-called Palaeolithic diet, perhaps the ultimately reductionist position, severely questioned by Marion Nestle, among others.[151] Less extremely, ecological nutrition can, however, explore the nutritional contribution of different diets and how they have been produced.[152]

The emergence of such debates illustrates the vibrancy of the nutrition–environment connection. In 2005, the President of the International Union of Nutrition Scientists and the editor of the journal *Public Health Nutrition*, and others, signed a Giessen Declaration at the world congress of nutritionists. This called for nutrition science to incorporate a more comprehensive understanding of food systems, which 'shape and are shaped by biological, social and environmental relationships and interactions. How food is grown, processed, distributed, sold, prepared, cooked and consumed, is crucial to its quality and nature, and to its effect on well-being and health, society and the environment.'[153]

Policy responses to nutrition evidence

The three nutrition traditions chart different trajectories ahead for nutrition science: different roles, relationships to the state and supply chain and to society.

The approaches differ conceptually while offering policy solutions that can appeal to different players in the food system. This has been true for obesity, for which a number of solutions are offered.[154] If one argues that there is a 'fat gene' predisposing a person to being fat (depending on nutrient intake and metabolic rate), the policy approach will be different to if one argues that obesity is shaped by an excess of cheap calories or formidable marketing.[9, 10, 53] Equally, policy on consumption of fish takes a different route dependent on whether one's priorities are preserving fish stocks,[155, 156] or consuming the essential fatty acids, which are so rich in fish oils.[157, 158] This can make for interesting tensions between policy advisors. In the UK, for instance, the Royal Commission on Environmental Pollution in 2004 gently urged the UK's Food Standards Agency to look again at its nutritional advice on fish consumption.[159] Until early 2008, FSA advice still was that: '[w]e should be eating at least two portions of fish a week including one of oily fish. But most people aren't eating enough fish. Fish and shellfish are rich in protein and minerals, and oily fish is rich in omega 3 fatty acids.'[160] Although this advice did not change, in February 2008—just prior to a report from the Sustainable Development Commission highlighting this intra-governmental conflict of advice[140]—a welcome announcement was made that a process would begin to address how nutrition might dovetail with sustainability issues (on-going as this book was completed).

Such lags between nutrition evidence, policy change and institutional development are not unknown. Evidence about diet's impact on health in general and NCDs in particular, as we noted above, is at least half a century old. Yet policy-makers are still struggling with how to address the issue. There are general statements or goals to alter diets but the means are somewhat vaguer. Within the three nutritions, there are divergent priorities and overall strategy. Life scientists might argue for new foods with more appropriate nutrient profiles. Social nutritionists might stress actions that flatten social gradients or inequalities in diet-related behaviour between social groups. Eco-nutritionists might point to the need to reconnect food culture with sustainable food systems, after a century that altered it through agricultural industrialization and the creation of 'cosmetic' foods. Table 4.2 provides some examples of the range of options in diverse policy sectors; they vary from 'hard' responses, such as bans or fiscal actions, to 'soft' ones, such as labelling or information. All of these might be appropriate and, collectively, they would be more coherent than any of them singly.[10]

The reality of policy-making is that paths have to be negotiated through such issues, designing options in politically feasible packages that policy-makers can translate into realizable objectives; but, inevitably, politics and non-nutrition

Table 4.2 Some possible policy responses to nutrition-related concerns

Policy sector	Goal is to ensure nutrition included in	Means available	Examples
Agriculture	Land-use policy.	Grants. Agricultural policy framework.	Animal and plant breeding.
Processing	Food supply.	Contracts and specifications.	Product reformulation. Change fat content in meat regulations.
Retail	Improving access to health-enhancing foods.	Retail and town planning.	Food pricing. Location of stores through town planning.
Culture	Change thinking about food to reshape demand.	Health education. Marketing. Social marketing.	Public education on obesity. Controls on marketing at children.
Society	Equitable access and re-balancing circumstances.	Welfare system.	School meals.
Economy	Macro-economic framework and fiscal measures.	Price signals. Taxation. Regulation and bans.	Taxing soft drinks. Banning TV advertising.

considerations can be a factor (see Chapter 3). Nevertheless at the global, regional, national and local levels, there is an impressive catalogue of policies, initiatives and experience in trying to address different aspects of the problems raised by nutrition. Over the last half-century, there has been a slow but persistent attempt to put nutrition issues centrally onto formal public policy. Table 4.3 itemizes some general nutrition policies at various governance levels: UN, Europe and the UK since World War II. It charts the slow but steady build-up of official positions.

As we noted earlier (see Chapter 2), the modern food policy framework really begins with post-World War II reconstruction. Within the productionist paradigm, social and life science nutritions were equal partners; ecological nutrition was absent. By the 1980s, certainly at international level, the environment received more general policy attention but not particularly in nutrition; the priority was still on quantity, development and agriculture. In theory, UN inter-governmental policy has long given equal emphasis to health, safety and environment but, in reality, responsibilities were addressed in separate policy boxes. Awareness of the obesity 'time-bomb' catalysed some movement. In 2003, the historic joint WHO and FAO review of evidence on diet, physical activity and health, asserted the need for wide-scale

Table 4.3 The evolution of nutrition-focused policies: World, Europe and UK

Date	Global	Europe	UK
1930s	League of Nations 'Mixed Committee on the Problem of Nutrition' [Burnet-Ackroyd] report (1936) maps nutrition as problems for social, agricultural and health policies.		British Medical Association Report (1933) highlights serious under-nutrition. UK focuses on feeding itself from the Empire. Hunger marches build argument for welfare.
1939–45	World War II total dislocation of supplies. Hot Springs Conference (1943) plans for creation of FAO and priority on rebuilding.	National Food Policies based on war-time (1939–). Famine in Netherlands (1944–45).	Introduction of rationing according to nutritional need.
1945–	Boyd Orr et al. vision of focus on rebuilding supplies + improved distribution via trade triumphs.	US Marshall Plan (1946) puts priority on aid to central Europe, as part of Cold War.	UK government passes Agriculture Act (1947) to rebuild supplies to feed people.
1950s		Treaty of Rome (1957) founds the Common Market and Common Agriculture Policy designed to feed people. Assumes market efficiencies provide adequate nutrition.	
1960s	UN General Assembly backs use of UN to transfer surpluses to 'food-deficient peoples' Resolution 1496 [XV] (1960).		
1970s	World Food Conference (1974).		Committee on Medical Aspects of Food Policy (COMA) published report on heart disease (1974)
1980s	World Commission on Environment and Development [Brundtland Report] (1987).		Committee on Medical Aspects of Food Policy (COMA) publishes stronger report on heart disease (1984)

Table 4.3 (continued) The evolution of nutrition-focused policies: World, Europe and UK

Date	Global	Europe	UK
1990s	WHO Technical Report 797 (1990). International Conference on Nutrition (1992) documents global problems in nutrition; no policy-follow up other than monitoring. World Food Summit (1996) returns to focus on developing world, ignores coincidence of over-, under- and mal-consumption.	Treaties of Maastricht (1992) and Amsterdam (1996) give health powers to the European Commission.	UK country report to UN's (1992) International Conference on Nutrition sees little problems in UK nutrition. Nutrition Task Force (1994–96) disagrees. James Report to Tony Blair (1997) calls for equal weight on nutrition and safety. 2nd James report on child health (1997) dismissed as too interventionist.
2000s	Commission on Nutrition Challenges of the 21st c. (2000) reports across entire UN, documenting complex picture. Joint WHO/FAO Technical Report TRS 916 (2003) repeats it. World Health Assembly (2004) agrees Global Strategy on Diet, Physical Activity and Disease (WHA 57.7).	Food Safety White Paper (2000) gives first mention to nutrition. Health Commissioner David Byrne expresses alarm about obesity threat (2002). Obesity Roundtable created (2005) to bring industry, consumers and health activists together.	Food Standards Agency created with small nutrition element (2000); it grows later. Chief Medical Officer warns about obesity 'time-bomb' (2003). School Food Trust created to tackle school meals following TV series by celebrity chef Jamie Oliver (2005). Public Service Agreement on obesity locks all Departments into tackling obesity (2005).

policy change.[6] It recommended restricting the intake of free (added) sugars to 10% or less of energy. Furious lobbying ensued from threatened food companies. The following year, at the World Health Assembly (the WHO's meeting of member states) a Resolution (57.17) was passed committing member states to act to improve diets, to build physical activity into daily lives and to achieve change by the food industry.[161]

Resolution 57.17 reflected the commitment of the then heads of the WHO, all political appointments through UN processes. Subsequent leadership did not give nutrition the same emphasis. Events moved on; the unfolding food commodity crisis of 2006–08 returned policy attention to under-consumption rather than inappropriate consumption and supply. An opportunity was dissipated. But a study funded by the WHO to assess how big food companies had responded to Resolution 57.17, found in 2005–06 a generally very low level of engagement in the world's top 25 companies, with retailers particularly weak.[162] At the EU level, the response was also slow, but deliberately so; it is not unknown for the EC to take the long view. The 'first get protagonists into the same room' principle has been a basis of member state engagement. In 2004, the Commission created a Roundtable on Obesity bringing together large companies, health professions and other stakeholders; this still meets and makes statements.[76] Within its powers, under the Maastricht Treaty, the EC's role is restricted to information and research. The health budget has been rising but from a low starting point. No transformation of obesity rates has thus far been detected.

A more interesting policy development has occurred in the UK, a country with a strong commitment to light-touch government. A 2-year investigation by the Chief Scientist's Foresight programme produced the best governmental systemic analysis of obesity to date.[13] Around the widely agreed 'engine' of obesity—too high calorific intake coupled with insufficient physical activity to expend it—the Foresight team developed a systems map with a complex web of interacting factors, in seven clusters: societal influences, food production, food consumption, individual psychology, individual activity, biology and activity environment. The Foresight report achieved a high international profile with its estimate that inaction on obesity would cost the UK economy £50 billion by 2050. A high-level ministerial team was appointed with two expert advisory groups. Having only had one nutritionist in its Department of Health (the others had been transferred to the Food Standards Agency after its creation in 2000), a team of more than 40 people were appointed to co-ordinate anti-obesity actions across Government. Time will tell if this yields change.

From the ecological public health perspective, no country or region yet appears to have developed an appropriately integrated framework, despite many useful commitments over the last three decades of the 20th century.[109] Table 4.4 details the gradual emergence of European policy across the WHO-E and the EU. At the global level, after 2 years of rising world food commodity prices, a long arranged High-Level Conference on Food Security in 2008 reasserted the 'old' interpretation of where nutrition problems lay: underconsumption. Rapidly rising prices had led 37 countries to experience some kind of food-related unrest from demonstrations to riots. Turbulence emerged in world commodity markets. Concern was expressed that the absolute figures of mal-nourished people was rising again; FAO estimated that 100 million more were likely to join the total due to the commodity price upsurge. $1.2 billion was offered by donors at the Rome Conference.[163] Warm words were expressed about the importance of agricultural development, after years

Table 4.4 Late–20th c. European nutrition policies: WHO-Euro and the EU

Date	Policy / initiative / action	Parent body	Comment
1988	Healthy Nutrition report to WHO-E	WHO-Euro (UN)	Documents Europe-wide nutrition-based problems and calls for government and supply change.
1992	Maastricht Treaty	EU	One section gave the European Commission powers to act on health, but primarily only on education and promotion.
2000	White Paper on Food Safety	EU	Introduced some focus on nutrition within what otherwise was overwhelmingly a safety focused policy.
2000	First European Food and Nutrition Action[a]	WHO-Euro (UN)	51 MS support resolution to tackle nutrition-based ill-health.
2005	European Charter on Counteracting Obesity	WHO-Euro (UN)	Meeting in Istanbul, MSs all acknowledge problems but are softer on what to do about it.
2005	European strategy for child and adolescent health and development[b]	WHO-Euro (UN)	
2006	European Strategy for the Prevention and Control of Non-communicable Diseases[c]	WHO-Euro (UN)	
2007	European framework for promotion of physical activity[d]	EU	
2007	Second Action Plan	WHO-Euro (UN)	Places more emphasis on physical activity, not just nutrition.

[a] WHO-E (2000). *Resolution: the impact of food and nutrition on public health: the case for a food and nutrition policy and an action plan for the European region of WHO 2000–2005*. Regional Committee for Europe, Fiftieth session, Copenhagen, 11–14 September 2000. EUR/RC50/R8 Copenhagen: WHO Regional Office for Europe.

[b] WHO-E (2005). *European strategy for child and adolescent health and development*. Copenhagen: WHO Regional Office for Europe. http://www.euro.who.int/document/E87710.pdf

[c] WHO-E (2006). *Gaining health. The european strategy for the prevention and control of noncommunicable diseases*. EUR/RC56/8 Copenhagen: WHO Regional Office for Europe. http://www.euro.who.int/Document/RC56/edoc08.pdf

[d] WHO-E (2007). *Promoting physical activity for health—a framework for action in the WHO European Region*. Copenhagen:WHO Regional Office for Europe.

of declining investment. But this was in some respects a return to familiar policy thinking, seeing nutrition as primarily a matter of under-nutrition.

And yet, the incremental institutional reform and development of the UN's food system is a real legacy of efforts to tackle famine, hunger and unmet need. The FAO's inception in the 1940s represents the success of politicking around farm reform and the triumph of the argument that hunger could be tackled if institutions were created to support new farming techniques and build capacity to increase output.[164–166] But the creation of other institutions under the FAO umbrella is testament to a continuing need. The World Food Programme was created in 1963 as a temporary programme of the UN body to get food to the needy in crises (see the longer account in Chapter 8); it is now permanent. The Food Insecurity and Vulnerability Mapping System (FIVIMS) was created after the 1996 World Food Summit to provide systematic information on the underlying causes of food insecurity, hunger and malnutrition, and to alert policy-makers about possible or likely crises. It integrates understanding of at-risk locations into national and regional databases for the UN system.

As has been noted, the policy responses to over- or mal-consumption have been slow and tentative (see Chapter 8). They draw from the same or similar approaches to those in the previous section. The focus may differ but the thinking or approach is the same. Product reformulation is one key commercial response to obesity, but is largely technocratic and suffers all the limitations of that approach. In the case of obesity, for instance, there was a flurry of interest from the commercial sector at the prospect that public health organizations might be interested to champion tough regulatory measures. Was food to be the new tobacco?[167] Were public health organizations, fresh from winning restrictions of consumer choice about whether and where to smoke, now turning attention to a similarly bitter struggle to restrict consumer access to fatty foods? There were heated debates in the media, but little tough action through public policy. Although food is not tobacco, there was and is some overlap in certain company portfolios.[168]

One particularly interesting approach has been the argument that, since so much food behaviour is shaped by price, then taxes and fiscal measures could be brought into play to address a range of NCDs by taxing fat, for example.[169] This has exercised health economists considerably.[170–172] There are some practical difficulties. Unlike the single product of tobacco, high fat and high calorie foods are ubiquitous. There are problems in measurement and setting thresholds. Yet the case for rebalancing intake is surely warranted by the cheapness of many fatty, sugary foods. The search for some kind of fiscal intervention is unlikely to dissipate.[173]

Another possible direction for nutrition policy is to focus on changing information flows that target consumers. Besides proposals to restrict information that targets children, a wider concern is about marketing and advertising generally. The dominant reflex of policy-makers has been to see nutritional challenges as ones that can safely be left to market forces and consumer choice. This assumes an omniscient consumer and perfect flows of information, neither of which conditions is necessarily valid or always true although in many societies there are articulate consumer and health groups. Worldwide, in developed and developing countries alike, the issues of food information, advertising and marketing have become highly contested policy battlegrounds.[53, 174]

For years, the marketing industry has dismissed the accusation that it moulds food tastes, arguing that there is little evidence of this being the case. Despite this being a surprising defence—one might wonder why, if marketing is so ineffective, companies expend such huge sums on it—it does seem to impress governments and stave off statutory controls or allow weaker forms of self-regulation. But that defence was firmly rebutted by a systematic review of the effects of advertising and marketing on the diet of young people, conducted for the UK's Food Standards Agency. This review by Hastings and colleagues found conclusive evidence that marketing does have measurable impact on diet.[175] Unsurprisingly, the UK food and marketing industries were disconcerted by this and complained that the Hastings review was biased. A further academic review was held but the industries' evidence was rejected as less comprehensive and systematic, and the complaint dismissed.[176] The Hastings review has been very influential around the world and has helped to engage policy-makers (governments) and companies to take the need for tighter controls on marketing more seriously, and has led to interest in such approaches as nutrient profiling and improved labelling.[177–179] But on their own, can these be effective?

Nutrition institutions and champions

Nutrition's leverage on policy can be weakened by its perceived contentiousness. Health bodies are nervous about being judged as too didactic, fearing the neo-liberal accusations of representing the 'nanny state' and unnecessary infringement of consumer liberty to choose. As a result there is some confusion among nutritionists about leadership and policy direction. Should they retreat to 'pure' science, leaving policy to the political process? Or should they redouble efforts to translate evidence into policy-friendly form? Whichever approach is adopted, the profound implications of nutrition for the relationship between supply chains, society and the state have to be addressed.

Firm advocacy can make a difference, just as hesitancy can hold it back. The UK's Food Standards Agency provided admirable, firm but fair leadership without compromising its commitment to best evidence in championing the implications of the Hastings Review, arguing for better controls and helping win some restrictions on food advertising on UK television. The Chief Medical Officer for England championed the urgency of obesity.[180] Building on the financial case made by the National Audit Office and the Parliamentary Health Committee's report,[71, 72] a cross-Government Public Service Agreement (PSA), a binding agreement between Treasury and other departments giving central funds for measurable action, was put in place for 'halting the year-on-year rise in obesity among children aged under 11 by 2010 in the context of a broader strategy to tackle obesity in the population as a whole'.[181] This formal commitment was shared across Government, but focused particularly on the ministries responsible for culture (advertising) and education, rather than food production or industry. Two years later, a report from three official watchdogs, the National Audit Office, the Audit Commission and the Healthcare Commission, was critical of performance for not meeting targets. In response, the Government retreated to the 'default' position, health education. Replying to the critics, it stressed the fact that its health education had increased awareness of the need to eat five portions of fruit and vegetables a day, and that it had increased investment in school food.[182] A year later, a powerful report from the Chief Scientist triggered another cross-government commitment.[183] This time there was to be some industry focus. The saga continues.

Too often, action—of even limited variety—is triggered by crisis. The UK created its Food Standards Agency in 2000 after a decade of food crises, transferring nutrition responsibilities there, away from central government. In 2001, when the Ministry of Agriculture, Fisheries and Food was replaced by a new Department for Environment, Food and Rural Affairs, the institutional restructuring was complete. But this left central government without core nutrition advice inside the central system. The institutional direction had been to put difficult areas at 'arms-length', and to weaken central institutions. Obesity, like other systemic issues, highlights the limitations of this contemporary organizational architecture. Co-ordination is essential, which is hard when there is a plethora of bodies.

At the international level, the capacity to address the complexity of the nutritional challenge is also not helped by institutional fragmentation. This assessment is not new. From the 1920s, the League of Nations' fledgling Health Organization (which post-war became the World Health Organization) sought an inter-governmental, common scientific position on nutrition.

Its policy ground was laid in a series of reports in the mid-1930s.[184–186] Viscount Astor, the liberal British thinker who played a central role in revitalizing policy formulation in the UK in the run-up to World War II and who helped to champion the importance of integrating agriculture, nutrition and health,[187] also championed the League of Nations' ponderously named 'Mixed Commission of the League of Nations on the relation of nutrition to agriculture, health and economic policy'.[188] These bodies were remarkably foresighted, arguing for the location of nutrition within labour, as well as supply and agricultural policies.

The close involvement of mid-20th century British nutrition scientists in policy thinking was significant. This was partly the legacy of the 'global' thinking that came with the management of the British Empire but partly from scientists' recognition that major change was needed and should be helped.[189, 190] Nutrition problems constantly troubled the British. One good thing that happened was cross-disciplinary involvement. The contribution of social science was brought home, literally, and applied to good effect in World War II, notably through the equitable rationing system, and also by the strong cultural appeals to the population to eat 'patriotically', cut waste and eat appropriately for the labour output.[191, 192] The British Empire also had a complex task in managing appropriate supplies for the diverse food tastes of different ethnic groups it had moved around the globe to suit its macro-economic goals of trade and imperial preference.[193]

While the British Government was struggling with its Empire, many of the 1930s generation of nutritionists' progressive thinking was halted by harsh, nationalist realities of the 1940s and its aftermath. But they seized the opportunity to push for structural change in the latter period of the war, and particularly around the creation of the post-war United Nations institutions. The WHO superseded the League's Health Organization. The FAO was created. Later, came Unicef, concerned about children, the UN Environment Programme (UNEP) and specific bodies such as Codex Alimentarius Commission, the inter-governmental body run by WHO and FAO from Rome, concerned about standards including nutrition and labelling. But this incremental growth has not so far yielded strong integrated traction, despite the role of the SCN, nominally the co-ordinating committee. Power lies with the Bretton Woods' institutions of the IMF and World Bank.

Why are the required quantum leaps in nutrition policy not forthcoming? Fine intentions are articulated but mass behavioural change is not following. Why is this? One answer is that institutions are not in themselves enough to deliver nutrition progress. In wars, the State is prepared to take draconian actions. In World War II, scientists and policy activists such as Boyd Orr,

Drummond, Titmus and le Gros Clarke, seized their chance to argue for policy refinement at the national level and for instruments to deliver equitable change.[165, 192, 194, 195] Good timing and energy also enabled Boyd Orr to champion the connection of nutrition to agricultural as the founding rationale for the FAO.[164] Seebohm Rowntree, scion of the chocolate firm in York, England, who had studied the nutritional status of his home town for half a century,[129, 196] turned his own firm's experience of having a system of works canteens to good effect in that war. His canteens taught him that they not only served wholesome food but improved time-keeping; the workers didn't go home for lunch or succumb to the temptation not to return.[197, 198] He helped roll out the social cafés, which Churchill, ever the nationalist and élitist, insisted be called British Restaurants, to raise the tone and remind users of the national emergency![199] In World War II, the British State recreated a nutrition-focused Ministry of Food (MoF), which gave room for academics such as Sir John Drummond and Dorothy Hollingsworth to turn their life-science orientation toward social nutrition.[200] A Ministry of Food had been created in World War I but was quickly folded afterwards, under pressure from industry. Sir William Beveridge advised that it ought to be recreated if conflict returned.[201] It did; MoF was. This development gave people like Hugh Sinclair, the far-sighted investigator of essential fatty acids (fish oils particularly), room to help develop nutrition monitoring.[157]

Why does it take a war before tough action is considered? In his memoirs, Lord Woolton, the UK Food Minister, gave a riveting account of deciding—illegally—to buy food on world markets, without Treasury approval; to have made this purchase openly would have alerted world markets that the UK, already fearful of a food blockade, was about to buy surpluses and signalled others to do the same and to raise prices just when hard-pressed national finances had rocketing war costs.[202] Such radical action would be unthinkable today, yet in 'peace' too, the evidence suggests it is needed. But the big lesson from nutrition is that multi-sectoral, cross-disciplinary action needs, not just good people but circumstances with room for manoeuvre.

References

1. Vernon J. *Hunger: a modern history.* Cambridge: Harvard University Press, 2007.
2. Nestle M, Dixon LB. *Taking sides: clashing views on controversial issues in food and nutrition.* New York: McGraw Hill, 2004.
3. Friedman M, Friedman RD. *Free to choose: a personal statement,* 1st edn. New York: Harcourt Brace Jovanovich, 1980.
4. Consumers International. *Consumer rights.* London: Consumers International, 2006.
5. Gribben C, Gitsham M. *Food labelling: understanding consumer attitudes and behaviour.* Berkhamstead (Hertfordshire): Ashridge Business School, 2007.

6. WHO/FAO. *Diet, nutrition and the prevention of chronic diseases*. Report of the joint WHO/FAO expert consultation. WHO Technical Report Series, No. 916 (TRS 916). Geneva: World Health Organization & Food and Agriculture Organization, 2003.

7. Cannon G. *Food and health: the experts agree*. London: Consumers' Association, 1992:230.

8. Nestle M. *Food politics*. Berkeley CA: University of California Press, 2002.

9. Rayner G, Hawkes C, Lang T, Bello W. Trade liberalisation and the diet and nutrition transition: a public health response. *Health Promotion International* 2006; 21(S1):67–74.

10. Lang T, Rayner G. Overcoming policy cacophony on obesity: an ecological public health framework for policymakers. *Obesity Reviews* 2007;8(Suppl.):165–181.

11. Rose G. *The strategy of preventive medicine*. Oxford: Oxford University Press, 1992.

12. Commission on the Social Determinants of Health. *Achieving health equity: from root causes to fair outcomes*. Interim Statement from the Commission. http://www.who.int/social_determinants/resources/interim_statement/en/index.html. Geneva: World Health Organization, 2007.

13. Foresight. *Tackling obesities: future choices*. London: Government Office of Science, 2007.

14. Scrinis G. On the ideology of nutritionism. *Gastronomica* 2008;8(1):39–48.

15. Pollan M. *In defence of food: the myth of nutrition and the pleasures of eating*. London: Allen Lane, 2008.

16. Vitti P, Rago T, Aghini-Lombardi F, Pinchera A. Iodine deficiency disorders in Europe. *Public Health Nutrition* 2001;4(2B):529–535.

17. FAO/WHO. *Vitamin and mineral requirements in human nutrition*. Report of a joint FAO/WHO expert consultation, Bangkok, Thailand, 21–30 September 1998, 2nd edn. Bangkok, Thailand: Food and Agriculture Organization and World Health Organization, 2004.

18. Allen L, de Benoist B, Dary O, Hurrell R (ed.) *Guidelines on food fortification with micronutrients*. Rome: World Health Organization and Food and Agriculture Organization, 2004.

19. Popkin BM. An overview on the nutrition transition and its health implications: the Bellagio meeting. *Public Health Nutrition* 2002;5(1A):93–103.

20. Popkin BM. The nutrition transition in low-income countries: an emerging crisis. *Nutrition Reviews* 1994;52:285–298.

21. Popkin BM. The nutrition transition and its health implications in lower income countries. *Public Health Nutrition* 1998;1(1):5–21.

22. Popkin BM. Urbanisation, lifestyle changes and the nutrition transition. *World Development* 1999;27(11):1905–1915.

23. Popkin BM, Nielsen SJ. The sweetening of the world's diet. *Obesity Research* 2003;11(11):1–8.

24. Hawkes C. The role of foreign direct investment in the nutrition transition. *Public Health Nutrition* 2005;8(4):357–365.

25. Millstone E. *Food additives*. Harmondsworth: Penguin, 1986.

26. London Food Commission. *Food adulteration and how to beat it*. London: Unwin Hyman, 1987.

27. Davidson J. *Courtesans and fishcakes: the consuming passions of classical athens*. London: HarperCollins, 1997.

28. Cannon G. The rise and fall of dietetics and of nutrition science, 4000 BCE–2000 CE. *Public Health Nutrition* 2005;**8**(6a):701–705.

29. Lind J. *A treatise of the scurvy. Containing an inquiry into the nature, causes and cure, of that disease. Together with a critical and chronological view of what has been published on the subject* (3 volumes). Edinburgh: printed by Sands, Murray and Cochran for A Kincaid and A Donaldson, 1753.

30. Hites RA, Foran JA, Carpenter DO, Hamilton MC, Knuth BA, Schwager SJ. Global assessment of organic contaminants in farmed salmon. *Science* 2004;**303**:226–229.

31. Bartholomew M. James Lind and scurvy: a revaluation. *Journal for Maritime Research: www.jmr.nmm.ac.uk/bartholomew* 2002(January).

32. Hutchison R. *Food and the principles of dietetics*, 2nd edn. London: Edward Arnold, 1901.

33. Garrow JS, James WPT, Ralph A (ed.) *Human nutrition and dietetics*, 9th edn. Edinburgh: Churchill Livingstone (Elsevier Health Sciences), 2000.

34. Geissler C, Powers HJ. *Human nutrition*, 11th edn. Edinburgh: Elsevier Churchill Livingstone, 2005.

35. von Liebig J. *Principles of agricultural chemistry, with special reference to the late researches made in England*. London: Walton & Maberly, 1855.

36. von Liebig J, Playfair LP. *Organic chemistry in its applications to agriculture and physiology*. London: Taylor and Walton, 1840.

37. Keys A, Brozek J, Henschel A, Mickelson O, Taylor H. *The biology of human starvation*. Minneapolis: University of Minnesota Press, 1950.

38. Keys Ae. Coronary heart disease in seven countries. *Circulation* 1970;**41**(Supple.1):1–211.

39. McKeown T. *The modern rise of population*. London: Edward Arnold, 1976.

40. McKeown T. *The role of medicine: dream, mirage, or nemesis?* Princeton: Princton University Press, 1979.

41. McKeown T. *The origins of human disease*. London: Basil Blackwell, 1988.

42. McKeown T, Lowe CR. *An introduction to social medicine*. Oxford: Blackwell, 1966.

43. Fogel RW. New findings on secular trends in nutrition and mortality: some implications for population theory. In: Rosenzweig MR, Stark O (ed.) *Handbook of population and family economics. Handbooks in economics*. Amsterdam; New York and Oxford: Elsevier Science North-Holland, 1977:433–81.

44. Fogel RW. *Nutrition, physiological capital, and economic growth*. Washington DC: Pan American Health Organization and Inter-American Development Bank, 2002.

45. Fogel RW. *The escape for hunger and premature death, 1700–2100: Europe, America and the Third World*. Cambridge: Cambridge University Press, 2004.

46. Szreter S. The importance of social intervention in Britain's mortality decline, c1850–1914. A reinterpretation of the role of public health. *Social History of Medicine* 1988;**1**(1):1–37.

47. FAO. *State of food and agriculture 2007*. Rome: Food and Agriculture Organization, 2007.

48. FAO. *World Food Security Summit, June 3–5 2008*. Rome: Food & Agriculture Organization, 2008.

49. WHO. Diet, nutrition and the prevention of chronic diseases. *Technical Report Series 797*. Geneva: World Health Organization, 1990.

50. WHO Europe. *Healthy nutrition: preventing nutrition-related diseases in europe.* Copenhagen: World Health Organization Regional Office for Europe, European Series, no 24. Copenhagen: World Health Organization Regional Office for Europe, 1988.

51. Maxwell S, Slater R. Food Policy Old and New. *Development Policy Review* 2003; **21**(5–6):531–553.

52. Lobstein T, Baur L, Uauy R, International Obesity Task Force. Obesity in children and young people: a crisis in public health. A report to the World Health Organization. *Obesity Reviews* 2004;**5**(S1).

53. Hawkes C. *Marketing food to children: the global regulatory environment.* Geneva: World Health Organization, 2004.

54. Hawkes C. *Marketing food to children: changes in the global regulatory environment 2004–2006.* Geneva: World Health Organization, 2007.

55. Nestle M. *What to eat.* New York: North Point Press (Farrar, Straus and Giroux), 2006.

56. COMA. *Diet and coronary heart disease: report of the Advisory Panel of the Committee on Medical Aspects of Food Policy (COMA).* Department of Health and Social Security, 1974.

57. WHO. *World Health Report 2002: reducing risks, promoting healthy life.* Geneva: World Health Organization, 2002.

58. WHO/IARC. *World Cancer Report World Health.* Geneva: World Health Organization/ International Agency for Research on Cancer, 2003.

59. International Diabetes Federation. *Diabetes atlas,* 3rd edn. Brussels: International Diabetes Federation, 2006.

60. Commission on the Nutrition Challenges of the 21st Century. Ending malnutrition by 2020: an agenda for change in the millennium. Final Report to the ACC/SCN. *Food and Nutrition Bulletin* 2000;**21**(3 Suppl.):Whole issue.

61. James WPT, Rigby NJ, Leach RJ, Kumanyika S, Lobstein T, Swinburn B. *Global strategies to prevent childhood obesity: forging a societal plan that works.* A discussion paper prepared for the Global Prevention Alliance McGill Integrative Health Challenge October 26–27, 2006. London: International Obesity Task Force/International Association for the Study of Obesity, 2006.

62. Murray CJL, Lopez AD (ed.) *The global burden of disease: a comprehensive assessment of mortality and disability from diseases, injuries and risk factors in 1990 and projected to 2020.* Cambridge MA: Harvard School of Public Health on behalf of the World Health Organization and the World Bank, 1996.

63. Wanless D. *Securing our future health: taking a long-term view.* London: H M Treasury, 2002.

64. Wanless D. *Securing good health for the whole population.* London: H M Treasury, 2004.

65. Sturm R, Ringel J, Andreyava R. Increasing obesity rates and disability Trends. *Health Affairs* 2004;**23**(2):1–7.

66. Surgeon General U. *A call to action to prevent and decrease overweight and obesity 2001.* Rockville, MD: US Department of Health and Human Services, Public Health Service, Office of the Surgeon General, 2001.

67. Sturm R. Increases in morbid obesity in the USA: 2000–2005. *Public Health* 2007; **121**(7):492–496.

68. Yach D, Stuckler D, Brownell KD. Epidemiologic and economic consequences of the global epidemics of obesity and diabetes. *Nature Medicine* 2006;**12**(1):62–66.

69. Witt L. Why we're losing the war against obesity. *American Demographics*. 2003; **25**(10):27–31.

70. Levy E, Levy P, Le Pen C, Basdevant A. The economic cost of obesity: the French situation. *International Journal of Obesity and Related Metabolic Disorders* 1995; **19**(11):788–792.

71. National Audit Office. *Tackling obesity in England*. London: Stationery Office, 2001.

72. Health Committee of the House of Commons. *Obesity*. Third Report of Session 2003–04, HC 23–1,volume 1. London: The Stationery Office, 2004.

73. Kemper HC, Stasse-Wolthuis M, Bosman W. *The prevention and treatment of overweight and obesity*. Summary of the advisory report by the Health Council of The Netherlands. *Netherlands Journal of Medicine* 2004;62(1):10–71.

74. Byrne D. Commissioner David Byrne says 'Time to take on obesity' as WHO debates worldwide strategy. *Speech 85/04*. Brussels: Commission of the European Communities, 2004.

75. Byrne D. *Enabling good health for all: a reflection process for a new EU Health Strategy*. Brussels: Commision of the European Communities, 2004:12.

76. European Commission Directorate-General for Health and Consumer Protection. *Summary Report: Roundtable on Obesity 20 July 2004*. Brussels: European Commission DG Sanco Directorate C, Public Health and Risk Assessment, 2004:7.

77. Asfaw A. Obesity and chronic diseases: not limited to the affluent. *IFPRI Forum* 2006:7.

78. Diabetes UK. *'Diabetes explosion—figures expected to soar'*. *Statement*. London: Diabetes UK, 2008.

79. International Diabetes Federation. *Diabetes epidemic out of control*. Press release, 4 December 2006. Brussels and Cape Town: International Diabetes Federation, 2006.

80. Robertson A, Tirado C, Lobstein T, Jermini M, Knai C, Jensen JH et al. *Food and health in Europe: a new basis for action*. Copenhagen: World Health Organization Regional Office for Europe, 2004.

81. Cattaneo A, Yngve A, Koletzko B, Guzman LR. Protection, promotion and support of breast-feeding in Europe: current situation. *Public Health Nutrition* 2005;**8**(1):39–46.

82. Palmer G. *The politics of breastfeeding*. London: Pandora, 1988.

83. WHO. *Global strategy on infant and young child feeding*. Geneva: World Health Organization, 2003.

84. Murton B. Famine. In: Kiple KF, Ornelas KC (ed.) *The Cambridge world history of food*. Cambridge: Cambridge University Press, 2000:1411–1427.

85. Dando WA. *The geography of famine*. London: Edward Arnold, 1980.

86. Dumont R, Rosier B. *The hungry future*. London: Deutsch, 1969.

87. Lappé FM, Collins J. *Food first: beyond the myth of scarcity*. New York: Ballantyne Books, 1977.

88. George S. *How the other half dies: the real reasons for world hunger*. Harmondsworth: Penguin, 1976.

89. Fogel RW. New findings on secular trends in nutrition and mortality: some implications for population theory. In: Rosenzweig MR, Stark O (ed.) *Handbook of population and family economics*. Handbooks in Economics, vol. 14. Amsterdam, New York and Oxford: Elsevier Science North-Holland, 1997:433–81.

90. The Hunger Project. *Ending hunger: an idea whose time has come*. New York: Praeger, 1985.

91. Rosset P, Gershman J, Cunningham S, Marilyn Borchardt. *Myths and root causes: hunger, population, and development* (reflections on 20 years of Food First). http://www.hartford-hwp.com/archives/28/079.html [accessed July 26 2007]. San Francisco CA: Food First, 1995.

92. Carefoot GL, Sprott ER. *Famine on the wind: plant diseases and human history.* London: Angus and Roberston, 1969.

93. Woodham Smith CBFG. *The great hunger: Ireland, 1845–9.* London: Hamish Hamilton, 1962.

94. Kinealy C. *The great Irish famine: impact, ideology and rebellion.* Basingstoke: Palgrave, 2002.

95. Sen AK. *Poverty and famines: an essay on entitlement and deprivation.* Oxford: Clarendon Press, 1981.

96. Drèze J, Sen AK, Hussain A. *The political economy of hunger: selected essays.* New Delhi; Oxford: Oxford University Press, 1999.

97. Sen AK. *Development as freedom.* Oxford: Oxford University Press, 1999.

98. Kent G. *Freedom from want: the human right to adequate food.* Washington, DC: Georgetown University Press, 2005.

99. Appleton J, SCF Ethiopia Team. *Drought relief in Ethiopia: planning and management of feeding programmes.* London: Save the Children, 1987.

100. Raikes PL. *Modernising hunger: famine, food surplus & farm policy in the EEC & Africa.* London: Catholic Institute for International Relations in collaboration with James Currey, 1988.

101. Kent G. *The political economy of hunger: the silent holocaust.* New York: Praeger, 1984.

102. Lappé FM, Collins J. *Food first: the myth of scarcity.* Revised updated ed. London: Souvenir, 1980.

103. Maxwell S. The evolution of thinking about food security. In: Devereux S, Maxwell S (ed.) *Food security in Sub-Saharan Africa.* London: ITDG Publishing, 2001:13–31.

104. Maxwell S, Smith M. Household food security: a conceptual review. In: Maxwell S, Frankenberger T (ed.) *Household food security: concepts, indicators, measurements: a technical review.* New York/Rome: UNICEF & IFAD, 1995.

105. Riches G. *First world hunger: food security and welfare politics.* London: Macmillan, 1997.

106. Dowler E, Turner SA, Dobson B, Child Poverty Action Group (Great Britain). *Poverty bites: food, health and poor families.* London: Child Poverty Action Group, 2001.

107. Eisinger PK. *Towards an end to hunger in America.* Washington DC: Brookings Institute Press, 1998.

108. Nord M, Andrews M, Carlson S. *Household food security in the United States 2002.* Food Assistance and Nutrition Research Report No. (FANRR35) Washington DC: Economic Research Service, US Department of Agriculture. October http://www.ers.usda.gov/publications/fanrr35/. Washington DC: Economic Research Service, US Department of Agriculture, 2003.

109. Lang T, Heasman M. *Food wars: the global battle for mouths, minds and markets.* London: Earthscan, 2004.

110. Watson JD, Crick FHC. A structure for deoxyribose nucleic acid. *Nature* 1953; **171**:737–738.

111. Wilkins MHF, Stokes AR, Wilson HR. Molecular structure of deoxypentose nucleic acids. *Nature* 1953;**171**:738–740.

112. Franklin R, Gosling RG. Molecular configuration in sodium thymonucleate. *Nature* 1953;**171**:740–741.

113. Watson JD, Crick FHC. Genetical implications of the structure of deoxyribonucleic acid. *Nature* 1953;**171**:964–967.

114. Human Genome Mapping Project. http://www.ornl.gov/sci/techresources/Human_Genome/project/about.shtml [accessed June 8 2008]. Washington DC: U.S. Department of Energy and the National Institutes of Health, 2008.

115. Heasman M, Mellentin J. *The functional foods revolution: healthy people, healthy profits?* London: Earthscan, 2001.

116. Chadwick R. Nutrigenomics, individualism and public health. *Proceedings of the Nutrition Society* 2004;**63**(1):161–166.

117. Kaput J, Rodriguez RL. Nutritional genomics: the next frontier in the postgenomic era. *Physiology & Genomics* 2004;**16**:166–177.

118. Lang T. Functional foods. *British Medical Journal* 2007;**334**:1015–1016.

119. Fieldhouse P. *Food and nutrition: customs and culture*, 2nd edn. London: Chapman & Hall, 1995 [1985].

120. MacDonald M. *Food, stamps, and income maintenance*. New York: Academic Press, 1977.

121. Leather S. *The making of modern malnutrition: an overview of food poverty in the UK*. London: Caroline Walker Trust, 1996.

122. Nelson M, Erens B, Bates B, Church S, Boshier T. *Low income diet and nutrition survey*, vols 1, 2 & 3. London: The Stationery Office/Food Standards Agency, 2007.

123. Bradshaw J, Middleton S, Davis A, Oldfield N, Smith N, Cusworth L *et al. A minimum income standard for Britain: what people think*. York: Joseph Rowntree Foundation, 2008.

124. Boyd Orr J. *Food, health and income: report on adequacy of diet in relation to income*. London: Macmillan and Co, 1936.

125. Mennell S, Murcott A, Otterloo AHv, International Sociological Association. *The sociology of food: eating, diet and culture*. London: Sage, 1992.

126. Boyle D. *Authenticity: brands, fakes, spin and the lust for real life*. London: Harper Perennial, 2004.

127. Engels F. *The condition of the working class in England in 1844*. London: Penguin Classics, 1987 (1845/1892).

128. Booth W. *In darkest England, and the way out*. London: International Headquarters of The Salvation Army, 1890.

129. Rowntree BS. *Poverty: a study of town life*. London: Macmillan, 1902.

130. Trowell H, Burkitt D (ed.) *Western diseases: their emergence and prevention*. London: Edward Arnold, 1981.

131. MacClancy J. *Consuming culture*. London: Chapman, 1992.

132. Berry V, Petty C (ed.) *The Nyasaland Papers 1938–1943: agriculture, food and health*. London: Academy Books, 1992.

133. Evans-Pritchard EE. *The Nuer, a description of the modes of livelihood and political institutions of a Nilotic people*. Oxford: Clarendon Press, 1940.

134. Leitzmann C. Nutrition ecology: the contribution of vegetarian diets. *American Journal of Clinical Nutrition* 2003;**78**(3):657S-659S.

135. *Nutrition Ecology: an integrative approach for problem-solving in the field of nutrition.* Poster presentation at FENS, Paris, 12 July 2007. Giessen: Justus-Liebig University of Giessen. European Conference on Nutrition; 2007; Paris.

136. Randolph TG. *Human ecology and susceptibility to the chemical environment.* Springfield, Ill.: Charles C. Thomas, 1962.

137. McMichael AJ. Integrating nutrition with ecology: balancing the health of humans and biosphere. *Public Health Nutrition* 2003;**8**(6A):706–715.

138. Chapagain AK, Hoekstra AY. *Water footprints of nations*, vols. 1 and 2. UNESCO-IHE Value of Water Research Report Series No. 16. Paris, 2004.

139. Stern N. *The Stern review of the economics of climate change. Final report.* London: H M Treasury, 2006.

140. Sustainable Development Commission. *Green, healthy and fair: a review of government's role in supporting sustainable supermarket food.* London: Sustainable Development Commission, 2008.

141. Haeckel E. *Generelle morphologie der organismen.* Berlin: G Reimer, 1866.

142. Haeckel EHPA, Lankester ER. *The history of creation or, The development of the earth and its inhabitants by the action of natural causes. A popular exposition of the doctrine of evolution in general, and of that of Darwin, Goethe and Lamarck in particular,* 2nd edn. London: Henry S. King & Co, 1876.

143. Lappé FM. *Diet for a small planet.* New York: Ballantine Books, 1971.

144. Gussow JD, Clancy KL. Dietary guidelines for sustainability. *Journal of Nutrition Education* 1986;**18**:1–5.

145. McMichael AJ. *Human frontiers, environment and disease.* Cambridge: Cambridge University Press, 2001.

146. Gluckman P, Hanson M. *Mismatch: why our world no longer fits our bodies.* Oxford: Oxford University Press, 2006.

147. *Ecological Public Health: new paradigms for old?* http://www.ukpha.org.uk/media/15thaphf/symposium/edinburgh%20ecopubhlth%20gr%2029%2003%2007.pdf. Health and Sustainable Development; 2007 March 30, 2007; Edinburgh International Conference Centre. UK Public Health Assocation.

148. Cohen JE. *How many people can the earth support?* New York: WW Norton, 1995.

149. *Our health, our environment: the ecological footprint of what we eat.* International Ecological Footprint Conference: *Stepping up the pace: new developments in ecological footprint methodology, applications,* 8–10 May 2007; Cardiff. http://www.brass.cf.ac.uk/uploads/Frey_A33.pdf.

150. Cordain L, Eaton S, Sebastian A, Mann N, Lindeberg S, Watkins B *et al.* Origins and evolution of the Western diet: health implications for the 21st century. *American Journal of Clinical Nutrition* 2005;**81**(2):341–354.

151. Nestle M. Paleolithic diets: a sceptical view. *Nutrition Bulletin* 2000;**25**:43–47.

152. Baroni L, Cenci L, Tettamanti M, Berati M. Evaluating the environmental impact of various dietary patterns combined with different food production systems. *European Journal of Clinical Nutrition* 2007;**61**:279–286.

153. Beauman C, Cannon G, Elmadfa I, Glasauer P, al. e. The Giessen Declaration. *Public Health Nutrition* 2005;8(6A):117–120.

154. Lang T, Rayner G. Obesity: a growing issue for European policy? *Journal of European Social Policy* 2005;**15**(4):301–327.

155. Defra. *Fisheries 2027: a long-term vision for sustainable fisheries.* London: Department for Environment, Food and Rural Affairs, 2007.

156. Porritt J, Goodman J. *Fishing for good.* London: Forum for the Future, 2005:60.

157. Ewin J. *Fine wines and fish oil: the life of Hugh Macdonald Sinclair.* Oxford: Oxford University Press, 2001.

158. Lang T. Food control or food democracy: re-engaging nutrition to civil society, the state and the food-supply chain. *Public Health Nutrition* 2005;**8**(6A):730–737.

159. Royal Commission on Environmental Pollution. *Turning the tide: addressing the impact of fishing on the marine environment, 25th report.* London: Royal Commission on Environmental Pollution, 2004.

160. Food Standards Agency. *Eat well, be well: fish and shellfish.* http://www.eatwell.gov.uk/healthydiet/nutritionessentials/fishandshellfish/ [accessed January 9, 2008]. London: Food Standards Agency, 2008.

161. WHO. Fifty-seventh World Health Assembly 17–22 May 2004, WHA57.17 *Global strategy on diet, physical activity and health.* Geneva: WHO, 2004.

162. Lang T, Rayner G, Kaelin E. *The food industry, diet, physical activity and health: a review of reported commitments and practice of 25 of the world's largest food companies.* London: City University Centre for Food Policy, 2006:80.

163. FAO. *Renewed financial effort in fight on hunger.* FAO press summary. June 5 2008 http://www.fao.org/newsroom/en/news/2008/1000858/index.html. Rome: Food and Agriculture Organization, 2008.

164. Boyd Orr J. *As I recall: the 1880's to the 1960's.* London: MacGibbon and Kee, 1966.

165. Boyd Orr SJ. *Food and the people. Target for tomorrow No 3.* London: Pilot Press, 1943.

166. Shaw DJ. *World food security: a history since 1945.* London: Palgrave Macmillan, 2007.

167. Daynard RA. Lessons from tobacco control for the obesity control movement. *Journal of Public Health Policy* 2003;**24**(3 & 4):291–295.

168. Hirschhorn N. *How the tobacco and food industries and their allies tried to exert undue influence over FAO/WHO Food and Nutrition Policies*, unpublished report to WHO. New Haven, Connecticut, 2002.

169. Marshall T. Exploring a fiscal food policy: the case of diet and ischaemic heart disease. *British Medical Journal* 2000;**320**(29 January):301–305.

170. Leicester A, Windmeijer F. *The 'fat tax': economic incentives to reduce obesity.* London: Institute for Fiscal Studies, 2004.

171. Strnad J. *Conceptualizing the 'fat tax': the role of food taxes in developed economies.* Working Paper, September 2002. *Working Paper.* Palo Alto, CA: Stanford Law School, 2004.

172. Loureiro ML. *The role of economic incentives to reduce obesity.* NOU 2007–8. Oslo: Finansdepartementet, 2007.

173. Mytton O, Gray A, Rayner M, Rutter H. Could targeted food taxes improve health? *Journal of Epidemiology and Community Health* 2007;**61**(8):689–694.

174. Hawkes C. Self-regulation of food advertising: what it can, could and cannot do to discourage unhealthy eating habits among children. *British Nutrition Foundation Bulletin* 2005;**30**:374–382.

175. Hastings G, Stead M, Macdermott L, Forsyth A, Mackintosh AM, Rayner M *et al.* *Review of research on the effects of food promotion to children.* Final Report to the Food Standards Agency by the Centre for Social Marketing, University of Strathclyde. London: Food Standards Agency, 2004.

176. Food Standards Agency. *Outcome of academic seminar to review recent research on food promotion and children, held 31 October 2003.* http://www.food.gov.uk/multimedia/ webpage/academicreview. London: Food Standards Agency, 2003.

177. Institute of Medicine of the National Academies. *Preventing childhood obesity: health in the balance.* Washington DC: Institute of Medicine of the National Academies, 2004.

178. Business in the Community. Responsible marketing to children: exploring the impact on adults' attitudes and behaviour. *Marketplace Responsibility Research.* London: Business in the Community, 2005.

179. WHO. *Marketing of food and non-alcoholic beverages to children.* Report of a WHO Forum and Technical Meeting, Oslo, Norway, 2–5 May 2006. Geneva: World Health Organization, 2006.

180. Donaldson L. *Annual Report of the Chief Medical Officer for England 2002.* London: Department of Health, 2003.

181. Department of Health. *Obesity public service agreement.* http://www.dh.gov.uk/en/ Policyandguidance/Healthandsocialcaretopics/Obesity/DH_4133951 [accessed June 20 2007]. London: Department of Health, 2004.

182. Department of Health. *Government response to report on tackling childhood obesity.* http://www.dh.gov.uk/en/Publicationsandstatistics/Pressreleases/DH_4130965 London: Department of Health, 2006.

183. Department of Health. *Healthy weight, healthy lives: a cross government strategy for England.* London: Department of Health, 2008:56.

184. Burnet E, Aykroyd WR. Nutrition and public health. *Quarterly Bulletin of the Health Organization* 1935;4(2):000.

185. League of Nations. *The problem of nutrition.* Interim Report of the Mixed Committee on the Problem of Nutrition, Volume 1. *A.12.1936.II.B.* Geneva: League of Nation, 1936.

186. League of Nations. *Final Report of the Mixed Commission of the League of Nations on the relation of nutrition to agriculture, health and economic policy.* Geneva & London: League of Nations & Allen and Unwin, 1937.

187. Astor WA, Rowntree BS. *British agriculture: the principles of future policy.* London, New York: Longmans Green, 1938.

188. Campbell JM. The nutrition report. *International Affairs (Journal of the Royal Institute of International Affairs 1931–1939)* 1936;17(2):251–253.

189. Smith DF. Nutrition science and the two World Wars. In: Smith DF (ed.) *Nutrition in Britain: science, scientists and politics in the twentieth century.* London: Routledge, 1997:142–165.

190. Ostry AS. *Nutrition policy in Canada, 1870–1939.* Vancouver: UBC Press, 2006.

191. Hammond RJ. *Food: the growth of policy.* London: HMSO/Longmans, Green and Co., 1951.

192. Titmuss RM. War and social policy. In: Titmuss RM (ed.) *Essays on the welfare state.* London: Allen and Unwin., 1958.

193. Economic Advisory Council. *Nutrition in the Colonial Empire.* First Report (Part 1) of the Committe on Nutrition in the Empire. Presented to Parliament July 1939. Cmd.6050. London His Majesty's Stationery Office, 1939:210.

194. Drummond JC, Wilbraham A. *The Englishman's food: a history of five centuries of English diet.* London: Jonathan Cape, 1939.

195. Le Gros Clarke F, Titmuss RM. *Our food problem and its relation to our national defences.* Harmondsworth: Penguin, 1939.

196. Rowntree BS. *Poverty and progress.* London: Longmans, 1941.

197. Rowntree BS. *How the labourer lives.* London: Thomas Nelson & Sons, 1913.

198. Rowntree BS. *The human needs of labour.* London: Longmans, 1921.

199. Driver C. *The British at table 1940–1980.* London: Chatto & Windus, 1983.

200. Drummond JC, Wilbraham A, with, Hollingsworth D. *The Englishman's food: a history of five centuries of English diet* (revised with new chapter by Dorothy Hollingsworth), 2nd edn. London Jonathan Cape, 1957.

201. Beveridge SW. *Food control.* Oxford: Oxford University Press, 1928.

202. Woolton TE. *The Memoirs of the Rt Hon. The Earl of Woolton.* London: Cassell, 1959.

Chapter 5

The supply chain

In the previous chapter, we reviewed the considerable challenges posed to and by nutrition. Translating nutrition's messages into coherent food policy is made more complex by the different conceptual approaches and traditions that we outlined: the three nutritions. But food policy, being a cross-sectoral policy 'live' area, is inevitably subject to such complexity. The real world of food is never, or only rarely, neat and orderly, which is why ensuring policy-makers have a good grasp of the realities of the food-supply chain, the subject of this chapter, is so important. The commercial world of growing, processing, trading, selling, cooking and marketing food is what gives shape to so much of what we discuss in this book. In this chapter we explore how and why the food system has the shape it does, in order to assess whether and how the various food sectors are rising to the ecological public health challenge; and if not, how to encourage or make them do so. For decades, centuries even, food producers have been locked into demands to increase output and to produce whatever they do more cheaply. Now, from health, environmental and societal interests, different urgent messages emanate, but can food businesses engage? Some argue that they can and must.[1-3] Others that they cannot and are locked-in.[4, 5]

The 21st-century ecological public health demands are to deliver quality, not just quantity; long-term planetary survival, not just feeding people here and now; complex rather than simple pathways between food and (ill) health; food justice within and between societies. In pursuit of this, new multiple, rather than single-issue, standards have to be met. Even the words have changed meaning in this transition. Whereas 'quality' fruit came to mean blemish-free in the 1960s, necessitating use of agri-chemicals to stop fungal growth and pest damage, now in the 21st century 'quality' may also mean good for the soil (and worker), and a supply chain that is both ethical and sustainable. Blemishes can be re-interpreted as a sign of being 'natural', but are still kept to a minimum. After years of draining wetlands and coastal areas for their fertile soils, now conservationists argue that this has led to biodiversity loss. Wildlife that was deemed predatory is now an indicator of biodiversity. Alongside these new demands, older political and economic realities have reared their heads too. The issue of corporate power is an example. In the 20th century the food system developed an unprecedented concentration of power. Huge new companies emerged in manufacturing, retailing and catering, dwarfing the influence of the state.

Due to these changes, the repertoire of policy instruments has been subject to heated ideological discussion with calls on governments to rein in industry damage.[6, 7] There are continuous debates, for example, about whether voluntarily, rather than compulsory, regulations on food companies can resolve health and environmental problems. The word 'protection' has negative connotations to neo-liberal economists, but is positive in environmental, health and social welfare policy, premised as they are on protecting and enhancing these features of life. The issue of food power, however, is thorny. Critics of corporations, mindful of experience in battling tobacco giants (one of which is also one of the world's largest food multi-nationals), are sober about how such powerful bodies can do anything other than look after their own corporate interests; profitability comes before people, surely. If this is so, critics argue, the chances of food-supply chains putting health and the environment at the heart of their business models are slim. Optimists counter that, given the urgency of the need to re-cast food supplies to help foster diets that are good for public health and for living within environmental limits, only powerful interests can make the necessary quantum leap to save planetary and human health.[3] Much depends on the outcome of this debate.

As we show in the next chapter, whichever way the word 'sustainable' is defined, food-supply chains are currently unsustainable; but what would a sustainable food system look like? This question increasingly troubles food companies, under pressure from civil society and sometimes governments. At present it is simpler to outline the criteria by which a sustainable food system might be judged than it is to point to perfect cases. Sustainability is not what the food system has been aiming for since the mid-20th century. World and national food systems are locked into the productionist paradigm. The economic signals and rules of engagement have encouraged a particular division of labour to emerge. More money is made from what happens to food after it leaves farming than by the people who grow it.

Sustainability used to be a fringe issue for food supply. For decades supply chain structures were wrapped up in their own internal business logic rather than meeting sustainability goals, which were restricted to niche products. But awareness of the enormity and urgency of addressing the ecological public health challenge has grown. Huge investments have been made into existing unsustainable food systems, such as distribution, factories and retailing.

Changing these will take time to change, but change they must. A system aiming to be low carbon and healthy is now required as the world edges towards existence after 'peak oil', the point at which half global oil resources has been used.[8, 9] For policy-makers faced with delivering this low carbon but healthy food system, a good understanding of the role, limitations and potential of food-supply systems is thus essential.[10] We now turn to describe what the food system and supply chains are, giving examples from the UK, Europe and world-wide. Supply chains, like governance, have to be located within a multi-level frame of analysis.

The structure of modern food-supply chains

One conventional way of describing how food gets to consumers is through a chain. Different sectors or links are joined together as a whole to transfer food along that chain. Particular foods and commodities have their own different supply chains, all within the overall food system or food economy. At its simplest, a food-supply chain is often depicted as a flow through farming, processing, distribution, retailing and catering. While farming is usually an initiator of this process, in that it creates plants and animals that are ultimately consumed, by managing the land (soil), water, energy (sunlight + oil) and biosphere, others take that raw food and perform actions that extend the chain. These are all multiple actions creating employment and adding further value. The simplest food-supply chain is when one grows one's own food and cooks it at home.

Different inputs feed into each sector. Farming, for instance, is underpinned by other links, such as finance, energy, transport, agri-chemicals, machinery, seeds and so on. Finance, energy, transport and many other economic activities underpin other sectors too. Models of food-supply chains that start off looking very neat and simple on paper can quickly start to look like a bowl of spaghetti or noodles! Economic and physical connections weave everywhere, with health, social and environmental outputs added as well. A balance has to be struck between realism and neat model-making. One way economists do this is to present how food flows along supply chains as a value-adding chain. Figure 5.1 uses UK data to illustrate this, derived from taxation, trade and other government sources.

The UK food system is clearly not a closed system; it imports and exports food, feed and drink, and has done for a long time.[11] It was last self-sufficient (with Ireland) in the mid-18th century.[12] With its colonies offering capacity for food from where land and labour were cheaper, UK imperial food policy did not favour self-sufficiency, although its experience in World Wars I and II, and the collapse of Empire (1940s on), shook that complacency. The original

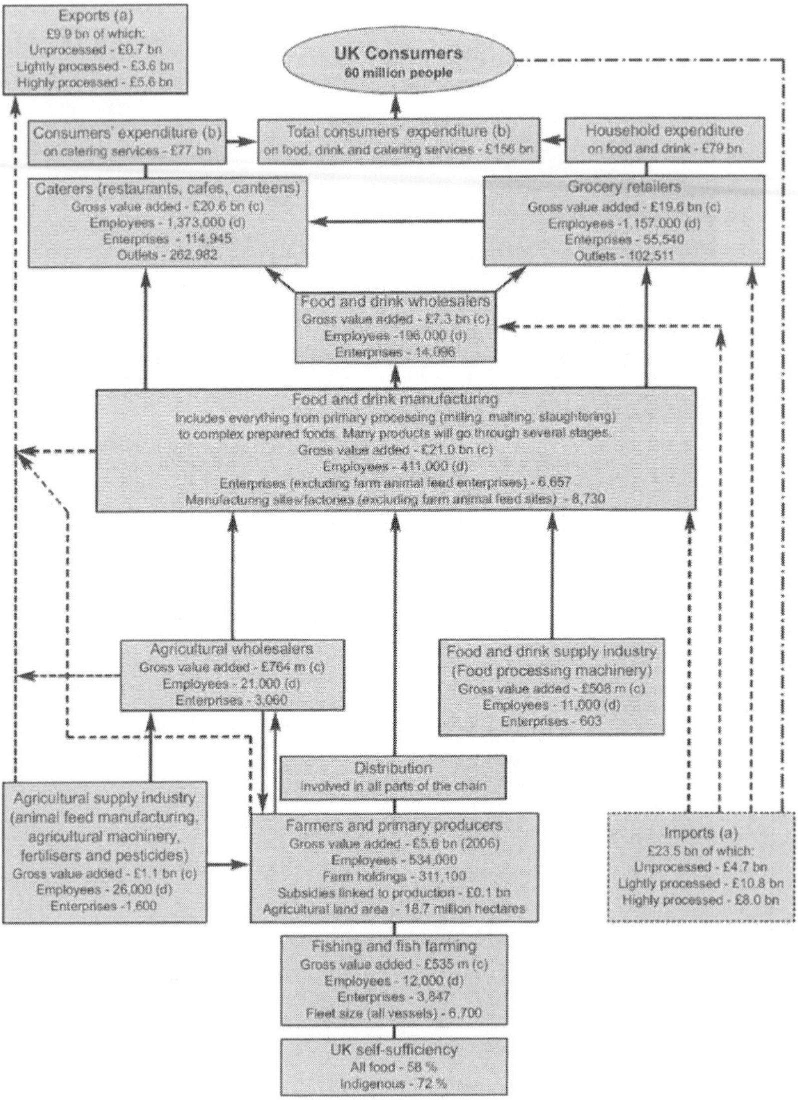

Fig. 5.1 A national food supply chain: the UK in 2007. Source: Defra 2007

policy tussle over whether to be fed by others or by oneself had been settled by the 1846 Repeal of the Corn Laws. These had imposed taxes on food imports to protect home producers, the big landowners. The Repeal represented the triumph of industrial over rural interests, winning the 'right' to aim for as cheap food as possible for the new urbanized (and restless) working classes. Progress was defined as cheap food (the complexity of what affordability actually meant was, and still is, fudged). Despite losing its Empire from the 1940s, that ideological legacy was hardwired into the UK state. In its own terms, the policy has been a success. By the 2000s, UK consumers spent on average 9% of household income on food, down from 25% in 1950. In 2006, the UK imported £23.5 bn of food in the year, exporting only £9.9 bn worth. This £13.6 bn deficit is known as the 'food trade gap'. In 1995–2006 it grew by 66%. By 2007, the UK produced only 58.8% of the food that it consumed, a proportion that was rapidly dropping from a high point in the 1980s. Proponents of ever more liberalization argue that this does not matter and point out that UK consumers eat a great deal, spending large sums on food in and outside the home and that, as an affluent society, the UK benefits from such a policy. But what is wise or sustainable and globally equitable is a politically charged question. What if supply chains are threatened? What if, as happened in 2006–08, world commodity prices rocket? What is sustainable and best land use? Policy varies across even developed countries; Australia, New Zealand, Brazil, Argentina, the USA all export heavily. China after the Maoist revolution aimed for self-reliance but is now importing heavily to feed its more affluent population. The USA, an agricultural powerhouse, has a balance between import and exports, while France fiercely maintains its farmers and has a trade surplus. The financial analysts Ernst and Young in 2008 judged that these latter two countries' policies were more resilient to external food shock than the UK's.[14]

The irony of such assessments is that they were not made for developing countries. Many developing countries dreamed of releasing spending power to spend on other economic activities in this way. For many it has long been a policy cornerstone.[15] The Washington Consensus (see Chapter 2) encouraged them to export rather than aim for self-reliance. That policy was associated with the past in the heyday of anti-colonial struggles.[16, 17] Far better, argued advocates of the Washington Consensus, that developing countries should specialize in what they are good at and purchase goods, including food if necessary, from the proceeds. Others decried this as re-colonization by agri-business and the desire of local, indigenous food systems.[18–20]

Returning to the supply chain and taking the UK as illustration again (Fig 5.1), we note that in 2006/07, total consumer expenditure on all food, drink and catering services was £156 bn. Out of this final spending, farming and primary producers had added only £5.6 bn, dwarfed by later sectors. Manufacturing added £21 bn, retailers £19.6 bn and catering £20.6 bn. Consumer spending by the UK's 60 million (human) mouths was split between catering services and retailers, in part reflecting a tension in lifestyles between eating 'in' or 'out'. Overall, the UK's 60 million citizens were 'fed' by 512,000 enterprises, run by 3.7 million employees.[11]

Such supply-chain analyses can be produced for any national food economy, also for particular product lines: meat, dairy, fruit, anything. Figure 5.2 gives

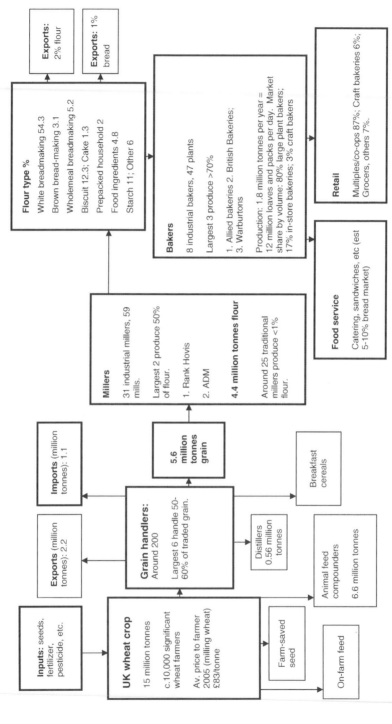

Fig. 5.2 UK wheat-flour-bread chain. Source: Sharpe et al. (2006)[21]

an example from a study conducted of the UK bread-supply chain.[21, 22] It illustrates how complex just one apparently everyday food product's supply chain can be, with many companies and different sub-chains behind multiple products under one heading: bread.

National policies within an international policy context

The UK is an EU member state, one of 27 member states, and therefore signed up to the Common Agricultural Policy (CAP) and CAP's complex political negotiation. CAP is sometimes described as an all-dominant policy framework, without flexibility. This is not true. It has in fact slowly evolved from its roots in reaction to the experience of extreme dislocation in World War II.[23–25] Member states interpret and apply its framework differently, particularly since member states agreed in 2003 to 'de-couple' subsidies from commodity support. Unlike France, Italy or Poland, the UK took a strategic position not to give high priority to keeping farmers on the land growing food.[26] It wanted its farmers to be more market-oriented. This policy was partly shaped by macroeconomic thinking and partly by Treasury exasperation with having to fund seemingly endless farm-based crises, from BSE in the 1980s to foot and mouth disease in 2001. Its argument was that agriculture in a rich service-based economy such as the UK only produces a fraction of gross domestic product and employs relatively few people, compared to retailing or catering. Tourism may be more important than farming.

Such thinking deems food just one commodity among many others. It is not special, and ought to be subject to common economic policy frameworks. Such views triumphed in 1994 when food and agricultural products came under new binding international trade rules signed at Marrakech and designed to lower tariffs and barriers to cross-border trade. The General Agreement on Tariffs and Trade (GATT) is an evolving inter-governmental trade framework created in 1948. Prior to 1994 it had not covered food and agriculture, but that agreement included a new Agreement on Agriculture (AoA) with related agreements on Technical Barriers to Trade (TBT) and sanitary and phytosanitary standards (SPS). The GATT secretariat became the World Trade Organization (WTO), a body first mooted in the 1940s but vetoed by the USA, which (perhaps rightly from its interests) saw an International Trade Organization, as it was to be called, as a potential threat to its emerging domination of world agricultural trade. When agriculture finally came under world trade rules half a century later, with the USA now signed up, proponents of development argued, as they do still today, that those rules favour rich, powerful, agriculturally advanced producer nations. The EU and USA could not just institute well-funded subsidy systems but pour out surpluses on to world markets.[25, 27] This focus on 'trade' became central in international dialogue about food policy in fundamental ways, marginalizing public health and environment. A policy fissure was created. On one side are those favouring liberalization; on the other are groups arguing for environmental and social justice. This debate hit official global politics with the riots at the Seattle meeting of the WTO when trade ministers were attempting to launch another round of trade talks in December 1999.[28]

Sensitivities about trade are not new; they are as long as history stretches and well-documented in the literature. Key episodes in UK food and trade history, for example, include the role of the (British) East India Company in annexing India,[29] the actions of sugar and slave traders in the West Indies,[30] and the geo-politics behind and after the creation of the Suez Canal.[31] To understand the impact of such events requires a dissection of motives, actors, opportunities and legacy, and is part of the richness of food policy studies. A case in point, at the international level, is the political argument over Structural Adjustment Programmes (SAPs), highly sensitive from the 1980s on. The World Bank and other international finance bodies had instituted SAPs to formalize and given intellectual coherence to what previously had been the use of financial terms and conditions for loans. The SAPs issue became an iconic debate about developing versus developed country food policy interests. [32, 33]

The basic purpose of SAPs was to impose conditions on loans. Developing countries could receive 'aid' or loans as long as they altered their policies in line with donor-approved economic goals. SAPs were used to wean developing countries off illusions of self-sufficiency. In practice, SAPs were often punitive, locking primary producing countries into raising food output in pursuit of foreign earnings, a policy goal outlined in the Washington Consensus. But they often met the reality of falling commodity prices.[32, 34] By the time commodity prices rose in the late-2000s, the damage was done, infrastructure had been altered, policy lock-in had occurred.[35] Coupled with the effects of the Green Revolution, which, whatever its success in raising gross output, was criticized for favouring affluent over small farmers, SAPs were attacked by development analysts, NGOs and also the UN's food rights watchdog (see Chapter 4).[36, 37] Their criticism was that SAPs locked countries into near fiscal serfdom. It might be acceptable for a rich country like the UK to choose not to grow as much food from its national resources as it could, but the similar strategy imposed by developing country leaders locked in by mighty international financial institutions meant something very different, and put them at risk of food insecurity. Either way—judged right or wrong, successful or not—SAPs locked countries into debt, with varying effects across countries.[38]

The world food supply

With this policy turmoil as background, what is the state of the world's food supply? According to FAO, between 1961 and 2005, the value of world agricultural production, i.e. food and non-food crop and livestock production, more than trebled in real terms.[39] This reflected a shift to higher value products. Measured in tonnage, the story is patchier. Successes have been cereals, oil crops, sugar, vegetables, eggs and meat, which all have seen output exceeding population growth rates. Production of pulses, roots and tubers, however, has declined. Since the 1990s, the rate of cereal output growth has also slowed, whereas that of oil crops has grown. Meat output has grown very fast, due to demand from urbanizing populations with greater spending power, but this has raised environmental concerns about livestock's use of cereals and water.[40] Livestock is the greatest user of agricultural land and represents nearly 40% of the value of all agricultural production world-wide. For developed countries, animals represent over half of farm output by value.[39]

In the latter part of the 20th century, most regions of the world saw growth in farm output; Sub-Saharan Africa was the general exception. Despite this, the FAO review for 2007 judged the last four decades a success, but exposed some paradoxes. One was that meat production is an indicator of affluence, and production should pursue that business opportunity. On the other hand, it acknowledged meat's deleterious environmental and health impact. Another was that lower prices made food affordable for people on low incomes but cheaper commodity prices meant less money for farmers, thus encouraging drift from the land and remaining farm sizes to get larger. Although larger farms are often more profitable, they do not necessarily maximize food output. For a century it has been recognized that market gardens and small-holdings can be more intensive in output than farms.[41] A policy counter-strand supports small and peri-urban farming, even within the FAO and certainly within thinking of research bodies such as the CGIAR and NGOs.[42–44] With energy prices fluctuating and rising, peri-urban agriculture and market gardening near urban centres of population become more logical, and are central to many community food-security movements' activities in rich and poor countries alike.[44–49] The Urban Agriculture Network (TUAN) has collated and co-ordinated that experience. When Cuba had its economic links with the old Soviet Russia severed in 1990, out of necessity it had to create a peri-urban and largely organic food system in dire circumstances but with some success.[50]

While urban agriculture represents a localist strand within primary production policy, championed by groups like TUAN, macro-economic policy has favoured formal cross-border trade for reasons already discussed. Between the early 1960s and early 2000s, in nominal terms, the value of global farm trade across borders rose 10-fold, but the share of agricultural products within total (not just food) world trade declined. It went from 25% in the early 1960s to less than 10% four decades later. Developing countries, committed to farm exports and aiming for surpluses from the 1960s, saw this reverse from the 1980s.[39]

This disjuncture helped spark the fair-trade movement, championing the need to get larger returns back to primary producers. What is fair about 'free' trade, NGOs asked? And they set up tiny alternative trading systems to make the point, promising higher returns to small farmers. From tiny beginnings a world system of audited standards has been developed, via the Fairtrade Labelling Organization International (FLO), now used by giant retailers.[51] From a health perspective, fair trade has some contradictions; many products are the legacy of colonial agriculture: coffee, tea, chocolate, cocoa, sugar. Giving better returns is a very important health boost—income improves health—but the majority of fair-traded goods are not noted for their health value. This is an issue being recognized, with the launch of fair-trade fruit and nuts.

Fair trade aside, however, the general trade situation is actually small. In 2002, only 10% of $3.2 trillion global processed food sales were traded across borders.[52] The majority of food produced and processed stays relatively regional. But that trade remains still grossly unfavourable. Back in the 1990s, this led to major political arguments at the UN, with its bodies such as the UN Conference on Trade and Development (UNCTAD) championing developing nations' case, whilst in the WTO those same nations, but via different Ministries, often were accommodating harsher economic realities. Institutions such as the FAO, as a result, had to look both ways. Exasperation resulted. Developing countries felt they had been asked to produce, which they had done, but they received small financial returns for their pains.[53] What they got for export crops rose but by less than the agricultural products they had to import to feed themselves.[39] Agricultural-exporting developing countries were on a treadmill, running faster to stay still (or go backwards). Even those who specialized in niche crops, such as Kenya with green beans, fared badly. The combination of squeezed trade and lower prices meant that after decades of decline, the number of malnourished people globally rose again from the mid-2000s.

Between 1990–02 and 2001–03, absolute numbers of the malnourished rose. In ascending order, the malnourished grew in Mexico, North Africa, Southern Africa, Central America, East Asia (except China), South Asia (except India), East Africa, the Near East and with Central Africa the worst. Numbers declined most dramatically in China, and less so in Southeast Asia, South America, India, the Caribbean, and West Africa. In this period the availability of supplies in fact improved considerably, but was not equitably distributed either within or between nations. In 1961–63, there were 2,280 kcal/person/day available; by 2001–03, this had risen to 2,800 kcal/person/day. The composition of diet changed over the same period. Meat, which provided about 3% of calorific value in 1961–63, had risen to 7% by 2001–03. Vegetable consumption went up by 50% but so too did sugar. But this overall situation is not necessarily translated to the household or local level. Inequalities distort the official global sufficiency of global supply. Some countries over-consume; others under-consume. The same is true within societies and households

Influence moves off the land

Off the land, the story—as with agriculture—is a divided one. In some parts, it is a tale of astonishing innovation and transformation. Scientists and technologists became key food actors in the 20th century. They helped shape the revolution in how food was processed, distributed and sold, and how this yielded lower prices, a remarkable growth of choice in urban food, flexibility in markets, food availability and a-seasonality, and increased output and productivity throughout supply chains. Against those criteria, food scientists and technologists could claim to be part of a great success story. They had delivered an unprecedented wave of change and response to problems inherited from pre-World War II, such as poor storage, waste, packaging, transportation, stock control, under-performance in factories, inappropriate variety, shelf-life. Yet in other respects, the tale is not so good, one of grossly unequal distribution, inefficiencies, under-investment, plainly unmet need and new forms of waste (plastic) replacing older ones (spoilage).

Explaining this picture, the conventional narrative is one of modernity and slow but incremental progress, with some failures too. But this rosy (Whig) interpretation of history sits uneasily alongside features already raised (Chapter 4), such as continued unmet need, new health problems (obesity), gross global inequality and environmental degradation. If science and technology claimed the former attributes, could they duck responsibility or collusion in the latter? New food critics argued that it is a myth that science and technology are neutral; their direction is framed by social assumptions. In the US, these arguments were articulated by civil society groups such as the Union of Concerned Scientists (created in 1969) and the Center for Science in the Public Interest (1971), and in the UK by the British Society for Social Responsibility in Science, launched at the Royal Society in 1969, spawning the specialist Agri-capital and Politics of Health Groups.[54, 55] Their case was that short-termism and pursuit of technical fixes limit science and tie it to commercial interests. This may be good for funding but is not necessarily good social mores. They argued that it is inappropriate to define food or any technologies as 'good' or 'bad', abused or properly used, because that implies science and technology are neutral. On the contrary, they are social projects and processes. From this perspective, science has to engage openly with political processes rather than subsume itself.

The impact and role of the oil-fuelled internal combustion engine on food illustrates these science politics. The effectiveness of engines in food-supply chains cannot be over-estimated; they underpin the growing, transportation and selling of food; they enable consumers to get to ever more distant food shops. Yet the oil-powered engine has come to symbolize the industrialization of food. It plays a part in the carbon footprint of food-supply chains, not least on the farm. In 1850, the USA had 6.6 million working animals providing motive power on farms, 4.3 million of them horses, the rest oxen and mules. As US farming moved West, the total rose rapidly to 13.1 million in 1880 and 21.8 million in 1910. But in that year, 10,000 tractors were present on US farms, heralding a rapid decline in working animals. By 1951 there were 4 million giant machines and barely any working animals.[56] Mechanization transformed everything. World-wide, the number of tractors went from 6 million in 1948 to 26 million 40 years later.[57] In North America and Europe, there are today more tractors than people working on the land, while in others there are very few, partly for difficulties of terrain (such as rice paddies). With mechanization, farms could get larger, new lands be worked, people, not just horses, be replaced. Investment in mechanization unfolded the productionist paradigm: efficiency, modernization, labour-saving, cheapness. Table 5.1 gives an overview of how dramatic this change was, using US agriculture as an example. Farm size went up (intensification); the number of crops each one produced declined (the rise of monoculture); the importance of farm work within overall national employment declined (industrialization); and the country de-ruralized (urbanization).

Similar technologies and scientific input yielded dramatic effects further down the food chain. Factories could be re-organized. Oil-driven equipment could move food further, faster, cheaper. A more complex food-supply chain could emerge. Early in the 20th century, highly concentrated combines had already begun to emerge. Some of those firms straddle the globe still today, such as Unilever, Nestlé, General Foods. Others are gone, merged or taken over. One such was the food empire of Thomas Lipton, a Scottish emigrant to the USA, who returned to Glasgow to take over his family shop. Before he died

Table 5.1 A century of structural change in US agriculture, 1900–2000

	1900	1930	1945	1970	2000/02
Number of farms (millions)	5.7	6.3	5.9	2.9	2.1
Average farm size (acres)	146	151	195	376	441
Average number of commodities produced per farm	5.1	4.5	4.6	2.7	1.3
Farm share of population (%)	39	25	17	5	1
Rural share of population (%)	60	44	36(1950)	26	21
				(%)	
Off-farm labour[a]	n/a	100 days	27	54	93

[a] 1930, average number of days worked off-farm; 1945, % farmers working off-farm; 1970 and 2000/02, % households with off-farm income.

Source: Effland A, Dimitri C, Conklin N. *The 20th century transformation of US agriculture and farm policy*. Washington DC, USDA Economic Research Service, 2005.

he had turned Liptons into an integrated supply chain, using his US contacts to provide food ever cheaper, and creating a network of hundreds of shops across the UK, many internationally source. All this was made possible by oil and refrigeration. Old techniques of preserving and storing food could be redesigned. Giant abattoirs and meat processing plants sprang up to feed the large new conurbations. But the human and social costs, and the effects on health and life, were constantly being exposed and criticized, providing a source of political agitation and calls for social reform.

In the USA, for instance, an outcry followed publication of Upton Sinclair's 1906 now classic novel *The Jungle*, which showed the dire conditions and quality of food.[58] He alleged that machinery was not even stopped when a worker fell in to machinery. So scandalized was President Theodor Roosevelt, let alone the US consuming public, that a secret inquiry was conducted, confirming Sinclair's dire account, which accelerated the passage of the US Food and Drug Act into statute. A now common dynamic can be detected: investment, innovation, speed-up, food adulteration and de-naturing, plus transformation of the labour process, then followed by reaction and reform. This happened in the UK in the mid-19th century; in the US in the early 20th. It has been repeated in many countries, again in the West in the mid- to late-20th century too; what else were the food safety crises of 1980–2000s? Demands for health and quality control inevitably become rallying cries for tighter regulatory control.[59–62]

The 20th century was a century of unprecedented change in food supply. Refrigerated train wagons enabled US meat packers to transport food on railways.

The first chilled meat came by sea from New Zealand to the UK in 1882. With its booming population, Empire and already highly urbanized working class, UK capital roamed the world seeking investment opportunities. Railways were laid across the Argentinan pampas to deliver meat to packing plants that became corned beef, a staple on working-class tables the other side of the world.[63, 64] Well before the age of flying food, early in the 20th century, food knew few boundaries or impediment to distance. Long before Chicago economists espoused it, or the Washington Consensus formalized it, globalization was underway, ushered in by vast investment into transportation systems, from the Great Lakes to Australia, from Argentina to India. Food moved in mass transit systems, and changed in its very nature. New foods, such as margarine, developed in 1869 to replace butter, became mass food products, sold on price.[65] The era of substitution had dawned, culminating in the routine use of additives, preservatives and colours, now normalized and legitimized in basic foods.[66]

As foods were increasingly processed, different dynamics up and down value chains emerged. Through purchasing scale, manufacturers could impose conditions on farming. Through communications, business networks could emerge, and divisions of labour be instituted. In the 20th century, such integration unfolded from plant breeding science right through to marketing departments. Artisan food crafts were routinized by factory systems, run on management systems learning from, but overtaking, Henry Ford's revolutionary car assembly line production. But as commentators have pointed out, food is not metal; it retains biological, perishable characteristics, which open it to risk.[67] But its nature was refashioned systematically throughout the 20th century first via processing, and latterly in the re-ordering of genes themselves and the emergence of life sciences nutrition, noted in Chapter 4, and in agriculture.[68]

Another remarkable feature of off-farm change in 20th century food-chains was the rise in importance of marketing and advertising. In some narratives, the impression can be given that consumers were, and are, all duped, putty in the hands of ruthless processors and traders; but there is always also a 'pull' as well as 'push'. Consumers saw identity opportunities from particular foods, and these were simultaneously fanned and targeted by marketers.[69, 70] Technical change offered opportunities for appellation of modernity. This happened with margarine in the late-19th century. It gave undoubted advantages to the retailer, of course; it could be stored, it had relatively long life, it was cheap, it opened up profitable markets among those who could not afford butter; but therein lay the 'pull'.

That said, consumer understanding is inevitably thin. If food-supply chains are so complex, can consumers be the omniscient beings market theory suggests they must be? Consumer exposés of quality and labour practices suggest not.[71]

The commercial pursuit of markets inevitably became psychological not just material or economic. Before World War II, the insights of psycho-analysis and psychology were quickly incorporated; after, they expanded. Consumers were studied, monitored, probed and their decision-making experimented on.[69, 72] But they could not be forced to buy foods; they, not the manufacturer, chose at the point of sale. The dynamic between supply chains and consumers can be re-balanced by sophistication within supply chains but cannot so completely be manipulated beyond it (see Chapter 7). Historians rightly show that marketing was known to the Romans, if only in the form of graffiti. What was new in modern times was the effort, the use of science to inform it, the scale and systematic nature. The two largest food-marketing budgets in the world are greater than the entire budget of the WHO for all health matters. Coca Cola and PepsiCo, both soft drink manufacturers but the latter also a snack manufacturer, spent, respectively, $US 2.2 billion and $US 1.7 billion on advertising in 2004, a combined level of spending exceeding the WHO biennial budget for 2002–03. No figures for the total global ad-spend on food are publicly available but total ad-spend is around $400 billion annually.[73] Advertisements bombard consumers via various media—TV, radio, printed, text, web. These media are the outlets of what is essentially a vast consciousness industry, attempting to shape culture and behaviour. To its 'old' channels of print, sound and moving picture are now added 'new' ones such as virtual, viral and social marketing.

In sum, the early 21st century food system is dramatically different to that of half, let alone a full, century or so ago. Our case is that the new ecological public health period has to address the fundamental nature of how food systems have been altered. Table 5.2 summarizes some features of modern food systems that now exist. On the positive side, it has been shown that relatively rapid change is possible; food systems are not fixed. More soberly, we now know that problems previously thought of as fixable are probably fundamental, and that current politics and frameworks might not be appropriate, nimble or daring enough to tackle what needs to be done. We now explore this further by discussing some particularly significant issues, policy responses to them and their implications.

Strategic problems arising for ecological public health

Risk and control

When a representative sample of consumers from across the entire EU was asked in 2006 for its first thoughts when thinking about food, taste came out as the top issue, then pleasure, hunger, health and necessity.[74] Such polls are salutary reminders that, although their behaviour is complex (see Chapter 7),

Table 5.2 Some features of rich society food purchasing in the 19th, 20th and 21st centuries

Factor shaping food purchasing	19th century	20th century	21st century?
Format	Markets plus small diverse speciality shops	Supermarket	Mixture of giant hypermarket + speciality stores
Transport	Walk or animal-drawn	From mass transit to personalized car	mixed
Energy source for logistics	Feedstuff (animals) + human	Oil	Hydrogen, electric, solar or human?
Majority food labour	Farm	Factory	Service
Retail experience	Service at front of shop counter	Self-service	Self-service plus speciality
Location	Local	Distant	Distant (time rich) + home delivery (affluent but time poor)
Food sourcing	Seasonal	A-seasonal	Return of 'seasonal'?
Food range	Limited within shops but variety of shops	Enormous	Shaped by climate change, energy and water costs
Where the consumer's money goes	Farmers	Processors	Retailers
Quality concerns	Crude adulteration	Scientific adulteration	Low carbon + high nutrient
Food market	Local	National/regional	Global, regional, local
Time taken	Daily local shopping	Weekly one-stop shop	Monthly + fresh weekly
Domestic expenditure	High percentage cost for majority	Falling costs	Cost internalization means price rises
Information sources	Print	Radio + TV	Text + internet
Characteristic technology	Margarine	Barcode scanning	Internet shopping
Contentious technology	Bread adulteration	Agri-chemicals + biotechnology	Nanotechnology
Food supply chain dominant player	Farming	Food manufacturers then retailers	Farming + retailers?
Overarching goal	Sufficiency	Value-for-money	Values-for-money

people eat food for remarkably simple reasons: enjoyment, bodily sustenance, health and sociability. These are the motives upon which marketing and product design build. If early in the last century, the food revolution was around its industrialization, today there is a more subtle engagement with, and probing of, the feelings and aspirations that consumers bring to the point of sale. This is not just by consumer psychologists, but by computers recording every purchase made at the check-out of supermarkets, using laser scanning.

The invention of the barcode is probably one of the most significant of the last half century. Its dissemination began extraordinarily. An Ad Hoc Committee of 10 US business executives took the embryonic technology and pushed it through the retail industry in 1971–73.[75] Not even they anticipated the adoption it received. Today it is the workhorse of the logistics industry, enabling instantaneous re-ordering of foods and the 'just-in-time' revolution. Replacements arrive on shelves just in time to stop them being empty. The warehouse, which used to be located behind the store, is obsolete. The motorway is now the warehouse, with contracted manufacturers delivering to strategically located regional distribution centres (RDCs) at a time dictated by the retailer. The rubric is 'efficient consumer response'. Yet the take-up of the barcode almost foundered on tensions between manufacturers and retailers. The former wanted it, the latter were more cautious; yet it was the latter that have benefited most. An early test convinced the sceptics that productivity gains of 44% could be achieved in a supermarket at the checkout.

The depth of the revolution in food-supply chains that technologies, such as barcodes and computerized inventory systems enabled, is remarkable. As little as possible is left to chance. Products are standardized, made predictable and reliable. Smooth flow through the supply chain is essential. Brand recognition is a goal; building brand values is a key commercial goal.[76–78] The brand value of Coca-Cola (and its subsidiaries) was estimated at $58.2 bn in 2008.[79] Not lightly is the word 'revolution' used to describe the fundamental transformation of the food, ingredients, methods of growing, manufacture, retailing, cooking, packaging, marketing, pricing. The nature of production to consumption has been analysed, transformed and re-designed. Table 5.3 summarizes some changes shaping food supply and their implications for state policy-makers, society and the environment

A study by Bill Pritchard and David Burch, of the tomato-processing industry, illustrates the extent to which this is not just a technological but geographical matter. One company, HJ Heinz, was not just a major force in the tomato-processing sector but also controls 30% of the global processing tomato-seed market. It began a seed programme in 1936 but only entered the seeds business commercially in 1992.[80] From a base in California, a 'globally

Table 5.3 Modern changes in food supply and implications for state, society and environment

	CHANGES HERE...		...RAISE KEY ISSUES HERE...	
Sector	Supply Chain	State	Society	Environment
Agriculture	1994 GATT. De-decline of farm numbers and labour employed. Biotechnology. Global sourcing. BSE and other crises.	Multi-level governance of farm trade. WTO. Regional Trade negotiations. Food safety crises. Intellectual property rights.	Crises over trust. Growth of organic food. Continued urbanization.	Environmental pressures. Pesticides. Water. Fuel dependency. Biodiversity loss. Climate change.
Fisheries	Stock crises. Pressures on farmed fish.	Failure of international stock control. Laws of the seas under pressure.	Employment. The sea as leisure rather than food source.	Pollution controls. Sustainability concerns. Effect of large scale fishing
Food processing	Squeeze on prices. Development of healthy 'niches'. Rise in energy costs. Risk analysis and rise of HACCP	Pursuit of product innovation. Focus on quality and safety standards.	Pursuit of 'natural' foods. Continued support for value-for-money consumerism but opposition emerges.	Energy constraints. Carbon auditing. Climate change. Packaging and waste.
Logistics	Application of 'Efficient Consumer Response' [ECR]. 'Just-in-time' management.	Road routes key to expansion (and congestion). Traceability systems.	Food miles debate. Electronic point of sale systems (EPOS).	Externalized costs. Fuel cost rises. Road policy becomes hot politics.
Retail	High concentration. Emergence of global food retailers. Decline of local independent shops.	Reliance on retailers to lower prices and arbiters of efficiency. Sensitivities about planning laws.	Decline of local shops. Changes in payment from cash to electronic. Changed tastes.	Rise in transport. Car use to shop. Re-emergence of home deliveries.

Table 5.3 (continued) Modern changes in food supply and implications for state, society and environment

CHANGES HERE...		...RAISE KEY ISSUES HERE...		
Sector	Supply Chain	State	Society	Environment
Catering	Growth of café/ restaurant numbers. Reliance on migrant labour.	Growth of catering employment as key economic policy. Safety controls.	Rise of eating out of home. Delivery of ready-to-eat meals.	Waste food. Energy use.
Marketing and cultural industries	Brand awareness. Value-adding. Intense marketing. Rise of health concerns (obesity). Market segmentation.	On-going politics of de-regulation vs. 'better' or light regulation. 'Choice' enshrined as key feature of policy.	Overall wealth and inequalities rise. Food spending drops relatively. Growth of concern about advertising.	Criticism for promoting consumerism and excess.

integrated seed research and development programs, co-ordinated via the company's seed technology headquarters has been created. In the northern summer months, the breeding programme is conducted in California and Ontario, and in the southern summer, in Victoria, Australia. Field trials are run globally in Portugal, Spain, Greece, Hungary, Chile, Venezuela, New Zealand, Australia, Canada and the USA. Commercial growing for seed extraction then takes place in Mexico, Thailand and India. A web of transactions occurs within a network of companies all owned by the parent.

From studies such as this, a picture of food production exhibiting classic features of industrialization emerges: standardization, a-seasonality, specialization, routinization, integrated planning, tight costs control, integration of specifications, and tightly controlled division of labour.[81] Many supply-chain studies have illustrated the remarkable effort and some commercial success of large companies in creating trans-national supply chains within the agri-food sector.[82–84] Not all do this, of course. Small companies, for example, have emerged with long supply chains, such as fair-traded chocolate or coffee.[85] Artisanal and local 'real' food stores have capitalized on the reaction; some of these are now themselves very large international players. The US retailer Whole Foods Inc. is an illustration; beginning in 1980 in Austin Texas as a 'natural' food retailer, by 2007 its sales were $6.6bn from only 276 giant stores overwhelmingly in the USA but also in Canada and UK.[86]

Risk is a major concern in food-supply chains. If something goes wrong with mass food, the consequences can be dramatic and life-threatening, not just a commercial or reputation loss. [87] Aberrant features have to be prevented, not least to protect brand reputation. Mass media can amplify any difficulties, with effects transmitted speedily. This happened in the 1960s with corned beef,[88] and again in the 1980s when food-poisoning concerns emerged on both sides of the Atlantic about salmonella in meat and poultry products, and again with BSE. Previously accepted high rates of contamination became contested; consumers demanded improvement. Industry reliance on consumers cooking meat 'thoroughly' to kill pathogens, a tacit policy until then, was heavily criticized by NGOs and ultimately government.[89] Demand for legislation and regulatory structures emerged, first resisted, but ultimately accepted by companies finally accepting the need to re-set the commercial 'level playing field' to higher standards.[90] In Europe, a decade of public contestation over food safety led to wholesale institutional reform, with many member states creating stand-alone food agencies and the EU itself creating an over-arching European Food Safety Authority coupled with a renewed and revised regulatory commitments.[91]

Social scientists, such as Ulrich Beck and John Adams, have argued that such public events illustrate the new cultural significance of public concern about risk following technical change.[92, 93] 'Big' technology, such as nuclear power, engenders existential worry about risk, whether real or perceived.[94] Proportionality of actual risk may not be what shapes cultural or political response to those risks. If food is perceived as a threat, that perception has to be met and lowered. Having initially tacitly blamed consumers for rising food poisoning in the 1980s, for example, when its systematic nature was exposed by public health proponents, companies went on the defensive. Faced by tougher regulation and renewed state commitment to defend consumer rights, one response was investment in public relations, corporate social responsibility, good media relations, and commitment to being good 'corporate community citizens'.

Another response was to change risk-control systems within supply chains. In the 19th and 20th centuries, food-risk control hinged on laboratory-based auditing and inspection, and the application of the then newly emerged science of food chemistry. But in the late-20th century, food safety crises, as we saw in Chapter 3, the new approach of Hazards Analysis Critical Control Point (HACCP) was introduced, putting the onus, not on the expert's occasional inspection or sampling, but on to the worker everyday. Public laboratories had been often sited next to public food sites such as markets, intending to facilitate regular food sampling and to send reassurance about quality control.

HACCP, by contrast, was designed first to assess where the greatest risks lay in supply chains and then to put preventive efforts at the critical points. Instead of focusing risk prevention where consumers met the food, it was more effective to focus on where risks originate, anywhere throughout potentially long supply routes; and to focus on the human determinants of risk, not just their biological or chemical vectors.

In theory, HACCP is an approach to managerial control premised on giving appropriate effort for maximum risk reduction. Food companies now write tight specifications about risk control into contracts, placing the onus on suppliers, right back to field level. If properly instituted, it can reduce risks considerably; too often, however, it becomes a box-ticking exercise. HACCP was designed for dealing with human–machine interfaces, but in the case of food, there is also the added difficulty of biological change. In the 1980s, new variants of *Salmonella* (phage types) spread. In the 1990s and 2000s, the greater concern was for *Campylobacter*. With more internationally sourced foods, weak points in supply chains might be far away. HACCP does not necessarily prevent risk. It was developed to ease out teething problems in complex engineering systems (space rockets). But what if the risks are structural, as is the case with climate change or water shortage, or fossil fuel reliance, as is the case with contemporary food systems? HACCP is fine in theory but requires total supply chain and transnational oversight.

Intellectual property rights (IPRs) are another policy 'hot-spot' concerning risk and control.[95] An important feature of late-20th century food, IPRs give inventors ownership of the design idea to control and profit from their work. The notion and legal right to ownership of an idea is centuries old, dependent on proof that the inventor invented the feature or object, and that it represented a genuine innovation, new idea, characteristic and performance. In the late-20th century, previously national patent systems came together in international accords, with food IPRs particularly sensitive due to biotechnology. IPR is now a fiercely contested area of food policy, with proponents seeking their extension under the WTO, and opponents resisting the encroachment by large companies on to what was previously deemed public space or 'commons'.[96] Many thousands of patent lawyers work on food, ensuring their products and brands are not infringed. A particularly contentious area has been plant rights, with developing countries alleging that IPRs were being used to privatise a formerly free gene pool.[95, 97]

Another technological and scientific issue on the mainstream food policy radar, and raising potential risk concerns is nano-technology, the manipulation of biological processes at the level of the nanometre, one billionth of a metre.[98] With many applications mooted for food and already receiving considerable financial investment, yet with so far low public awareness, this might follow the path of other big investments that met trouble, such as GM or irradiation. Policy structures so far are driven by need to keep up with the speed of technical possibility rather than potential social response of consumers. In 2004, the US Patent and Trademark Office, for instance, created a new classification for nanotechnology.[99] Ethical questions are raised by nanotechnology's invisible food characteristics.[100, 101] The science leaps ahead and the ethics lag behind.[102]

Power, concentration and control

The food system is highly concentrated. In meat, seeds, agri-chemicals, food processing, now even retailing, relatively small numbers of companies have emerged with high market share. By 2005, the top 10 companies accounted for 55% of the commercial seed market; the top 10 publicly-traded biotech companies accounted for three-quarters of that market; the top 10 agri-chemical companies had 84% of the pesticides' market; the top 10 foods companies had 24% of the estimated $1.25 trillion global market for packaged foods; and the top 10 retailers had an estimated 24% of the $3.5 trillion world market.[99, 103] And within countries, concentration had reached remarkable levels too. In the USA, the top four beef packers, for example, have 81% of the market.[104, 105] In the UK, four retailers have three-quarters of all sales, with one accounting for one-third of national food sales. Concentration levels are higher in Western Europe than in Eastern Europe.[106] Ratios vary considerably. In 2002, the top three retailers in Sweden had 95% of the national retail market; in the Netherlands 83%, France 64%, Spain 44% and Greece and Italy 32%.[107]

The trend over the past century has been for a power to shift along food-supply chains, from farmers to manufacturers and ultimately, and over the last 30 years, to retailers and traders, with the wholesalers also seeing an erosion of their position in many product-supply chains. Food service (catering) changed from being primarily a domestic service for the rich and the new 19th-century middle classes to being a massive high street global presence, with by far the largest employee force. The consciousness industries, such as marketing and advertising, have grown in influence dramatically. The sectors jostle for influence as they pursue the consumer's spending. One feature of this power transfer is the shift from producer-driven to buyer-driven supply chains. Value has become increasingly captured near the consumer by retail buyers rather than the primary producer, the farmer/grower. However, there has been a further shift in the buyer-driven aspects in that the dominant position of food manufacturers has given way to the retailers/supermarkets, which have been able to dictate the terms of contracts and act as gatekeepers to the large majority of food consumers, threatening non-compliant suppliers with de-listing and the ending of access. Using a shorthand developed by von Schirach-Szmigiel,[108] a table can be generated to summarize these relative shifts across the supply chain over the 20th century (see Table 5.4). A number of factors may transform where power goes in the present century.

Liberal economic theory proposes that optimal benefits accrue in perfect markets, when many producers or sellers vie for the attention of many consumers. Free-flow of goods relies on open information. In fact, food sectors are like many others–they exhibit signs of considerable concentration. The emergence of giant companies is not new; none perhaps ever will achieve the dominance of the East India Company. But all food sectors have witnessed accelerated growth of large companies, which dominate particular markets. Over time, accompanying the gradual shift across the supply chain from farm to seller, there has been a shift from national to regional to global supply chains. The term globalization is perhaps over-used. Food systems are not by any means fully globalized in that most food is produced, processed, transported and sold within continents; food is regionalized in this sense, rather than globalized.

David Goodman and others have argued that trends towards globalization are detectable but take different forms in various products. Some are made from internationally sourced ingredients; many are not. New, uneven, unequal relationships are formed.[109] Food manufacturers, retailers and food-service companies all vary in the international scope of their operations, both by sector and by company.[73] The McDonald's Corporation, for example, is a highly globalized food-service company, which doubled in size from the late-1990s into the 2000s, with around 30,000 restaurants world-wide; much of this growth was outside its home market. Supermarkets, in contrast, have been less internationally spread, although their supply chain undoubtedly is. Wal-Mart, the world's largest food retailer, dominates its US home market but its geographical presence was limited to nine countries in the mid-2000s; it even sold up and left one, Germany. On the other hand, a number of global players in the food retail sector have emerged. The presence of supermarkets world-wide is increasing. The US, which invented the supermarket self-service format for food retailing, has the highest concentration of supermarkets, but growth rates in some regions, such as Latin America and China, have expanded rapidly.[110]

Some global players have high profiles. Fast-food companies, such as KFC and McDonalds, are global presences with high international marketing presence. But others have low public profiles. One German company, for instance, has been estimated to have 68% of the world market in the genetics

Table 5.4 Shifting domination in 20th century Western food value added chains

Period	Farmers	Manufacturers	Wholesalers	Logistics	Retailers	Foodservice	Marketing
≤ 1900	**Dominant**	Minor	Major in a few trades	**Dominant**	Very Minor	Dominant (domestic)	Minor
1900 1950	Declining (except WWII)	**Dominant**	Major in many trades	Declining	Minor	Declining (except WWII)	Emerging (USA only)
1960 1970	Rebuilding (subsidized)	**Dominant**	**Dominant**	Rebuilding	Emerging	Minor	Emerging
1980 2000s	Declining	Declining	Rapidly Declining	Linked to retail dominance	**Dominant**	Emerging	Important
2000– 2010	Returning?	Uncertain	Minor	Squeezed	**Dominant**	Uncertain	Important

Source: authors, informed by von Schirach-Szmigiel (2005).[108]

for white-egg layer hens. A Dutch company has around two-thirds of the genetics for the brown-egg layer hen market. Each was second player in the other's top market.[111] In food manufacturing, top companies include well-known brands such as Nestlé, Unilever, Archer Daniels Midland, Kraft (Altria), PepsiCo, Tyson, Cargill, Coca-Cola, Mars and Danone. Calculating concentration figures relies heavily on commercially confidential information and informed estimates. Different research groups come up with different league tables, but they agree on the high level of concentration. Leatherhead International, one such company research group, estimated that in 2004 the top 10 food manufacturers accounted for 24% of total sales of world packaged foods, with the top 100 accounting for two-thirds.[112] These are remarkably high presences.

Different measures of the reach of big food companies are possible: sales, presence, capitalization, employees, growth and profitability. For illustration, Table 5.5 gives a picture of the world's top 10 food manufacturers, top 10 retailers and the top 5 food-service companies, by capitalization rather than by sales. It gives where the parent company is headquartered, how many countries they are present in and the extent of their global reach.[73] The food-service is in fact really two separate markets: one is fast food with ubiquitous outlets, the other is within mass contract catering.

The growth of big retailing started later and more slowly than in food manufacturing, but from the 1980s, it developed rapidly. It has been marked within the EU member states, North America and Australasia. From the 1990s, supermarkets have spread rapidly through to Latin America, Asia, and parts of the Middle East and Africa.[113] The result is that developing countries, including more advanced ones in Eastern Europe, are experiencing supermarketization and hypermarketization even more rapidly and over a shorter period, than North America and Western Europe before them.[106]

As buyers at the end of supply chains, supermarkets are in a position to demand and set exacting standards and contract specifications from their suppliers. They can seek to extract value from the products supplied, which is what is happening in Europe with own-brand goods, branded manufactured goods and fresh produce (milk, fruit and vegetables, and meat) alike. Traditionally, the producer and the processor/manufacturer have battled over the capture of value. These new buyer–supplier relationships, however, represent the emergence of private systems of governance along supply chains. They take two forms. The largest supermarket chains are huge power blocs in their own right, but smaller chains have created cross-border buyer alliances to extract maximum discounts from processors. There are no shops with those names, they are consortia behind the chains. In 2007 two of these, EMD and

Table 5.5 The global top 25: the market capitalization (US $ 2004), headquarters and presence of the largest 10 food manufacturing, 10 food retail and 5 food-service companies

Food Manufacturers	Market capitalization, bns	Headquarters	Countries present in
Cadbury Schweppes	$21.179	London, UK	Not given
Coca-Cola	$101.027	Atlanta, USA	Over 200
Conagra	$12.104	Omaha, USA	11 (Americas, China, Europe, Australia)
Danone	$29.634	Paris, France	120
Kraft	$51.19	Northfield,Illinois, USA	Over 155
Masterfoods/Mars	N/A (private)	McLean,Virginia, USA	Over 100
Nestlé	$117.256	Vevey, Switzerland	Not given
Pepsico	$92.024	Purchase, New York, USA	Over 200
Tyson	$5.96	Springdale Arkansas, USA	Over 80
Unilever	$126.045	London, UK & Rotterdam, NL	Over 150
Food Retailers			
Ahold	$7.088	Zaandam, NL	6
Aldi	N/A (private)	Essen, Germany	Not given
Carrefour	$31.65	Paris, France	32
Ito-Yokado	$15.038	Tokyo, Japan	18
Kroger	$14.802	Cincinnati, USA	1
Metro	$16.007	Düsseldorf, Germany	30
Rewe	N/A (co-operative)	Köln, Germany	14
Schwarz	N/A (private)	Neckarsulm, Germany	Not given
Tesco	$43.452	Cheshunt, UK	13
Wal-Mart	$179.412	Bentonville, Arkansas, USA	9
Foodservice			
Burger King	N/A (private)	Miami, USA	60
Compass	$8.858	Chertsey, UK	Over 90
McDonald's	$41.264	Oak Brook, Illinois, USA	119
Sodexho	$5.908	Montigny-le-Betonnexus, France	Over 76
YUM!	$13.731	Louisville, Kentucky, USA	Over 100

Source: Lang, et al. (2006).[23]

Coopernic, had the largest food sales, by turnover, in Europe, greater than Carrefour or Tesco. [106]

Another manifestation of the new buyer-power within supply chains has been the emergence of corporate systems of standards setting. These have now become very powerful. The two main examples are GlobalGAP and Global Food Safety Initiative (GFSI). GlobalGAP was an initiative by 13 European retailers; the GAP stands for good agricultural practice.[114] It was originally EurepGAP but changed its name to Global-GAP when so many companies around the world had to, or began to, meet its standards. It was founded to try to create a shared approach to pesticide use, on flowers initially, but then developed into a complex set of standards across the entire food range.[115] GFSI was another body of standards set up by 50 retailers by CIES an international food business association in 2000. As its name implies, its starting point was food safety and the fact that food businesses were not content to leave standards development to the European Commission, although it too was in the throes of publishing its White Paper on Food Safety, which announced the setting up of the European Food Safety Authority (EFSA).[91] GFSI's aims were to create convergence across companies, to share benchmarks (standards) and to cut costs.[116]

Policy-makers' response to the rising expression of retail and buyer control varies. On standards, a dual structure now operates. On competition policy, as lawful entities, companies are in the hands of their home base governments or other international bodies. Western governments all have competition policies with regulators to oversee whether markets are working fairly, variously defined. The EU is exceptional in that it has a regional policy and authority over and above national interests, though there is obviously liaison. The US and many OECD countries have strong anti-monopoly regulators. Whatever format, their workings are subject to much debate. Critics argue that competition policies are narrowly defining, down-playing health, social and environmental considerations;[117–119] in the main, they do not. Market efficiencies tend to be economically defined in terms of profits, market share, prices, contractual relations and so on. Pressure to inject wider criteria has been voiced over recent years. One particularly sensitive area has been retail concentration and whether this disadvantages people on low incomes. In the UK and US, community food-security movements and environmental organizations have resisted the continued growth of large superstores on cultural, aesthetic, health and environmental impact grounds (see Chapter 8).[120]

Costs, subsidies and economic drivers

One of the great successes of the post war food revolution has been lower prices. In the UK, the average household expenditure dropped from around a quarter of average disposable income to less than a tenth. There are consider-able differences, of course, between socio-economic groups, with the top-tenth of income earners' spending merely a twentieth and the poorest people spending a sixth, but the general trend for all social groups has been down-wards. International figures suggest a similar direction. It is one of the reasons, at the macro-economic level, that international investment in agricultural development declined from its high point in the 1980s (itself a legacy of the early 1970s food crisis).[39, 121] Off the land, the squeeze on prices was an incen-tive for mergers, acquisitions and further concentration of market share; this happened across the food chain.[122] This led to a number of financial policy hot-spots of direct importance for food and ecological public health policy.

The first was mounting evidence about the gap between and within countries. Life-expectancy and the nature of dying from food-related illnesses follow a social gradient; this is partly material, partly social status and partly diet.[123] Food price signals do not help. Sugary, fatty foods and soft drinks are often cheap. Fruit and vegetables can be relatively expensive for low-income households. Energy-dense foods are cheap. In the USA, socio-economic status predicts the range and type of foods consumed. Higher socio-economic groups eat more whole grains, lean meat, low-fat dairy products, fresh vegeta-bles and fruit. Lower income groups eat less of those and eat more refined grains and added fats.[124] Food prices send the wrong signals. But this raises thorny issues for policy-makers, implying a moral role to redirect behaviour through fiscal measures.[125] Public health proponents accept that food is not tobacco but its health burdens may be as extensive.

The second price hot-spot has concerned subsidies and income transfers. These went overwhelmingly from the state (tax-payer) to farming and were a significant policy instrument for governments in directing productionist agricultural development and intensive fishing systems. Rich countries poured huge sums into nurturing agricultural change. Beneficiaries from subsidies were not just farmers but a whole army of infrastructure and support indus-tries from equipment manufacturers to land-owners.[126] Similar dynamics were exposed for fishing. Artisan fisher-folk were swept aside by large-scales destructive fish-farming and trawling.[127–129] Nutritionists advised consump-tion but stocks faced collapse.[130, 131]

By the 1980s, cash transfers and hidden support were under attack from a variety of quarters. Neo-liberals did not like them, on principle, for distorting markets. Developing countries argued that rich-country subsidies were unfair and that they acted as barriers to entry and led to surpluses being dumped on them, undercutting their production, thereby giving wealth to traders (via export refunds) and processors (via cheap food ingredients). Environmentalists accused them of intensifying environmental damage and, in the case of EU fisheries, leading to stock decline. Consumer bodies argued that they were hidden and kept food prices artificially high. Health groups attacked how subsidies gave plentiful fat and sugar to processing industries, harming health. Social justice groups argued that they doubly penalized the poor who paid proportionately more as tax-payers and when purchasing food. The OECD, the rich countries research think-tank, monitored and agitated among its member states, embarrassing them with annual audits of consumer subsidy equivalents and producer subsidy equivalents, measures for who gained and lost.[132, 133]

These arguments had come to a head at the 1994 Marrakech GATT talks, which first persuaded the USA and EU to lower their producer subsidies. The EU and USA were the largest subsidizers by total amount, although some countries actually give greater subsidies (e.g. Japan) but without the impact on world trade.[133] New Zealand cut its farms subsidies in 1986, giving farmers just 8 months' notice.[134] Its subsidy rate is now the OECD's lowest, barely registering. Fiscal policy arguments such as these have dogged the EU's CAP, with clear political divisions emerging between the founding members, such as France, who fiercely promote their farm interests, and the liberalizers led by the UK, Sweden and, when it joined latterly, Poland. Low-subsidy countries organized in a coalition known as G-21 kept up pressure at the Doha Round of WTO talks, which replaced the attempt to start a new round at Seattle in December in 1999 but which was brought to disarray amidst riots.

Alongside this top-level political clash over subsidies, another rather more academic issue emerged but which has a slow-burning fuse. This is about whether food prices reflect the full cost of production or whether cheap food policies have externalized public health and environmental costs on to other budget headings, or indeed whether they are paid at all and not just dumped on to the planet or society collectively.[135, 136] The post-war food-policy package (outlined in Chapter 2) had promised lower prices, but from the 1980s, environmental economists in particular began to argue that the environment picked up the additional costs from the squeeze. The cost of cleaning up residues from pesticide or nitrogen fertilizer added direct costs to water consumers (see Chapter 6 for a full discussion). NGOs championed this argument effectively. As a major road transport user, was it the food industry (particularly retailers) or the taxpayer who paid the full cost of motorway building, oil use, pollution, noise, loss of habitat and biodiversity?[117] The externalities argument is a broad attack on neo-liberal policy thinking. From agriculture to retailing, the economic system reinforces cheapness but mines (literally) the earth. The costs of damage to environment and health are not included in the cost of food.[137] A 2005 UK study found that such externalities contributed an additional 12% on top of consumer bills.[138]

The powerful evidence of diet's impact on health shows that healthcare costs are a hidden externality and questions the domestic politics of cheap food for the consumer. Two reports for the UK Treasury on healthcare by former banker, Sir Derek Wanless, produced huge estimates of the value of preventing diet-related ill-health by changing diet.[139, 140] The Review of the Economics of Climate Change conducted by former World Bank economist, Sir Nicholas Stern, articulated similar arguments.[141] But despite the neatness of such evidence, governments have not fully been persuaded of the case for better internalizing full costs, with three notable exceptions. Fuel taxes in some countries are overtly justified on climate-change grounds to discourage car owners from using their vehicles, as are tax duties on alcohol and tobacco on health grounds. Generally, however, finance ministers draw a distinction between food production, where they desire cheapness and conventionally defined efficiency, and the social costs of healthcare or environmental protection. These are deemed to come under different budget headings.

Despite this general resistance, strongly supported by food-industry interests, NGOs and food and health analysts have begun to deploy and refine the externalities argument.[142–144] One particular debate goes under the heading of 'fat taxes', the argument being that, since productionism has made fat so cheap, its health costs should be added via taxation.[145–147] The debate has been given particular focus in the EU over obesity and the consumption of not just cheap fat but cheap calories.[135, 145, 148–150] But practicalites as to how and where to levy a fat tax remain.

Our final example of a price and cost policy hot-spot is the issue of corporate auditing. As evidence mounted of the huge environmental burden of food-supply chains (see Chapter 6), companies became sensitive to reputational risk and to the potential for taxation. As we have noted above, one response was to begin labelling for food products' greenhouse gas emissions (GHGs) using life-cycle assessment methodologies (see Chapter 6).[151–153] Another response was to conduct whole company audits, treating the company as though it was a supply chain. Of all the food-chain sectors, agriculture is widely agreed to be the heaviest source of greenhouse gases. But since they sell its products, might not retailers or caterers also be implicated? In a pioneering move in 2007, Tesco, the third biggest food retailer in the world, published its own carbon audit, using guidelines laid down by the World Business Council for Sustainable Development. These included into the company's direct CO_2 equivalent (CO_2e) the following: its offices, business travel, the stores, home delivery, primary distribution, distribution centres (RDCs) and refrigerant emissions. However, the methodology defined other factors as not the retailer's responsibility which are surely significant and within its sphere of influence.

These include: the production of goods, international freight, supplier transport, asset sites, waste recycling and disposal, employee commuting, customer transport and consumption and disposal of the goods (see Chapter 6 for a full discussion).[154] Getting full agreement about auditing approaches is likely to be a significant policy issue in the future. Where does responsibility for GHGs lie along the supply chain?[155] On the other hand, a supply-chain approach would surely imply shared responsibility for full cost inclusion.

The labour process

An issue that receives too little policy attention within health, environmental or social policy analyses of food, is the issue of labour. Yet it is clear that the remarkable transformation of food systems (Table 5.4) has altered the labour process between the 19th century and today. But this impact has not been even. In Western societies, domestic food labour has largely gone. Only very wealthy homes have living-in cooks. Yet service is hidden; the take-away, the pizza delivery and the catering trades are the modern equivalent, all huge employers, as we saw for the UK (see Fig. 5.1). Conditions are variable but characterized generally by low pay. Farm labour may have declined rapidly with the advent of mechanization but as global trade in agricultural products grows and food chains have come under the tight control of large companies, so modern food systems have been able to incorporate a larger hidden labour force in the developing world. The vast plantations growing citrus and other fruit in Central America for health-conscious Western consumers have been the subject of considerable study and campaigning by development NGOs. Oxfam Germany in 2008, for instance, showed how German supermarkets were selling bargain fruit from there, but behind the bargain were examples such as workers at pineapple farms in Costa Rica working 12-hour shifts for pay of €9 per day or 75 cents an hour ($14 per day/$1.19 per hour).[156, 157]

In Africa, European retailers have helped foster new large-scale farming to provide out-of-season fresh vegetables for affluent consumers.[71] Kenyan and Gambian horticulture, for example, have been heavily shaped by European supermarkets.[158, 159] Low food prices disguise the cost to the health of workers, particularly women workers, and to the environment.[160] Migrant labour can also be a key factor, with workers from poorer countries being brought in as temporary or seasonal workers in packing stations or as pickers on fields in North America and Europe.[161] This is a global phenomenon, long an object of campaigning for worker and human rights. Migrant farm labour suffers poor pay, conditions and harassment; illegal migration provides a ready labour pool but at some human cost. It is to combat the developing country end of the danger of labour exploitation that the ethical and fair-trade movements have linked up with trade unions, arguing that consumers need to know and act responsibly towards small family farmers and the labour on giant fruit plantations, who are both low-waged food workers in a global food system.

The banana trade was the subject of particularly relevant but protracted trade dispute between the US and EU from the early 1990s to the mid-2000s. The US favoured 'dollar' bananas grown on historically US company-dominated vast plantations, whilst the EU favoured its former colonies, such as the Windward Islands, where small farm labour predominates.[162, 163] The dispute illustrated a downside of trade liberalization for labour. Undercut by the cheaper dollar bananas, the small producers faced either leaving the land or being reduced to penury.[163] This happened to many, until fair-trade commitments intervened following hard work by Western NGOs to persuade retailers to stock fair-trade bananas in their stores. Nurtured by global umbrella NGOs, like FLO, and in the UK by the Fairtrade Foundation, the non-profit Co-operative Group pioneered the sector but total market share rocketed in 2007 when one of the top three UK food retailers went entirely fair-trade. Welcome though such moves are, the majority of bananas sold world-wide are not grown under these better labour conditions. Even the biodiversity of bananas has a labour impact. Of the world's 300 varieties, the vast bulk of international production is of one variety, the 'cavendish'.[164] Grown in mono-cultural situations, agri-chemicals are required to keep pests at bay, and workers experience health and safety problems as a result.[164, 165]

Food workers often experience dangerous conditions. Misuse of agri-chemicals is a particularly well-documented trouble, highlighted by long-term campaigning and monitoring by international NGOs such as the Pesticides Action Network and Oxfam.[166, 167] Trades unions have doggedly acted to rein in worst practices.[168–170] The UN's International Labour Organization esti-mates that each year there are approximately 70,000 acute and long-term poisoning cases leading to death and a much larger number of acute and long-term non-fatal illnesses due to pesticides.[171] Each year world-wide, half the estimated 355,000 fatalities in, or due to, the workplace are in agriculture.[172] In the UK, agriculture is among the worst industries for fatal accidents and occupational ill-health records of any major employment sector. Agriculture employs only 1.7% of the British workforce but in 2005–06 had 16% of the fatal injuries to workers.[173]

The discussion earlier in this chapter (Table 5.1 and 5.2) stressed how, in developed countries, labour has moved away from the land, and this trend is evident in developing countries too as they became locations for cheap manufacturing. World-wide, however, agriculture is still the largest labour force. 1.1 bn people work in agriculture, half the world's workforce.[171] Of those, 450m (40%) are waged labour, 170 million are children; and the remaining 20–30% are women.[172] Wages and conditions, of course, vary. The best are admirable; the worst are disgraceful. A 1996 ILO study of the worth of agricultural wages calculated how many hours it took for farm workers on the average wage to buy a kilo of their local/staple cereal. It took 5 minutes in Sweden, 37 minutes in India and 6 hours in the Central African Republic.[174]

When financial journalists cover the many mergers and acquisitions (take-overs) in the food sector, it reads like sport; but for workers, such transactions are a threat. As retailing has grown, jobs among independent stores declined. The restructuring of European food manufacturing— squeezed by increasingly powerful retailers and subject to leveraged buy-outs from private equity firms—also saw a serious decline in jobs. In the period 1999–2004, there was an overall employment decline of 15.2%, from 4.4 to 3.9 million workers, despite this being a time of rising turnover. Only 5% of these job losses were due to companies relocating abroad.[175] In other words, this was an intra-supply chain squeeze on labour. The European food processing market being highly concentrated has the top 10 food companies accounting for nearly half of turnover. Yet most remaining employment is in the large number of small and medium-sized (SME) companies.

Are supply chains addressing ecological public health?

The answer to this question has to be 'not thus far'. Progress is slow. Engagement is patchy. This state of affairs is not just the responsibility of companies. State bodies, with few exceptions, have not yet given the required strong lead, and public health is often weak or poorly represented at political tables where fundamental decisions are made about food policy and implementation. Nor is there enough pressure from the bulk of consumers despite good intentions and campaigns by NGOs. But this chapter has underlined how important a sound understanding of the food system and supply-chain dynamics is for the ecological public health challenge. A number of conclusions may be drawn.

Firstly, there is a general nervousness within supply chains about ecological public health. This varies between countries and by how well-organized or ideologically located their industries are. US companies tend to be more confrontational than most on health, for example, but so are its NGOs; a certain culture has been created.[176] Generally, environmental and health issues are seen as threats rather than opportunities, and certainly to be addressed separately. When they do engage, food companies' reflex tends to be to address issues on a step-by-step basis. Product reformulation is preferable to regulation. For years the population approach to food and health was seen as a threat by commercial interests but functional foods, for example, offered opportunities to create individualistic, profitable niche markets. But adding health-enhancing ingredients to foods is hardly a fundamental response to NCDs.[177, 178] Too often, the onus is put on to consumers to eat healthily or save the planet. Even labelling can become contentious. Governments seem wedded to the view that front-of-pack labelling and carbon labelling are key policy initiatives. They might be useful but are unlikely to deliver the big changes needed to create a genuinely low-carbon, low-calorie food system. The resistance of powerful sections of the food industry to clear labelling, as was shown by the 2006–09 battle over the 'traffic lights' and Guideline Daily Amount (GDA) schemes, suggests the limits to how for it is prepared to engage with public health. Corporate responsibility and niche marketing are no substitute for proper food policy and implementation.

Secondly, macro-economic and corporate considerations shape choice. Politicians and economists love to talk of consumer choice as the main driver of food supply, but the reality is that choice is only one feature among many shaping what is produced and how. Choice is not a fixed entity but a range from unrestricted to constrained. It is rare that choice is not possible; even prisoners get a choice of food. Yet the ideological discussion mostly assumes people have unrestrained choice. The reality is that it varies according to a household's class, income and geographical location. In truth, food companies conduct behind the scenes 'choice-editing', a phrase used to describe the process of 'pre-selecting the particular range of products and services available to consumers'.[179] They routinely choice-edit through contracts and specifications, framing what consumers then 'choose'.[7] Within food policy generally, frameworks are the result of considerable negotiation, formal and informal. At the international level, for example, commercial interests have been effective in ensuring that their interests are served.[96] Trade rules and IPRs have illustrated their effectiveness in lobbying for sympathetic structures.

Thirdly, the growth of corporate food power raises problems with institutional architecture (see Chapter 3). Are institutions appropriate, too light or too old? A 2008 study by the UK's Sustainable Development Commission found that the entire UK central and devolved state related with supermarkets on food matters via 19 ministries, agencies or government bodies, and at 100 different points of policy; yet the state's policy reflex was to imply that food policy was a matter best left to 'markets'.[7] In the name of marketisation state governance has moved into 'hands-off' mode, and corporate policy nominally but inadequately fills the vacuum. This split between public and corporate policy is not helpful just when a cross-sectoral, multi-dimensional approach is needed. In the 1970s and 1980s, some advocates of improved diet-related health championed the view that, since the retail sector was now so concentrated, it offered the best route to tackle the huge and costly NCD health problem. Much as the 1930s social nutritionists looked to agriculture to provide the building blocks for health—good, accessible nutrients—some late-20th century health advocates sought alliances with retailers. They still do but alliances for health have not reduced over-production of fats and sugars, nor delivered low fossil-fuel food economies.

Two traditions of critical analysis are at odds. One argues that the public good is not the same thing as corporate good. For the other, since the corporate sector has an interest to feed people, government should leave it to whoever is most powerful in the chain. This argument is now fought out not just in national but in multi-level systems of governance. Take obesity, in 2003 at the global level, WHO and member governments sent strong signals to companies to act urgently to reduce obesity.[180] Partly driven by reputational risk, some companies began to reformulate and wanted to be seen to respond, but it remains to be seen if such limited, product-specific actions will transform food culture. At the EU level, since 2007, companies sit with other sectors on an EU Roundtable; this begins engagement but has not been a source of radical change or urgency. Nationally, in the UK, company reaction to the powerful 2007 Foresight report was muted, accepting its logic but unsure what to do. This is not a happy situation, but is replicated in other areas. If society is serious about tackling major issues such as obesity or climate change, quantum leaps not tweaks are needed.[181]

This raises a fourth issue, the question of policy direction. For last 30 years, as evidence of the looming ecological public health challenge deepened, policy has remained fairly weak. Strong signals of the need for radical changes have been sent from Brundtland in 1987 to the IAASTD in 2008.[6, 182] But like an oil tanker in mid-ocean, the food supply chain appears slow to turn round. How can change be speedier? Does it need crises? Is long-term action by civil society and professions only marginally effective in restructuring supply chains? Policy structures have a tendency to lag behind technical development; and companies are often exasperated by slow state action or mixed signals.[7] But equally a lesson from studying food companies' slow progress towards ecological public health is that the old consumerist mantra *caveat emptor*, let the buyer beware, is unlikely to deliver sufficient change. Certainly, good supply chains require a new emphasis on citizenship, *caveat cives*, food citizens rather than consumers, but the rules of the market, too, need to be changed. The next chapter explores a prime reason why: the difficulties light-touch markets have in protecting the environment.

References

1. Hawken P. *The ecology of commerce: a declaration of sustainability*, 1st edn. New York, NY: HarperBusiness, 1993.

2. von Weizacher EU, Lovins AB, Lovins LH. *Factor four: doubling wealth—halving resource use: the new report to the Club of Rome*. London: Earthscan, 1996.

3. Porritt J. *Capitalism as if the world matters*. London: Earthscan, 2005.

4. Karliner J. *The corporate planet: ecology and politics in the age of globalization*. San Francisco CA: Sierra Club Books, 1997.

5. Monbiot G. *Captive state: the corporate takeover of Britain*. Basingstoke: Macmillan, 2000.

6. IAASTD. *Global Report and Synthesis Report*. London: International Assessment of Agricultural Science and Technology, 2008.

7. Sustainable Development Commission. *Green, healthy and fair: a review of government's role in supporting sustainable supermarket food*. London: Sustainable Development Commission, 2008.

8. Leggett J. *Half gone: oil, gas, hot air and the global energy crisis*. London: Portobello Books, 2005.

9. Mobbs P. *Beyond oil*. Leicester: Matador, 2005.

10. Cabinet Office Strategy Unit. *Food: an analysis of the issues*. http://www.cabinetoffice.gov.uk/strategy/work_areas/food_policy.aspx. London: The Strategy Unit of the Cabinet Office, 2008:113.

11. Defra. *Food statistics pocketbook 2007*. London: Department for Environment, Food and Rural Affairs, 2007.

12. Defra. *Food security and the UK: an evidence and analysis paper*. Food Chain Analysis Group. London: Department for Environment, Food and Rural Affairs—Food Chain Analysis Group. http://statistics.defra.gov.uk/esg/reports/foodsecurity/foodsecurity.pdf [accessed 22 Dec 2006], 2006:96.

13. Chatham House. *UK food supply: storm clouds on the horizon?* Preliminary findings of the Food Supply in the 21st Century Project. London: Royal Institute of International Affairs, 2008.

14. Ernst and Young. *Food for thought: how global prices will hit uk inflation and employment*. Report of the Item Club, May. London: Ernst & Young, 2008.

15. Timmer CP, Falcon WP, Pearson SR. *Food policy analysis*. Baltimore, Maryland: Johns Hopkins University Press & World Bank, 1983.

16. Dumont R, Rosier B. *The hungry future*. London: Deutsch, 1969.

17. Amin S. *Unequal development: an essay on the social formations of peripheral capitalism* (trans Brian Pearce). New York: Monthly Review Press, 1976.

18. Dinham B, Hines C. *Agribusiness in Africa*. London: Earth Resources Research, 1983.

19. Raghavan C. *Recolonization: GATT, the Uruguay Round and the Third World*. London: Zed Press, 1990.

20. Coote B. *The trade trap: poverty and the global commodity markets*. Oxford: Oxfam, 1992.

21. Sharpe RP, Barling D, Lang T. *Final report on the investigation into ethical traceability in the UK wheat–flour–bread supply chain*. Report to DG Research. Framework 6: Science & Society. London: Centre for Food Policy City University, 2006.

22. Sharpe RP, Barling D, Lang T. Ethical traceability in the UK wheat-flour-bread chain. In: Coff C, Barling D, Korthals M, Nielsen T (ed.) *Ethical traceability and communicating food*. New York: Springer, 2008:125–165.

23. Fennel R. *The Common Agricultural Policy of the European Community*. London: Granada, 1979.

24. Tracy M. *Government and agriculture in Western Europe, 1880–1988*, 3rd edn. New York, London: Harvester Wheatsheaf, 1989.

25. Neville-Rolfe E. *The politics of agriculture in the European Community*. London: Policy Studies Institute, 1984.

26. HM Treasury and Defra. *A vision for the Common Agricultural Policy*. London: HM Treasury and Dept for Environment, Food and Rural Affairs, 2005:76.

27. Knutson RD, Penn JB, Flinchbaugh BL, Outlaw JL. *Agricultural and food policy*, 6th edn. London: Prentice Hall, 2007.

28. Jawara F, Kwa A. *Behind the scenes at the WTO: the real world of international trade negotiations*. London, Bangkok: Zed Books, Focus on the Global South, 2003.

29. Robins N. *The corporation that changed the world: how the East India Company shaped the modern multinational*. London: Pluto, 2006.

30. Mintz SW. *Sweetness and power: the place of sugar in modern history*. Harmondsworth: Penguin Books, 1985.

31. Pudney J. *Suez: de Lesseps' canal*. London: J.M.Dent & Sons, 1968.

32. Watkins K. *Rigged rules, double standards*. Oxford: Oxfam Publications, 2001.

33. World Bank. *World Development Report 2008: Agriculture for Development*. New York: World Bank, 2007.

34. Stiglitz JE. *Globalization and its discontents*, 1st edn. New York: WW Norton, 2002.

35. Bello W, Cunningham S, Rau B. *Dark victory: The United States, structural adjustment and global poverty*. London: Pluto Press with Food First and the Transnational Institute, 1994.

36. Barratt Brown M, Tiffen P. *Short changed: Africa and World Trade*. London: Pluto Press & Transnational Institute, 1992.

37. UNCESCR. General Comment 12: *The right to adequate food* (article 11). Substantive issues arising in the Implementation of the International Covenant on Economic, Social and Cultural Rights. Committee on Economic, Social and Cultural Rights, 20th session, Geneva, 26 April–14 May 1999. E/C.12/1999/5, CESCR. Geneva: United Nations Committee on Economic, Social and Cultural Rights, 1999.

38. George S. *The debt boomerang: how Third World debt harms us all*. Boulder, Colo: Westview Press, 1992.

39. FAO. *State of food and agriculture 2007*. Rome: Food and Agriculture Organization, 2007.

40. FAO. *Livestock's long shadow—environmental issues and options*. Rome: Food and Agriculture Organization, 2006.

41. Kropotkin PA. *Fields, factories and workshops: or industry combined with agriculture and brain work with manual work*. London: S Sonnenschein, 1901.

42. Garnett T. *Growing food in cities*. London: National Food Alliance/SAFE Alliance (now Sustain), 1996.

43. van Veenhuizen R. Stimulating Innovation in Urban Agriculture. *Urban Agriculture* 2007(19):1–7.

44. Pretty J. *The living land: agriculture, food and community regeneration in the 21st century.* London: Earthscan, 1999.

45. Smit J, Ratta A, Nasr J. *Urban agriculture: food, jobs and sustainable cities.* New York: UN Development Programme Habitat II Series, 1996.

46. Dahlberg KA. World food problems: making the transition from agriculture to regenerative food systems. In: Pirages D (ed.) *Building sustainable societies.* Armonk, NY: M.E. Sharpe, 1996:257–274.

47. Minnesota Food Association. *Strategies, policy approaches, and resources for local food system planning and organizing.* Minneapolis, MN: Minnesota Food Association, 1997.

48. Allen P. *Together at the table: sustainability and sustenance in the American Agrifood System.* University Park, PA: Penn State Press, 2004.

49. Koc M, MacRae R, Mougeot LJA, Welsh J (ed.) *For hunger-proof cities: sustainable food systems.* Ottawa: International Development Research Centre (IDRC), 1999.

50. Funes F, García L, Bourque M, Pérez N, Rosset P. *Sustainable agriculture and resistance: transforming food production in Cuba.* Oakland CA: Food First Publications, 2002.

51. Lamb H. *Fighting the banana wars and other fairtrade battles.* London: Rider/Ebury, 2008.

52. Regmi A, Gehlhar M. *New directions in global food markets.* Washington DC: United States Department of Agriculture Economic Research Service, 2005.

53. Barratt Brown M. *Fair trade: reform and realities in the international trading system.* London: Zed Press, 1993.

54. BSSRS. *Bread: who makes the dough?* London: British Society for Social Responsibility in Science Agricapital Group, 1977.

55. Lang T. Going public: food campaigns during the 1980s and 1990s. In: Smith D (ed.) *Nutrition scientists and nutrition policy in the 20th century.* London: Routledge, 1997:238–260.

56. Pyke M. *Technological eating: or where does the fish finger point?* London: John Murray, 1972.

57. Millstone E, Lang T. *The Atlas of Food: who eats what, where and why.* London/Berkeley: Earthscan/University of California Press, 2008.

58. Sinclair U. *The jungle.* Harmondsworth: Penguin, 1906/1985.

59. van Zwanenberg P, Millstone E. *BSE: risk, science, and governance.* Oxford: Oxford University Press, 2005.

60. Paulus I. *The search for pure food.* Oxford: Martin Robertson., 1974.

61. Lang T. Food, the law and public health: tree models of the relationship. *Public Health*, 2006;**120**:30–41.

62. Wilson B. *Swindled: from poison sweets to counterfeit coffee—the dark history of the food cheats.* London: John Murray, 2008.

63. Knightley P. *The rise and fall of the House of Vestey: the true story of how Britain's richest family beat the taxman—and came to grief.* London: Warner, 1993.

64. Woods A. *A manufactured plague: the history of foot-and-mouth disease in Britain.* London: Earthscan 2004.

65. van Alphen J, Boldingh J, Feron R, Frazer AC, Hoffman WG, Hunt KE *et al. Margarine: an economic, social, and scientific history, 1869–1969.* Liverpool: Liverpool University Press, 1969.

66. Millstone E. *Food additives*. Harmondsworth: Penguin, 1986.

67. Fine B, Heasman M, Wright J. *Consumption in the age of affluence: the world of food*. London: Routledge, 1996.

68. Goodman D, Redclift M. *Refashioning nature: food, ecology and culture*. London: Routledge, 1991.

69. Gabriel Y, Lang T. *The unmanageable consumer: contemporary consumption and its fragmentation*. London: Sage, 1995.

70. Brewer J, Trentmann F (ed.) *Consuming cultures, global perspectives: historical trajectories, transnational exchanges*. Oxford: Berg, 2006.

71. Lawrence F. *Not on the label*. London: Penguin, 2004.

72. Conner M, Armitage CJ. *The social psychology of food*. Buckingham: Open University Press, 2002.

73. Lang T, Rayner G, Kaelin E. *The food industry, diet, physical activity and health*. A review of reported commitments and practice of 25 of the world's largest food companies. London: City University Centre for Food Policy, 2006.

74. DG Sanco. *Risk Issues: Special Eurobarometer 238*. Brussels: Commission of the European Communities' Health and Consumer Protection Directorate General, 2006.

75. Brown SA. *Revolution at the checkout counter*. Cambridge, Mass: Harvard University Press, 1997.

76. Davidson MP. *The consumerist manifesto: advertising in postmodern times*. London: Routledge, 1992.

77. Lury C. *Brands: the logos of global economy*. London: Routledge, 2004.

78. Boyle D. *Authenticity: brands, fakes, spin and the lust for real life*. London: Harper Perennial, 2004.

79. Partos L. *Coca-Cola brand value tops $58.2 bn, claims report*. http://www.foodanddrinkeurope.com/news/ng.asp?id=85240-coca-cola-pepsi-brands [accessed June 14 2008]. Food&DrinkEurope. com

80. Pritchard W, Burch D. *Agri-food globalization in perspective: restructuring in the global tomato processing industry*. Aldershot, Hants: Ashgate Publishing, 2003.

81. Clunies-Ross T, Hildyard N. *The politics of industrial agriculture*. London: Earthscan, 1992.

82. Friedland WH, Barton AE, Thomas RJ. *Manufacturing green gold: capital, labour and technology in the lettuce industry*. Cambridge: Cambridge University Press, 1981.

83. Bonanno A, Busch L, Friedland W, Gouveia L, Migione E (ed.) *From Columbus to ConAgra: the globalization of agriculture and food*. Lawrence: University Press of Kansas, 1994.

84. Goodman DE, Watts MJ (ed.) *Globalizing food: agrarian questions and global restructuring*. London: Routledge, 1997.

85. Sams C, Fairley J. *Sweet dreams: the story of Green & Blacks*. London: Random House, 2008.

86. *Whole Foods Markets*. 2007 Annual Report. Austin, Texas: Whole Food Markets Inc, 2007.

87. Penningon TH. *When food kills*. Oxford: Oxford University Press, 2003.

88. Smith DF, Diack HL, with, Pennington TH, Russell EM. *Food poisoning, policy and politics: typhoid and corned beef in the 1960s*. London: Boydell Press, 2005.

89. Phillips (Lord), Bridgeman J, Ferguson-Smith M. *The BSE Inquiry report: evidence and supporting papers of the Inquiry into the emergence and identification of Bovine Spongiform Encephalopathy (BSE) and variant Creutzfeldt-Jakob Disease (vCJD) and the action taken in response to it up to 20 March 1996.* London: The Stationery Office, 2000:16 volumes.

90. London Food Commission. *Food adulteration and how to beat it.* London: Unwin Hyman, 1987.

91. Commission of the European Communities. *White paper on food safety.* Brussels: Commission of the European Communities, 2000.

92. Beck U. *Risk society: towards a new modernity.* London: Sage, 1992.

93. Adams J. *Risk.* London: UCL Press, 1995.

94. Adam B, Beck U, Loon Jv. *The risk society and beyond: critical issues for social theory.* London: SAGE, 2000.

95. Tansey G. Patenting our food future: intellectual property rights and the global food system *Social Policy and Administration* 2002;**36**(6):575–592.

96. Tansey G, Rajotte T (ed.) *The future control of food: a guide to international negotiations and rules on intellectual property, biodiversity and food security.* London & Ottawa: Earthscan & IDRC, 2008.

97. Yamin F. Intellectual property rights, biotechnology and food security. *IDS Working Paper 203.* Brighton: Institute of Development Studies University of Sussex, 2003.

98. Council for Science and Technology. *Nanosciences and nanotechnologies: a review of government's progress on its policy commitments.* Chaired by Professor Sir John Beringer. London: Council for Science and Technology of H M Government, 2007.

99. ETC. Oligopoly, Inc. 2005. *Communiqué* 2005(91):1–16.

100. UNESCO. *The ethics and politics of nanotechnology.* Paris: United Nations Educational, Scientific and Cultural Organization, 2006.

101. Korthals M. The naked Emperor: bioethics today and tomorrow. In: Marcus Düwell CR-SaDM (ed.) *The contingent nature of life: bioethics and limits of human existence.* Amsterdam: Springer, 2008:221–232.

102. Mnyusiwalla A, Daar AS, Singer PA. 'Mind the gap': science and ethics in nanotechnology. *Nanotechnology* 2003;**14**(3):R9–R13

103. ETC. *The world's top 10 seed companies—2006.* http://www.etcgroup.org/en/materials/publications.html?pub_id=656 [accessed July 12 2007]. Amsterdam: ETC Group, 2006.

104. Hendrickson M, Heffernan W. *Concentration of agricultural markets (USA).* Columbia, MO: Department of Rural Sociology University of Missouri, 2002.

105. Hendrickson M, Heffernan WD, Howard PH, Heffernan JB. *Consolidation in food retailing and dairy: implications for farmers and consumers in a global system.* Report to National Farmers Union (USA). Columbia, Missouri: University of Missouri Department of Rural Sociology, 2001.

106. Barling D, Lang T, Rayner G. Current trends in food retailing and consumption and key choices facing society. In: Rabbinge R, Linnemann A (ed.) *Forward look on European food systems in a changing world.* Final report to European Science Federation (ESF/COST), April 2008. Strasbourg: European Science Foundation, 2008:166–199.

107. *The changing face of the global food-supply chain.* Paper to OECD Conference 6–7 February 2003, The Hague. Changing Dimensions of the Food Economy; 2003 6–7 February; The Hague. OECD.

108. von Schirach-Szmigiel C. *Who is in power today and tomorrow in the food system.* Paper to conference 'Policy and Competitiveness in a Changing Global Food Industry', April 28 Washington DC: USDA Economic Research Service, 2005.

109. Goodman DE. Rethinking Food Production-Consumption: Integrative Perspectives. *Sociologia Ruralis* 2002;**42**(4):271–277.

110. Reardon T, Timmer PC, Berdegué JA. Supermarket expansion in Latin America and Asia: implications for food marketing systems. In: Regmi A, Gehlhar M (ed.) *New directions in global food markets.* Washington, DC: Economic Research Service/USDA, 2005.

111. Gura S. Livestock breeding in the hands of corporations. *Seedling* 2008:2–9.

112. Etc Group. Oligopoly, Inc. 2005. *Communiqué* 2005(91):1–16.

113. Reardon T, Timmer P, Barrett C, Berdegué J. The rise of supermarkets in Africa, Asia and Latin America. *American Journal of Agricultural Economics* 2003;**85**(5):1140–1146.

114. GlobalGAP. *What is GLOBALGAP?* http://www.globalgap.org/ [accessed June 15 2008]. Cologne Germany: GLOBALGAP, 2008.

115. GlobalGAP. *Eurepgap becomesGlobalgap on Sept 7 2007 at Bangkok conference.* http://www.globalgap.org/cms/front_content.php?idcat=9&idart=182 [accessed Sept 23 2007]. Cologn Germany: GLOBALGAP, 2007.

116. GFSI. *Global food safety initiative: the mission.* http://www.ciesnet.com/2-wwedo/2.2-programmes/2.2.foodsafety.gfsi.asp [accessed June 15 2008]. Paris: CIES-GFSI, 2008.

117. Raven H, Lang T, with, Dumonteil C. *Off our trolleys?: food retailing and the hypermarket economy.* London: Institute for Public Policy Research, 1995.

118. Simms A. *Tescopoly: How one shop came out on top and why it matters.* London: Constable & Robinson, 2007.

119. Vorley B. *Food Inc: corporate concentration from farm to consumer.* London: UK Food Group, 2004.

120. Lang T, Barling D. The environmental impact of supermarkets: mapping the terrain and the policy problems in the UK. In: Burch D, Lawrence G (ed.) *Supermarkets and agri-food-supply chains.* Cheltenham: Edward Elgar, 2007:192–219.

121. FAO. *Food Price Index* (May 2008 report). http://www.fao.org/worldfoodsituation/FoodPricesIndex. Rome: Food and Agriculture Organization, 2008.

122. Dobson PW, Waterson M, Davies SW. The patterns and implications of increasing concentration in European food retailing. *Journal of Agricultural Economics* 2003;**54**(1):111–126.

123. Marmot MG. *The status syndrome: how our position on the social gradient affects longevity and health.* London: Bloomsbury, 2004.

124. Darmon N, Drewnowski A. Does social class predict diet quality? *American Journal of Clinical Nutrition* 2008;**67**:1107–1117.

125. Haddad L. Redirecting the diet transition: what can food policy do? *Development Policy Review* 2003;**21**:599–614.

126. Body R. *Agriculture: the triumph and the shame.* London: Temple Smith, 1982.

127. Kurlansky M. *Cod.* London: Jonathan Cape, 1998.

128. Porritt J, Goodman J. *Fishing for good*. London: Forum for the Future, 2005:60.

129. Clover C. *The end of the line: how overfishing is changing the world and what we eat*. London: Ebury, 2004.

130. Crawford M, Marsh D. *The driving force: food, evolution and the future*. London: Heinemann, 1989.

131. Pew Oceans Commission. *America's living oceans: charting a course for sea change*. Washington DC: Pew Charitable Trusts, 2003.

132. OECD. *Evolution of agricultural support in real terms in OECD countries from 1986 to 2002*. Paris: Organization for Economic Co-operation and Development, 2003.

133. OECD. *Agricultural policies in OECD countries: monitoring and evaluation*. Paris: Organization for Economic Co-operation and Development, 2005.

134. Walker AB, Bell B, Elliott REWE. *Aspects of New Zealand's experience in agricultural reform since 1984*. Wellington NZ: Ministry of Agriculture and Forestry, 1997.

135. Variyam JN. The price is right. *Amber Waves (USDA ERS)* 2005;**20**(3):20–27.

136. Barling D. Food-supply chain governance and public health externalities: upstream policy interventions and the UK State *Journal of Agricultural and Environmental Ethics* 2007;**20**(3):285–300.

137. Pretty JN, Brett C, Gee D, Hine R, Mason CF, Morison JIL *et al*. An assessment of the total external costs of UK agriculture. *Agricultural Systems* 2000;**65**(2):113–136.

138. Pretty JN, Ball AS, Lang T, Morison JIL. Farm costs and food miles: an assessment of the full cost of the UK weekly food basket. *Food Policy* 2005;**30**(1):1–20.

139. Wanless D. *Securing our future health: taking a long-term view*. London: HM Treasury, 2002.

140. Wanless D. *Securing good health for the whole population*. London: HM Treasury, 2004.

141. Stern N. *The Stern Review of the economics of climate change*. Final report. London: HM Treasury, 2006.

142. Elinde LS. *Public health aspects of the EU Common Agricultural Policy*. Stockholm: Statens Folkhalsoinstitut/National Institute of Public Health, 2003.

143. Veerman JL, Barendregt JJ, Mackenbach JP. The European Common Agricultural Policy on fruits and vegetables: exploring potential health gain from reform. *European Journal of Public Health* 2006;**16**(1):31–5.

144. Birt C. *A CAP on health? The impact of the Common Agricultural Policy on public health*. London: Faculty of Public Health (of the Royal Colleges of Physicians), 2007.

145. Marshall T. Exploring a fiscal food policy: the case of diet and ischaemic heart disease. *British Medical Journal* 2000;**320**(29 January):301–305.

146. Rayner G, Rayner M. Fat is an economic issue: combating chronic diseases in Europe. *Eurohealth* 2003;**9**(1, Spring):17–20.

147. Institute of Contemporary Arts (ICA). *Should we introduce a fat tax?* Institute of Contemporary Arts/The Economist Debate; 13 May 13, 2004.

148. Leicester A, Windmeijer F. *The 'fat tax': economic incentives to reduce obesity*. London: Institute for Fiscal Studies, 2004.

149. Strnad J. *Conceptualizing the 'fat tax': the role of food taxes in developed economies*. Working Paper, September 2002. *Working Paper*. Palo Alto, CA: Stanford Law School, 2004.

150. Foresight. *Tackling obesities: future choices.* London: Government Office of Science, 2007.

151. Tukker A, Huppes G, Guinée J, Heijungs R, de Koning A, van Oers L *et al.* *Environmental Impact of Products (EIPRO): analysis of the life cycle environmental impacts related to the final consumption of the EU-25.* EUR 22284 EN. Brussels: European Commission Joint Research Centre, 2006.

152. Carbon Trust. *Carbon Trust launches carbon reduction label.* Press launch, London, March 15 2007. http://www.carbontrust.co.uk/about/presscentre/160307_carbon_label.htm [accessed March 18 2007]. London: The Carbon Trust, 2007.

153. Carbon Trust. *Tesco and Carbon Trust join forces to put carbon label on 20 products.* http://www.carbontrust.co.uk/News/presscentre/29_04_08_Carbon_Label_Launch.htm [June 3 2008]. London: Carbon Trust, 2008.

154. Tesco plc. *Measuring our carbon footprint.* http://www.tesco.com/climatechange/carbonFootprint.asp [accessed June 12 2008]. Cheshunt: Tesco plc, 2007.

155. Stern SN. *The economics of climate change. The report of the Stern Review.* Cambridge: Cambridge University Press, 2007.

156. Wiggerthale M. *Last stop—supermarket: the scoop on tropical fruit.* Berlin: Oxfam Germany, 2008.

157. McGroarty P. *Oxfam claims low prices terrible for laborers, April 15.* http://www.spiegel.de/international/germany/0,1518,547550,00.html [accessed June 14 2008]. *Spiegel online* 2008.

158. Barrett H, Browne A. Export horticultural production in Sub-Saharan Africa: the incorporation of the Gambia. *Geography* 1996;**81**(350):47–56.

159. Barrett H, Illbery B, Browne A, Binns T. Globalization and the changing networks of food supply: the importation of fresh horticultural produce from Kenya into the UK. *Transactions of the Institute of British Geographers* 1999;**24**:159–174.

160. Kuye R, Donham K, Marquez S, Sanderson W, Fuortes L, Rautiainen R et al. Agricultural health in The Gambia 1: agricultural practices and developments. *Annals of Agricultural and Environmental Medicine* 2006;**13**:1–12.

161. Dench S, Hurstfield J, Hill D, Akroyd K. *Employers' use of migrant labour.* Main report. London: Home Office, 2006.

162. Josling TE, Taylor TG (ed.) *Banana wars: the anatomy of a trade dispute.* Wallingford CAB International Publishing, 2003.

163. Myers G. *Banana wars: the price of free trade: a Caribbean perspective.* London: Zed Press, 2004.

164. Banana Link. *Social and environmental impacts: how are bananas grown?* http://www.bananalink.org.uk/content/view/77/37/lang,en/ [accessed June 14 2008] 2008.

165. Harari R. *The working and living conditions of banana workers in Latin America.* Quito (Ecuador): Corporation for the Development of Production and the Working Environment (IFA), 2005.

166. Bull D. *A growing problem: pesticides and the Third World poor.* Oxford: Oxfam, 1982.

167. Jacobs M, Dinham B. *Silent invaders: pesticides, livelihoods, and women's health.* London: Zed Books, 2003.

168. Hurst P, Hay A, Dudley N. *The pesticide handbook.* London & Concord, Mass: Journeyman, 1991.

169. Dinham B. *The pesticide hazard: a global health and environmental audit.* London; Atlantic Highlands, N.J: Zed Books, 1993.

170. Lang T, Clutterbuck C. *P is for pesticides.* London: Ebury, 1991.

171. International Labour Organization. *World Day for Safety and Health at Work 2005.* A Background Paper. Geneva: International Labour Organization of the United Nations, 2005.

172. Hurst P, with, Termine P, Karl M. *Agricultural workers and their contribution to sustainable agriculture and rural development.* Rome & Geneva: Food and Agriculture Organization, International Union of Foodworkers, International Labour Organization, 2005.

173. Health and Safety Executive. *Health and safety in agriculture.* http://www.hse.gov.uk/agriculture/hsagriculture.htm [accessed June 15 2008]. London: Health and Safety Executive, 2008.

174. International Labour Organization (UN). *Wage workers in agriculture: conditions of employment and work.* Geneva: International Labour Organization, 1996.

175. International Union of Foodworkers. *Private equity funds: the harsh realities.* Summary of Seminar held at the European Parliament, 19 April 2007. Geneva: International Union of Foodworkers, 2007.

176. Brownell KD, Horgen KB. *Food fight.* New York: McGraw-Hill, 2003.

177. Heasman M, Mellentin J. *The functional foods revolution: healthy people, healthy profits?* London: Earthscan, 2001.

178. Lang T. Functional Foods. *British Medical Journal* 2007;**334**:1015–1016.

179. National Consumer Council and Sustainable Development Commission. *I will if you will.* Report of the Sustainable Consumption Roundtable. London: Sustainable Development Commission, 2006.

180. WHO. Fifty-seventh World Health Assembly 17–22 May 2004, WHA57.17 *Global strategy on diet, physical activity and health.* Geneva: WHO, 2004.

181. Cabinet Office Strategy Unit. *Recipe for success: towards a food strategy for the 21st century.* London: Cabinet Office, 2008.

182. Brundtland GH. *Our common future.* Report of the World Commission on Environment and Development (WCED) chaired by Gro Harlem Brundtland. Oxford: Oxford University Press, 1987.

Chapter 6

The environment and ecosystems

The problem

The natural environment is under severe stress from the cumulative effects of human activity. The ecological footprints of human activity accelerated dramatically with industrialization and urbanization. These processes are still unfolding, as we are witnessing currently in the major emerging economic nations, such as Brazil, China and India. Major public policy priorities have emerged over the past 40 years around the effective means of managing and alleviating the more harmful effects of human and industrial activity on the environment—not least those impacts generated by our food supply. In turn, the healthy state of the natural environment is a key component of food policy. Human health is closely connected to the stability and the sustainability of the natural environment and of the plant and animal species and of the air, water and soil. As explained in Chapter 2, the move to a more holistic and integrated approach to food policy will be based on the firm inter-connections being made by policy-makers and by the public of the symbiotic nature of the relationship between human health and the health of our natural environment. To this extent, food is a touchstone of the inter-connectedness of human health with the environment.

The production of food is dependent upon the interactions of biophysical and climate features, hence production features vary between temperate and tropical regions, and within regions according to features such as soil type, water-table availability and altitude. Nonetheless, a feature of the industrialization of food production has been ongoing attempts to engineer the management of food cultivation through: chemical inputs, the properties of seeds and the development of animal genetics and pharmaceutical applications. Also, there has been the simulation of different growing conditions, such as those conditions engendered by large-scale greenhouse production of fruits and vegetables, which have loosened seasonal and temperature constraints. The biological nature of food and the processes of human digestion are still constraints upon the extent of industrial substitution of the natural environment for food production and its subsequent consumption. However, the industrialization of food production and its exchange have wrought environmental costs in their wake. This chapter explores the environmental impacts of our food production and our contemporary supply chains and the policy responses that have emerged to address these impacts. These policy responses are still quite hesitant and the environmental impacts are still unfolding as we complete the first decade of the new millennium. In policy terms, our food supply can act as the proverbial canary warning of the potentially serious consequences of de-stabilizing and damaging our natural environment. The Millennium Ecosystem Assessment has warned that 15 out of the 24 of the world's ecosystem services are being degraded or used unsustainably.[1] Climate change is bringing in its wake sudden and unexpected variations in climate resulting in weather extremes in terms of severe drought or storms and flooding, which can decimate harvests and widen the spread of insect-borne animal disease dislocating upon food supply. The impacts of dislocated food supply affect the poorest nations and the poorest within individual national economies most severely.

The adverse impact of modern food production and supply systems upon the environment is one side of the coin; on the other are the constraints that environmental damage and dislocation are bringing to the current ways of producing and supplying food. Can the current trajectories of food production and consumption continue? In addressing these challenges, the nature of the policy responses that have emerged to deal with these challenges are considered. There is a clear inter-dependency, both in terms of the impacts of production, delivery and consumption of the food supply upon the environment, and in terms of how loss and damage to natural resources and environmental change are in turn impacting upon the sustainability of the food supply.

A key concern for this exposition of these inter-dependencies is the response of public policy-makers and other key actors in the food sector in addressing these relationships between the food-supply chain and the natural environment. The immediacy of these environmental impacts and the need for adequate policies to address them are urgent. Agricultural pollution, biodiversity, water and soil, fisheries stocks, levels of waste are all deteriorating; and the impacts of climate change and energy-use threaten society. The impacts upon the environment and our ecosystems are explained in more detail in the next section; followed by a more detailed explanation of the development of environmental policy and the particular policy-responses to these impacts in the areas of agriculture and fisheries and the food-supply chain post-farm-gate.

In the case of the policy responses for food and the environment, the international contexts are presented, globally and at EU levels. At national level, particular attention is paid to the experiences and policies of the UK. The picture that this chapter paints is one of emerging actions: from international regimes to national programmes and regulation, to stakeholder engagement and participation. Internationally, for example, there is division around the appropriate technologies and farming strategies for the best sustainable development of agriculture, particularly in the developing world. The setting of targets in international regimes, such as on climate change, is weak and compromised by national economic interests. Equally, the lead from governments and public policy-makers is still unsure and relatively hesitant. The setting of some national targets and policy inducements in the UK has been weak in terms of generating behaviour changes right along the supply chain, from producers to consumers and in-between. The tools of contemporary governance are being deployed by the state to engage industry and the market-place and consumers. However, the ecological stability needed for a successful food policy will need more substantial advances than are being achieved at present.

The impacts of our food supply on the environment and the ecological constraints

An overview

The workings of the contemporary food supply are having a significant impact upon our natural environment. These impacts can be identified along the whole length of the supply chain, notably in terms of the generation of pollution and depletion of natural resources, energy use, and waste from production through to consumption. An overview representation of the impacts of the food-supply chain is portrayed for agriculture (see Table 6.1) and the post-farm-gate food-supply chain post (see Table 6.2). The latter covers from food processing and manufacturing to retail, catering and home consumption. This configuration of the food-supply chain, and of the food sector, is linear, which belies the complex realties of the food trade where ingredients and indeed livestock may be bartered, traded and moved between a range of locations before finally entering the food processing and manufacturing stages. However, adopting this rather linear supply-chain approach allows some key dimensions to be identified, both in terms of the impacts of our systems of food supply and the food sector on our ecosystems; and, the constraints that these impacts are in turn applying to the productive resources necessary to produce, manufacture and consume our food. These impacts are summarized below. The subsequent narrative also identifies some of the major resource constraints that our contemporary food supply is facing, both currently and into the near future.

Agricultural production and fisheries

There has been a long exploitation of natural food supplies, notably wild-catch fisheries, and strong evidence that ecological limits are being reached.

Table 6.1 Environmental impacts and ecological and constraints on agricultural production

Inputs	Activity	Adverse environmental/ ecological impacts	Environmental/ ecological constraints
Inorganic fertilizers	Application to crops and horticulture	Nitrates in water courses Eutrophication Loss of soil fertility Ammonia emissions → acidification and acid rain	Oil-based Depletion of water ecosystems and fisheries Air pollution
Pesticides	Applied to crops and horticulture; and to preserve foods in supply chain	Persistent organic pollutants in water supply and food chains	Petroleum derived Loss of biodiversity, e.g. habitats for wildlife food chains → farmland birds
Machinery	Tractors, harvesters, etc.	CO_2 emissions Soil compaction	Oil (and diesel) based Contribute to climate change
Plough	Tillage	N_2O emissions. Loss of water holding capacity → water run off	Mechanised and oil-based Contribute to climate change
Feed—grass and/or feed inputs	Livestock production	Over grazing and land use change → biodiversity loss, e.g. change of pasture to grass silage production CH_4 emissions Animal faecal pathogens, e.g. *Cryptosporidium* and *E. Coli* in water supply Soil compaction	Destruction of natural habitats inc. forests and bush Contribute to climate change
Deforestation	Deforestation for new land → agricultural use	Loss of biodiversity Loss of carbon sinks Loss of landscape and recreational value	Loss of major forest and bush ecosystems
Water	Water abstraction and irrigation for growing	Depletion of natural aquifers; aridity of land and soil Embedded water in food products	De-stabilising of existing ecosystems

Table 6.2 Environmental impacts and ecological constraints on post-farm-gate food-supply chain

Activity	Stage(s)	Adverse environmental/ ecological impacts	Environmental/ecological constraints
Food distribution	Between and within all stages form production to household use	Energy use	Oil based energy use
		Emissions	Air pollution
		Refrigeration and refrigerant GHG gases	Contribution to climate change
Large site energy use	Processing mills, and manufacturing plants; distribution centres; large retail stores	Food and packaging waste	Oil based energy use
		CO_2 emissions	Air pollution
		Waste water streams	Contribution to climate change
Packaging (plastics glass, etc.)	All stages	Waste	Land
		Landfill space	Pollutants
		Energy use	Contribution to climate change
		CH_4 emissions	
		Incineration—pollutants/ CO_2 emissions	
Refrigeration	All stages	Emission of refrigerant GHGs.	Oil based energy use
			Contribution to climate change
Water	All stages— especially large site use	Water use	Impacts on natural water resources
		Waste water	Water course pollution
		Embedded water in food products	
Cooking	Most stages—but particularly catering and household	Use of energy	Depletion of oil stocks
		Food waste	Contributions to climate change
		Packaging waste	

Note: the post-farm-gate food-supply chain is deemed here to be: food processing (first stage) ⟶ food manufacturing and second stage processing ⟶ retailing and catering ⟶ home consumption.

The FAO calculates that fish is a significant part of the animal protein diet at almost 20% of the average per capita for more than 2.8 billion people.[2] Industry, in turn, is increasingly focusing on sources of fish rich in omega 3 oils; both in terms of species' capture and farming for retail, and for oil extracts, which are in high demand from food manufacturers as a value-added ingredient for the functional foods market.[3] Yet the majority of wild fish stocks are depleted, with 52% of wild stocks being 'fully exploited' according to the FAO's classification. The FAO points out that this means that they were 'producing catches that were at or close to their maximum sustainable limits, with no room for further expansion'.[2] In addition, another 25% of wild stocks:[2]

> were either overexploited, depleted or recovering from depletion (17 percent, 7 percent and 1 percent, respectively) and thus were yielding less than their maximum potential owing to excess fishing pressure exerted in the past, with no possibilities in the short or medium term of further expansion and with an increased risk of further declines and need for rebuilding.

Furthermore, most of the top 10 marine fish species, which together account for about 30% of all capture-fisheries' production, are fully exploited or over-exploited.[2] One result has been an increasing reliance upon aquaculture for human consumption. By 2004, 32.4% of the world's fish provision by weight came from aquaculture, with that share expected to rise over the next decades.[2] However, aquaculture is in turn fed by meal from wild-catch fisheries, reinforcing the depletion of the ecological food-chains for wild fish species; estimated as taking from 2 to 5 kg of wild fish to feed 1 kg of farmed fish. In addition, large-scale fish farming had generated further adverse impacts in terms of disruption of coastal zones and tropical mangrove ecosystems (in the case of shrimp farming), as well as disrupting native biodiversity, polluting waters and spreading disease into wild species.[4–9]

The modern processes of growing food through agriculture and horticulture produce a wide range of external impacts. The productionist drive towards more intensive and higher yielding grain and oil-seed crops, and livestock for meat and dairy, have been dominating features of agriculture and food production from the middle years of the 20th century onwards. Underpinning these advances has been the increased mechanization of agriculture (see Chapter 5), reducing farm labour and increasing airborne pollution and oil-based energy use in food production.

Greater yields from arable crops are the result of both enhancements in plant genetics and breeding, and the application of inputs, notably artificial inorganic fertilizers (primarily nitrogen, phosphate and potash based) and synthetic chemical pesticide application. The combination of plant genetics and the application of inorganic fertilizers were part of the 'green revolution' that led to rapidly increased yields in the developing world agriculture from the 1960s through to the 1990s. The production of artificial fertilizers is a highly energy-intensive process and synthetic pesticides are manufactured from oil-based petroleum, which is a key stage in their production. It has been estimated that these applications account for almost 40% of the energy used in USA agriculture, although fertilizers are by far the dominant user at around 37%.[10] Both fertilizers and pesticides are major contributors to groundwater pollution. The entry of nitrates from fertilizers (including from organic sources such as livestock manure) into water courses incurs damage to water ecosystems through eutrophication, which is the growth of dominating plant life and algae that absorb the oxygen and so damage marine ecosystems and their resident fisheries. A notorious example was along the Gulf of Mexico, where coastal fisheries were devastated in a 'dead zone' created by agricultural run-off from the Mississippi Basin in the USA.[11] Pesticide run-off pollutes groundwater and some of the chemical ingredients, notably persistent organic pollutants, enter the food chain with damaging effects.[12] Farming in the UK contributes 87% of the ammonia emissions to the atmosphere, from fertilizers and organic manures, which contribute to both water eutrophication and to acidification of the land, including via acid rain.[13] OECD monitoring at agricultural sites in its member states of industrialized countries from 1990 to 2006 showed that high levels of water pollution from farming practices persist.[14]

The productionist drive in agriculture included a move from mixed cropping and livestock systems on land to larger scale crop production and successive cropping supported by pesticide and inorganic fertilizer applications. Critics have identified the creation of a technological treadmill of continuous application to control pests, which in turn develop resistance, promoting the need for further new chemical applications.[15] The spread of large-scale crop plantings meant increased tillage of soil, resulting in increased water run-off and the ecosystem impacts previously mentioned. Repeated inorganic fertilizer applications have masked the declining fertility and productivity of the soil. The decline in soil fertility is enhanced by soil erosion, which is caused almost entirely by agriculture in the UK.[13, 16] A UK Government assessment identified significant levels of soil erosion and attributed the contributory factors to: increased use of inorganic fertilizers at the expense of organic fertilizers, poor soil-management practices, fewer fallow periods and compaction by heavy machinery and increased livestock.[13] Both lowland and upland grasslands have experienced more intensive grazing adding to soil erosion. Also, the increased run-off has exacerbated the flooding impacts of heavy rainfall. For example, in the summer of 2007, heavy rains in the east of England badly affected the harvests of one of the main vegetable growing areas of the UK. In addition, globally, 70% of our freshwater is used by agriculture.[17] In the UK, agriculture accounts for 742 million m^3 of water compared to the food and drink industry's 155 million m^3 used.[18] In areas where there have been extensive irrigation systems put in place to support production, there has been accompanying stress on aquifers adding to their ecosystem vulnerability.

The drive to greater arable crop production has been stimulated, in no small part, by the expansion of modern livestock production, whereby crop products and their by-products are turned into industrialized feed products and supplements for livestock, from cattle to pigs to chickens. Modern livestock production has been achieved through selective and intensive breeding, hormone and antibiotic use, and increased herd and flock sizes. Large units for dairy production, feed lots for cattle fattening, huge pig-breeding units and broiler chicken units increase the need to manage effluents entering into water-courses. Animal welfare concerns have arisen over these industrial-scale techniques, including the use of hormones and antibiotics to aid production. Also, there are human health concerns about the impacts of such liberal uses of drugs used in combating human disease and infection, in terms of the development of resistance and the disruptive effects upon humans' biological development of such chemicals entering the food chain. Intensive livestock production has magnified the water run-off pollution and added bacterial contamination into the water system and the food supply through the spread of animal faecal pathogens, such as *Cryptosporidium* and *Escherichia coli*.[13]

The demand for more animal feed has been another link in the chain leading to the destruction of ancient forests, jungle and bush, rich in its own biodiversity, in order to provide virgin grazing lands for livestock or to plant industrial-scale crops for feed and other industrial food purposes, such as with soybean and maize and palm oil plantations.[19] For example, in Malaysia, 87% of de-forestation from 1985 to 2000 was to convert land to palm oil production for use in food processing and manufacture, as well other industrial products.[20] The destruction of Amazonian forests in Brazil and of rain forests in South-East Asia in recent decades, echoes earlier destruction of native flora and fauna to create grazing and planting lands for agriculture from North America to Australia and New Zealand, the so-called white settler colonies of the 18th and 19th centuries. Modern agricultural production has had adverse effects on biodiversity. The FAO estimates that three-quarters of the world's agricultural biodiversity was lost in the 20th century, as varieties across food crops from potatoes to wheat to apples have disappeared.[21]

In the UK, three-quarters of the land cover is farmed and a great deal of the biodiversity has evolved or adapted within agricultural systems.

However, intensive agricultural practices, notably mono-culture crop planting and upland grazing, have reduced species diversity. The move from spring-sown to autumn-sown cereal crops has impacted upon the decline in numbers of some species of farmland birds, with nine species falling by more than a half from 1970 to 1995.[22] Studies of the grey partridge found that crop weeds provided herbage and seeds for bird feed and act as hosts to insects, an important food source in raising young chicks.[23] Herbicide application can remove such important ecological habitat support. The numbers of farmland birds has been adopted by policy-makers (not least in the UK Treasury) as an indicator of the state of farm biodiversity and the agri-environment. While farmland bird populations had declined by 60% between 1970 and the late-1990s, the levels subsequently stabilized up to 2006.[24] This stabilizing is related to the variety of agri-environment related measures introduced under the CAP since the late-1980s, including set-a-side, as discussed further below. Conversely, a decline in bird life has been reported from 1990 to 2006 across the wider industrialized countries of the OECD.[14]

The quantifying of the costs of such environmental impacts upon our ecosystems, and to human health, and the costs of clearing up such environmental damage has been developed over recent years. The damage to the public good, i.e. the environment and the benefits that other activities bring that are not presently reflected in the price of goods in the market-place, can be given a value and measured. In this way the environmental externalities of a product—both negative and positive—are quantified providing a truer cost of food production and transfer to price in the market-place. There are problems with agreeing the value of some impacts—such as the value of individual wildlife, and the relationship to the willingness of the public to pay these costs. Hence, attempts to assess the annual costs of pesticides in the USA undertaken in the early 1990s varied from $1.3 billion to $8 billion.[25] Work has been done on costing the environmental impacts of UK agriculture.[13] One study estimated the costs, by analysing what is spent to deal with the externalities of production, and reached a figure of £1.566 billion.[22] Another study sought to estimate the depreciation of the stocks of natural capital associated with agriculture and the environmental services generated, and then arrived at costs by matching values to evidence from willingness to pay studies.[26] This latter study came up with a total of £1.072 billion, but taking away the benefit value of carbon sinks raised the external costs to £1.432.[13] This work also highlights the environmental and ecosystem benefits that the farmed landscape can provide, both in terms of biodiversity support and habitats and maintenance of soil and water properties of the land, as well as landscape value and carbon sequestration (or carbon sinks). Hence, policy-makers have paid more attention to promoting agri-environmental management and improvement over the past two decades or more, and are now turning more attention to the role that agriculture can play in mitigating climate change.

Costing the water used in bringing a product to market, a concept termed as embedded water, is another way to assess the ecological impacts of food production. So, according to work done from the Netherlands, the embedded water taken to produce 1 kg grain-fed beef takes 15 m^3 of water, 1 kg of lamb from a sheep fed on grass needs 10 m^3 and 1kg cereals needs 0.43 m^3— although such calculations would vary according to the climate and growing conditions of the particular location chosen.[27] These calculations reinforce the high land-use costs of meat production, both through grazing pasture and for growing crops for feed. The large ecological footprint of meat production is reinforced by livestock contribution to global climate change, which we turn to next.

The food sector and greenhouse gas emissions

Global climate change has emerged as the most far-reaching threat to the stability of our ecosystems and as an environmental constraint to the current workings of the agri-food sector, which covers both agriculture and food production and the whole food sector beyond the farm-gate. The Intergovernmental Panel on Climate Change (IPCC) is unequivocal that the scientific evidence shows that climate change through atmospheric warming is taking place.[28] The main indication of climate change is the warming of the earth's atmosphere caused by increased concentrations of greenhouse gases (GHGs) emitted, largely due to human activity. The major greenhouse gas is carbon dioxide (CO_2) but there are others in smaller atmospheric concentrations with a proportionately greater warming potential (gwp). These are: methane (CH_4) at 23 times gwp; nitrous oxide (N_2O) at 296 times gwp, and refrigerant gases at thousands' times gwp.[28] The impacts of climate change upon food production are, and as they increase in the future will be, widespread and vary from location to location. The commonly presented scenarios include impacts such as an increase of extreme climate events and rising sea levels and shifting temperature zones. Agriculture and food impacts include some regionally specific advantages, such as increased rainfall or milder temperatures and longer growing seasons, but the overall picture is negative. There will be more extreme weather events from drought to flooding, and so harvest loss, increased and wider spread of crop and livestock diseases (currently witnessed with blue tongue disease and avian flu), water loss, and shifts in optimum growing areas for particular crops. Particularly at risk are those parts of the world where populations and their agricultures are already highly vulnerable to disruption, notably in areas prone to flooding, such as estuarial zones.[28] Along the supply chain there will be disruption to sourcing of foods, unexpected shortages, and transport and supply dislocations. There will be impacts at the consumption level in areas such as household energy use.

The agri-food sector is a major contributor to all GHG emissions. In terms of EU consumption, it is estimated that the sector contributes 31% of total GHG emissions.[29] In the UK, with its comparatively smaller agricultural sector and larger industrial sector, one estimate of the contribution is put at around 19%.[30] Of this, the approximation for the UK is that agriculture contributes 38%, transport-related 16%, with around 10.5% each from food manufacture, household food activity and fertilizer manufacture. Retail, catering and packaging approximate at 5% each.[30]

Agriculture is a major contributor to both methane emissions, from ruminant livestock such as dairy cows, beef and sheep, and to nitrous oxide emissions, largely from fertilizer use (both inorganic and organic) but also from tillage of soil and deforestation for farming use. In 2006, the FAO reported that the livestock sector generated more greenhouse gas emissions, 18% as measured in CO_2 equivalent, than transport. It accounts for 9% of anthropogenic CO_2 and 37% of anthropogenic methane, and 65% of anthropogenic nitrous oxide.[31] However, the carbon figures were based on including the estimated carbon loss of de-forestation for livestock rearing. This raises questions about the boundary setting for such calculations and substitution. For example, what would be the costs of alternative sources of protein to replace meat in diets?[32] Life-cycle analysis (LCA) of food products and their supply chains is a rapidly emerging tool to aid policy-makers in decisions around the environmental impacts of particular food and food supplies. The differentiation of the boundaries and the criteria of the LCA can lead to very different results and implications. Food-supply chains post farm-gate make a substantial contribution to climate change and energy use, and LCA has been applied to identify the environmental hot-spots in such chains. For example, for bread production, the prime hot-spot is at the baking stage.

The fundamental importance of ecosystems to economic well-being was quantified in respect of global climate change with the findings of the Stern Review commissioned by the UK Government. This put the costs of inaction over GHG emissions at the equivalent to losing between 5% and 20% of global GDP each year, against an estimated cost of acting immediately at 1% global GDP per year.[33] The Stern review put forward an economic framework for action based upon the three strategies of carbon pricing, the draw-through of new technologies and tackling market barriers. The UK Government began pricing carbon, albeit at the lower end of the Stern estimates of what was needed.[34]

The food-supply chain beyond the farm-gate

The shift in focus to beyond the farm-gate highlights a range of key environmental impacts from our contemporary systems of food supply. The complexity of specific supply chains and of manufacturer, wholesaler, retailer and caterer sourcing for food ingredients and products, reflects both a wider geographical range in the supply of foods and more sophisticated logistical arrangements (such as just in time ordering and delivery systems) and more demanding standards setting by buyers from these organizational positions (see Chapter 5). There are environmental benefits and dis-benefits to these complex but logistically integrated supply-chain methods. For example, in the developing world up to 40% of food harvested can be lost before it is consumed due to the inadequacies of processing, storage and transport.[35] Better logistically-integrated and supported supply-chain systems, alongside better infrastructure (such as roads), would bring marked improvement to such food supply. Nonetheless, as Table 6.1 indicates, two environmental impacts that run throughout the modern efficient supply chains are transportation and resultant emissions, and energy use, to which transport is a significant contributor.

In the case of the UK, transport is the biggest user of energy in the food chain and accounts for a third of all 20.6 million tonnes of oil used in the food chain each year.[36] Food transport's externalities are identified as including: GHGs, air and noise pollution, congestion, accidents and infrastructure impacts.[37] Attempts to cost these externalities for the UK have been priced variously at £1.9 billion and £4 billion.[38] The biggest external cost to society of food transport is congestion, not emissions; this is reflected in the statistic that food transport accounts for 25% of UK Heavy Goods Vehicle (HGV) movements.[18] Air-freight is the fastest growing mode of transporting food, trebling in vehicle kilometres over the period 1992 to 2004.[39] However, air-freight accounts for only 1% of food tonne kilometres and 0.1% of vehicle kilometres, but for 11% of food transport emissions on a CO_2-equivalent basis.[37] The breakdown in terms of CO_2 emissions from food transport is: HGV transport 45%, air and sea transport 11–13% each and consumer shopping car transport 21%.[37] Emissions of CO_2 from food transport totalled almost 18 million tons in 2004, an increase of 19.4% since 1992. Food transport by car accounts for 50.2% of food vehicle km, predominantly consumer shopping.[36]

The complexity of contemporary supply chains, as food ingredients and final products are increasingly moved around geographically, reinforced by the increase in counter-seasonal sourcing of food and ingredients for manufacturers and to fill retailers' shelves year round, has contributed to the distances travelled by food to reach the consumer in affluent developed nations markets such as the UK. The term 'food miles' was coined in 1992 to capture both the complexity of these supply chains and to question the rationale for such complexity in our food supply and the large distances of travel before reaching the final consumer.[40] The refrain of food miles has been taken up both by: environmental organizations concerned about the energy, and other environmental and social implications,[41] as well as producers seeking to promote domestic-produced foods in their own markets over imported alternatives.[42] In terms of food transport, the food-miles concept is better understood as a short-hand for a variety of different externalities.[37] A result of the adoption of food miles by policy protagonists around the costs of local, as against imported, food has been a fresh wave of work investigating the energy embedded within differing foods, drawing on developing LCA methodologies for food products.

The emerging work on LCA studies, especially around imported versus domestically produced food, is still developing the boundaries and the criteria for accurate comparisons. For example, a New Zealand study found imported apples and lamb grown in New Zealand for sale in the UK, to be more energy efficient than UK produce.[43] The study failed to distinguish between UK lamb reared and fed on lowland grasslands (more energy intensive) versus hill-fed lamb (less intensive) and the energy figures have been challenged.[44] Likewise, the New Zealand study failed to allow for seasonality in the UK apple crop—where the greatest domestic energy use is from cold storage for consumption beyond the natural season. Here the evidence can show that at some times during the year, transporting produce from other countries may have a lower environmental impact than refrigerating produce grown in the UK, but not at other times of the year.[30]

There are other examples of comparing domestically produced food in the UK with imports sold in the UK, in energy terms. Tomatoes produced in UK hothouses use 10 times the energy and emit nearly four times as much CO_2 as the same quantity produced in unheated polytunnels in Spain and road-freighted to the UK market. Conversely, UK tomatoes are often grown using fewer pesticides and closed-irrigation systems to minimize the release of excess nutrients to the environment.[37] In short, studies need to be: spatially precise, adjusted for growing conditions, seasonality and inputs; and to factor in the variety of supply-chain logistics, such as refrigeration and storage time and period between harvest and placement in the retail market, alongside mode and costs of transport.[45] In addition, a key component in the LCA along the food chain is the domestic consumer. For consumers, driving six and a half miles to a shop to buy food produces more carbon than air-freighting a pack of green beans from Kenya to the UK.[46] LCA accounting can be extended to consider the social (and health) dimensions in addition to environmental aspects.[47] For example, UK imports of fresh produce grown in sub-Saharan

Africa (excluding South Africa) have been estimated to support over 700,000 workers and their dependents.[48] A further form of environmental externality auditing of food products, mentioned previously, is embedded water. It is estimated that it takes 13 litres(l) of water to produce a 70 g tomato, 200 l to produce a 200 ml glass of milk, and 2,400 l of water to produce a 150 g hamburger.[27] The notion of 'virtual water' has been introduced to capture the embedded water in internationally traded foods.[49]

Along the food chain, and particularly at the consumption, as well as food transit, product packaging and food waste are two further identifiable environmental impacts for action. In 2006, evidence from the UK estimates that consumers contribute to throwing away 6.7 million tonnes of food that could have been eaten and 5.2 million tonnes of packaging waste. The value of edible food waste is calculated at £250–£400 per UK household. The food waste is equivalent to 15 million tonnes of CO_2 emissions, and the vast majority goes into landfill, where it generates methane.[50] It is estimated that as much of 40% of packaging in a shopping basket cannot be recycled.[51] For consumers, food packaging and waste are causes of environmental impacts that are more visible in their daily lives.

What is clear from the foregoing discussion of measuring environmental impacts and the costing of externalities along the food-supply chain, is that policy advocacy, such as around the benefits of domestically grown food against imported food, has the policy advocates searching for new evidence. In turn, this is generating a policy-oriented research agenda. Also, the costing of externalities is only beginning to be properly developed, although it is a rapidly moving area methodologically. The accuracy of such evidence, or, more importantly, the acceptance of its validity, is only one piece in the policy process, however. The next stage is turning the evidence into realizable and effective policy actions, either by governments with and/or by other actors in the food system. In the case of the evidence of ecosystem stress and collapse, and the environmental impacts of modern food production, the need for serious policy response is compelling.

Reframing environmental policy and food

Establishing environmental policy

The environmental impacts and the ecosystem constraints that have emerged around the workings of the contemporary food sector are demanding both multi-level governance and multi-actor responses. Food policy in this regard sits within the environmental policy domain, and so the policy responses to these environmental and ecosystem challenges have to be interpreted within the wider arena of environmental policy. Environmental policy as a distinct policy area within the apparatus of the state is relatively young. It can be marginalized by governments in the face of more traditional high-policy areas, such as foreign affairs, defence, economic policy as well as the imperatives of agricultural policy and the need for a secure food supply. In the case of a secure food supply, the irony is that agricultural policy-makers have had to be convinced of the importance of the environmental and ecosystem redress to ensure that such a supply proves to be sustainable in the future. Indeed, environmental policy cuts across other established policy sectors. Consequently, as well the emergence of a distinctive environmental policy domain, progress in environmental and ecosystem protection is dependent upon the integration of these priorities into the other relevant policy sectors. Environment policy has remained on the agendas of the state, both domestic and international, as the evidence for the need for continuing and greater action on the deteriorating state of our environment and ecosystems, and the threats of climate change, have accelerated. The evidence itself has generated advocacy and so support for more detailed research. Advocacy has come from both professions in the sciences and from the growth of social activism around environmental pollution issues and the limits of economic and industrial growth from the 1960s onwards. Earlier forms of environmental activism emerging from the late-19th century had focused on conservation and landscape issues. This resulted in the setting-up of wildlife and bird protection societies and to heritage preservation bodies such as the UK's National Trust, as well as the creation of the USA's substantial system of national parks to preserve the natural wilderness. Major policy initiatives for the better management of environmental pollutants and natural resource degradation emerged in the late 1960s and early 1970s onwards.

The first phase of modern environmental policy response from developed countries bore remarkable similarities, not withstanding the differing policy styles and political and socio-economic circumstances and structures. Governments responded with a combination of: legislation specifying more stringent controls on pollutants and toxic substances, and regulating the use of the air and the water; creation of new organizations and either new institutions or the adaptation of existing ones to new responsibilities such as Departments of Environment and Environmental Protection Agencies; and the creation of expert panels or bodies to provide high-level technical and scientific advice.[52] The basic approach was the identification of the problems of pollution and the setting of targets for its reduction across different media (air, water and soil) based on an essentially command and control approach. However, the targets set were not met as policies ran into 'implementation deficit' or failure. Not only were the targets often over-ambitious in the time frames set, but there was a lack of engagement by key stakeholders across different policy sectors, such as industrial policy or energy policy and so on. There was a lack of policy integration, where environmental objectives struggled to compete with, or address, existing and ongoing policy priorities in these other established policy sectors with their often settled policy communities. New approaches to actor engagement and policy integration were needed. Two guiding concepts for policy that emerged from these experiences were those of sustainable development and the related concept of ecological modernization.

Within the emerging environmental critique, a broader division has been identified between what we might term environmental management approaches, which entered the main policy discourse, and the more radical green critiques of contemporary capitalist economies. This broad division has been cast variously as: dark green and light green, eco-centric and techno-centric, and environmentalism and ecologism.[53, 54] Within the environmental movements that emerged from the 1960s, a more radical approach eschewed environmental management based upon technocratic solutions and posed more fundamental questions about industrial, or indeed post-industrial, trajectories based upon continued economic growth. In these critiques lay a more fundamental challenge to modern market capitalism and its anthropocentric design.[54] They ranged from economic-based, such as the work of Schumacher (1974) and the Club of Rome's Limits to Growth study;[55] to the more holistic and mystical Gaia hypothesis (1979), and the philosophical Deep Ecology.[56] This more radical Green thinking has clear overlaps with the concerns of managing our ecosystems more effectively to allow for our food supply to survive and prosper. The prescriptions within this broad range of thinking remain to the edge of the main political stage but an underlying refrain within environmental policy discourse is the extent to which contemporary governance and environmental management strategies can generate the step changes in policy needed to address adequately the litany of environmental and ecosystem problems. This continuing and steadfast policy advocacy calls for a more radical and fundamental turn in policy towards an alternative Green political agenda for solutions.

Sustainable development and ecological modernization

The term sustainable development in policy debate emerged in the 1980s, from earlier origins, when it was famously coined in the Brundtland report of the World Commission and Environment set up by the United Nations

Environment Programme (UNEP) in 1987. The oft-quoted definition of sustainable development used was: 'development that meets the needs of the present without compromising the ability of future generations to meet their own needs'.[57] Sustainable development was to be a different pathway for development, one that promoted social justice alongside protection of the environment for future generations and that aspired to build environmental and social externalities into sustainable economics. Policy and politics, viewed through this lens, are to accord equal emphasis to: the environment, society and economy; three foci commonly found in contemporary policy use of the term. To this extent, sustainable development embraced the environmental management approach of seeking to harness economic progress in a more harmonious manner. Sustainable development was conceptualized in the context of international development and the environment with the Brundtland report, and subsequently with the UN Conference on the Environment and Development (UNCED) at Rio in 1992. From this so-called Earth Summit came the International Framework Conventions for Biodiversity and Climate Change (see below), and Agenda 21, which sought to engage civil society and grassroots action. The common concern was to take actions to address the erosion of the world's sustenance base while allowing for the economic development of less-developed nations. Policy integration of environmental priorities into other policy areas (industry, energy, transport, agriculture and tourism) was a focus of the EU's interpretation as manifest in the 1992 Fifth Environmental Action Programme 'Towards Sustainability'.[58, 59] Sustainability is a highly contested concept, nonetheless, and the debates about what sustainable development means reflect differing visions and priorities about how society, economy and the environment can sustain life for many generations.

Alongside sustainable development, the concept of ecological modernization was developed in response to the perceived regulatory failures of the 1970s and 1980s. Mike Jacobs points out that: 'Ecological modernization effectively reinterprets the idea of sustainable development within a broader understanding of political economy'.[60] The focus is not just measuring environmental improvements in a scientific sense, as it is on finding social, economic and political processes and instruments that will help lead to environmental improvement. That is a focus on 'environmental reforms in social practices, institutional designs and societal and policy discourses to safeguard societies' sustenance bases'.[61] The drive is to situate ecological principles at the heart of economic, social and policy thinking and actions. The environmental challenges are seen as opportunities for economic growth and economic competitiveness; through adoption of new and cleaner technologies, such as in energy generation (wave, wind and solar), to replace reliance on the carbon economy. An increased importance is attached to market dynamics and economic agents as ways of shaping public behaviour and so meeting environmental conservation and management policy goals. Pricing in the externalities of food production and distribution are examples. Labelling and eco-labelling schemes provide another market-based approach for providing economic agents (consumers) with information for purchasing choice, reinforced by traceability schemes for food and feed. The aforementioned incorporation of environmental priorities within other governmental departments, and so across the range of governmental departments, is stressed. In addition, the role of the nation-state should be transformed from above through membership of collaborative multi-level international environmental agreements and regimes. Also, from below, through the devolving of more responsibility to local and regional levels, as with the Local Agenda 21 initiatives of the 1990s, allowing more grass-roots participation in formulating policy solutions. In turn, more participatory policy processes are encouraged in policy implementation, technology assessment and so on. A more socially responsive science and technology is sought, where expert opinion can be challenged by lay opinion through new participatory procedures. Such processes provide for the wider public discursive practices to be aired and to feed into policy debate.

This work emerged in the Northern and Western European countries and has remained embedded in the developed world. However, the global nature of many third-generation environmental challenges (such as ozone layer depletion, global climate change and biodiversity loss), and the ongoing impacts upon ecosystems and natural resources, mean that these approaches are also of importance to developing countries and their food producers. The embrace of discourse practices suggests the need to consider indigenous forms of environmental knowledge and practices found in developing country settings within policy formulation, not least at the farmer-grower stage. The ensemble of policy practices and instruments, as identified under ecological modernization policy, are being deployed in the advanced industrial nations. For example, there is the reappraisal of the externalities of the contemporary food system and its costs, and of the processes necessary to make it more sustainable. The question remains as to whether an ecological value set can become ascendant in these contemporary processes of policy-making change and innovation. Will there be significant change in policy and social discourses to embed the cultural values necessary for a more sustainable society?[62, 63] This question has been explored in relation to society's interaction with risk in contemporary times, where both environmental risk and food risk have been at the forefront of the policy agenda.

Technology, the environment and risk

The importance of discursive practices and widening participation in policy-making over the future directions for society, and the challenging of expertise by lay opinion, are vividly illustrated over food and risk governance. One line of work has examined the importance of the assumptions that inherently frame the scientific assessment of risk. Here there has been a lack of openness and lack of clarity with the political risk managers seeking to promote scientific opinion as a concrete basis for policy decisions, while failing to acknowledge the uncertainties that may be involved in the scientific opinions given. In this sense science is poorly served by its political masters. This has been identified as a continuing weakness of the risk governance around food safety in recent decades, most clearly illustrated by the problems over the management of the BSE epidemic and its human health consequences.[64]

Another critique has been around the relationship of expert opinion *vis-à-vis* lay opinion, where the technocratic and bureaucratic attempts to manage risk through expert advisory and regulatory systems have been challenged by social groups. Ulrich Beck identifies 'reflexive modernization' as the process by which society questions and challenges the traditional rationales and expertise of modernity as key institutions lose their historical legitimacy.[65] Instead, modern societies face increasing uncertainty and are increasingly aware of this. Beck is quite explicit that reflexive modernization 'does not mean… reflection, but rather self-confrontation and self-transformation'.[66] Hence, society and its members have become more critical of expert opinions. This rise of social reflexivity 'entails fundamental questioning of the forms of power and social control implicated in contemporary conflicts over risk'.[67] The emergence of the social movement of environmentalism arose, in part, in the 1960s and 1970s, around a lack of faith and questioning of technological interventions and advances, notably as nuclear power generation, which had potentially devastating health and environmental side-effects, but also interventions in food production and agriculture. This theme of public distrust has become increasingly vocal around a range of technological innovations in the food chain from pesticides to additives to animal feeding practices to the genetic modification of food and feed crops.

A recent and complex manifestation of the governance of risk and its democratization has occurred around the introduction of genetically modified (GM) crops into the food chain. The major commercial applications in the first wave of GM crops from the 1990s were to allow for further applications of agri-chemicals for herbicide resistance in the crop and to insert pesticide attributes. The potential production savings for farmers were off-set by a range of environmental concerns around agronomic practice and potential environmental contamination, such as the widening of resistance across related wild species and other related adverse biodiversity impacts. These potential biodiversity and ecosystem risks attracted increasing regulatory attention at European level and in the form of the International Biosafety Protocol.[8, 69] However, the refinement of environmental regulation was only part of the regulatory response. The introduction of GM crop derivatives into the European food and feed chains from 1996 onwards, became a focus for opposition from civil society and environmental groups. The opposition campaigns and accompanying media attention ignited consumer anxiety and mistrust around the interventions of technologies, in this case from the life sciences, into food production. The result was a rapid response from the consumer end of the food chain as retailers led the way in segregating foods with GM derivatives from the main supply of food products in their supply chains. There followed a range of market regulations from the public authorities, led at the EU level, to assure the consumer and provide a form of choice over the consumption of GM food. This was sought with regulations introducing traceability and labelling-regulation of foods containing or made from (but not with) genetically modified organisms (GMOs).[70] The risk response was a combination of environmental regulation on the one hand, with corporate and market response, and EU market and food safety regulation on the other.

The International Biosafety Protocol, which came under the Biodiversity Convention, incorporated the precautionary principle, which had already been written into European law. The precautionary principle was a policy tool that had been put forward for risk managers in areas of scientific uncertainty. The precautionary principle can be applied in circumstances of scientific uncertainty reflecting the need to take action in the face of potentially serious harm in the absence of scientific proof.[71] The precautionary principle is not a matter for science alone, as it is a political and a value-laden statement expressing a fundamental shift in the attitude of the general public to the environment and risk.[72] The application of the principle raises a set of questions as to when such harm is potentially serious and what is regarded as uncertainty and what is deemed a lack of scientific proof. Answers to such questions may be contested and so become matters of political judgement. The incorporation of the principle into public policy is one response to the advent of the risk society and the need to allow for wider societal discourse around new and innovative applications, not least to our food.

Policy and governance responses to food, the environment, and ecosystems

International regimes and multi-level policy frameworks

The workings of the contemporary food supply and the activities of the agri-food sector to the environment and the earth's ecosystems have promoted policy responses at multi levels from global to regional, to international and sub-national and local. The formation of international regimes through framework conventions, with subsequent binding protocols containing multi-lateral legal instruments, have set frameworks for both regional (such as EU) and national state regulation and sub-national and policy initiatives. International regimes extend to embrace the involvement of wider actors adding epistemic communities of experts, international organizations, trade associations and civil society organizations and alliances (see Chapter 3). International regimes around natural resource protection rapidly expanded from the mid-20th century. From the 1960s and 1970s the common cross-border problems of acid rain and ozone depletion saw nation states further pooling their sovereignty to tackle these shared concerns. The aforementioned UNCED summit of 1992, and the resultant international regimes for biodiversity and climate change, were followed by the World Summit on Sustainable Development (WSSD) in Johannesburg in 2002. The WSSD called for significant improvements in: the supply and quality of water; the use and generation of energy, health and agriculture; and the conservation of biodiversity. At the Johannesburg meeting, the FAO and the World Bank announced a global consultative process on a proposed international assessment of the role of agricultural science and technology for development (IAASTD) which reported its conclusions in 2008.[73]

The existence of these regimes provides an international framework for policy response at the member-state level within the sustainable development discourses. Furthermore, as elaborated in Chapter 3, the WTO agreements, such as the Agreement on Agriculture, and the SPS and TBT agreements, provide a further policy framework for food standards, agricultural policy supports and subsidies, and trade-related issues such as product and process standards and labelling, including food and feed production processes, such as from GMOs. There are unresolved tensions between the terms of the International Biosafety Protocol and the WTO agreements over the reporting demands of the importation of GMOs, for example.

For EU member states, most environmental legislation originates from the EU inter-governmental level. The EU regulations and directives also provide a framework for national policy decisions; or a further stage in the framing of international regime commitments, as with biodiversity and climate change. The policy responses to the agri-environment are also found within the CAP and in the case of Fisheries management within the Common Fisheries Policy (CFP). The dynamics of what has been explained as multi-level governance were explained in Chapter 3, and shape the responses at national and sub- national levels to food and the environment. Other environmental impacts of the agri-food sector are regulated at EU level, including packaging and waste and nitrate and other pollution of water-courses. The regulation and management of the agri-environment and fisheries are considered next.

International regimes provide a framework for national-level policy actions. At the national level, engagement by the main participants along the supply chain is crucial to food policy: from farmers, growers and fisherfolk at one end, to consumers at the other end. The next sections focus on these policy responses with particular attention paid to the UK to illustrate national policy responses. The picture that emerges is one of hesitancy but increasing engagement. But there is a lack of policy integration and of clarity in policy direction. These weaknesses have to be addressed in order to meet the step changes necessary in the state of the environment and the ecosystems for a food policy that is appropriate for the 21st century.

Improving the agri-environment and fisheries

The main direction of agricultural policy has focused for the greater part of the past 60 years on improving levels of production, not only by offering support for technological applications and extension service advice but also through agricultural subsidies for farmers, offering protection in the market-place. In EU member states, the CAP provided market protection for producers through a combination of: guaranteed minimum prices for selected commodities, and tariff protection by taxing imports, and, finally, through intervention to buy up surplus production, thus maintaining price levels. The surplus was put into store, hence the so-called butter mountains and the milk lakes, or was subsidised and sold overseas depressing world prices at the expense of producers from other countries. The export-led support for agricultural production had been a feature of US agricultural subsidies from the mid-20th century, and were increasingly focused on the production of selected commodities produced on a large scale. In the case of the CAP, subsidies began to be dismantled slowly under the disciplines of the WTO policed Agreement on Agriculture, leading to reforms that switched supports to 'green box' compliant schemes that were increasingly de-coupled from production (see Chapter 3 for more detail). The core of the most recent reform is a single farm payment, whereby farmers are paid for the provision of agreed public goods. In general terms, this means the maintenance of agricultural land, including permanent pasture, in good agricultural and environmental condition. Payment support is dependent upon cross-compliance with a range of regulations covering environmental protection, animal and plant health, animal welfare and food safety. Some national exemptions allow production supports for politically sensitive produce to be more slowly decoupled.

In an earlier phase of subsidy reform, the agri-environment measures (Regulation 2078/92) were introduced—but these were only about 5% of the CAP budget before the 2003 reforms. Another, albeit inadvertent, benefit to biodiversity and farmland birds, was the related introduction of payments for a limited amount of land to be set-aside from production as part of the reforms of the early 1990s.[74] However, this programme is due to be ended from 2008. Also, biodiversity conservation has been targeted under EU and national responses to the Convention on Biodiversity. In the case of England in 2008, less than 40% of species and habitats were stable or improving, reflecting 50 years of adverse impacts that have stabilized only over the past decade.[75] Regulatory measures have been introduced, which impacted upon the management of the agri-environment, such as the EU Nitrates from Agricultural Sources Directive (91/676), which has spawned successive action plans for managing agricultural run-off, including the identification of Nitrate Vulnerable Zones where intensive farming practices seriously affect water-courses. Progress in ameliorating such pollution problems has been slow.[14] In addition, there are the measures that have evolved under the more general EU Water Framework Directive, which apply along the length of the food-supply chain and address areas of water catchments. Farming's role in reducing climate change and GHGs has also been signalled in the UK's Rural Climate Change Forum, set up under Defra in 2005, composed of key stake-holders from the farming industry, landowners, conservation and wildlife institutions and groups. The forum has focused on communicating research to farmers about reducing GHG emissions, mitigation strategies, and harnessing farm waste into energy sources through anaerobic digestion.[76]

The dominant form of agriculture in developed countries, and increasingly in developing countries, has been described as industrial or productionist agriculture, although in policy discourse the term conventional agriculture is used, reflecting the pre-eminence of this approach to farming in public policy. The term conventional agriculture also allows for other farming systems to be categorized, usually under the title of alternative agriculture. In response to concerns about the adverse impacts of the conventional model, a variety of different approaches to farming have emerged. The FAO has promoted an approach termed as 'conservation agriculture' based upon the principles of: minimal soil disturbance, permanent soil cover and crop rotations. Conservation agriculture is targeted, in particular, at smallholder farmers as a method for achieving profitable agricultural production alongside environmental and ecological goals.[77] Conventional agriculture has adopted management strategies to mitigate specific problems, such as nitrates regulation and agri-environment schemes, to protect areas vulnerable to intensive farming practices. Strategies to reduce pesticide use at the farm level, for example, have led to the introduction of integrated farm management (IFM) and integrated pest-control techniques and grower protocols. These protocols have been certified for the market-place through schemes such as Linking the Environment and Framing (LEAF), set up 1991 in the UK, and promoted by the larger scale retailers. Similarly, individual retailers have taken initiatives around phasing-out some pesticides from use in their food suppliers ahead of public regulation (see Chapter 3).

The market initiatives utilize a combination of standards setting and accreditation, backed by audit and traceability, and labelling instruments, which shift more responsibility to the consumer as a method of achieving policy outcomes. To a large extent, the private corporate managers of supply chains amongst the large food manufacturers and retailers, have led this approach. Private governance of supply chains, as identified in Chapter 5, is a key component of the retailer and buyer ascendancy over the terms of trade over suppliers along food-supply chains. Private governance has burgeoned from farm and food assurance schemes, to segregation of GM from non-GM food ingredients, and, from intervention and purchasing of organic foods to IFM protocols with growers. These protocols include international and collaborative corporate-led standards, such as the European Retailer Good Agricultural Practice standards (EUREPGAP)—later renamed GLOBALGAP to signify its reach. The large European food manufacturers, in turn, have also set up collaborative compliance schemes for suppliers such as the Sustainable Agriculture Initiative (SAI) platform created by Unilever, Danone and Nestle in 2002.[78]

The most developed amongst the alternative agriculture approaches is organic farming, which sees 'the farm as an organism... a coherent, self-regulating and stable whole' rather than seeing farming in terms of external inputs to be applied and managed in a more environmentally beneficial manner.[79] Organic agriculture offers some clear environmental advantages in terms of not applying inorganic fertilizers or most synthetic pesticides; but, with reduced production levels, it does not necessarily make it more efficient in terms of land to energy input ratios or in terms of GHG emissions.[44] The EU agri-environment supports have recognized the environmental benefits of organic farming, with specific financial supports for conversion to organic farming and subsequent environmental stewardship. Organic food has seen remarkable growth in market demand, and has been probably the most successful of the farming marques amongst consumers, but remains a very small percentage of overall agricultural production.

A related theme being highlighted within conventional and alternative farming systems are the attempts to make agriculture more sustainable. Pretty has identified the key components of sustainable agriculture, as needing to draw upon, and in turn sustain, both natural capital and social capital.[25] Natural capital (including soil, water, air, plants, animals and ecosystems) has to be integrated in agricultural systems in the form of regenerative technologies, such as: use of nitrogen-fixing plants for soil conservation, use of natural predators for pest control, integration of animals into cropped systems. Social capital entails utilizing: farmer and community labour, and knowledge and experience; and underpinning community cohesion. The aim is to achieve enhancement of both the quality and quantity of wildlife, water, landscape and other public goods of the countryside. The importance of greater reliance upon natural organic inputs, farmer participation and reduction of external and non-renewable inputs, is also reflected in the emergence of the principles of agro-ecology as a model for small and peasant farmers, particularly in developing countries.[80] The principles of agro-ecology have been embraced by the food sovereignty movement of peasant farmers' organizations movements. The concept of food sovereignty was launched by Via Campesina (the small and peasant farmers' organization) at the World Food Summit in Rome in 1996, and called for the 'rights of peoples, communities and countries to define their own agricultural, labour, fishing, food and land policies, which are ecologically, socially, economically and culturally appropriate to their unique circumstances'.[81]

The IAASTD was initiated by the World Bank in open partnership with a multi-stakeholder group of organizations, including FAO, GEF, UNDP, UNEP, WHO and UNESCO and representatives of governments, civil society, private sector and scientific institutions. It depicted its process of gathering evidence and opinions as being 'a strongly consultative "bottom-up" process that recognizes the different needs of different regions and communities'.[73] However, missing from the signatories to the IAASTD's report were some of the major large-scale agricultural commodity exporting countries. Amongst the stakeholders, the biotechnology companies withdrew before the conclusion of the process. The report warned that: 'Degradation of ecosystem functions (e.g. nutrient and water cycling), constrains production and may limit the ability of agricultural systems to adapt to climatic and other global changes in many regions' and it identifies that 'sustainable agricultural practices are part of the solution to current environmental change'.[82] In particular, emphasis is placed on the role of smallholder farmers in these processes, not least because 'agriculture provides a livelihood for 40% of the global population and 70% of poor in developing countries live in rural areas and are directly or indirectly dependent on agriculture for their livelihood'.[82] Examples of practices that will abate climate change include: 'improved carbon storage in soil and biomass, reduced emissions of CH_4 and N_2O from rice paddies and livestock systems, and decreased use of inorganic fertilizers'.[82] Public policies are identified as key in providing the frameworks for these solutions. Conversely, the example of the rush to replace food and feed crops with crop plantings for bio-fuels that was incentivized by some governments (including the USA and the EU) as a green solution to carbon-based fuels, has been widely criticized as being poorly thought through.[82] Not least, this is due to the impacts of large-scale bio-fuel plantings upon global food supply and food commodity prices, and so food availability for the world's poor. In this case, the win-win approach of economic gain through environmental innovation has not been achieved.

The policy response to resource management of fisheries has been mixed. International law has been based on open access to the seas and fisheries. The result has been a complex iteration of changes to the Laws of the Sea over time. This included granting of national rights for exclusive fishing or economic zones up to 200 miles off national shores. The collapsing state of many natural fisheries led the FAO to propose a responsible fisheries code in the mid-1990s.[2] The FAO has put particular emphasis upon regional fisheries management organizations as the way forward to manage the conservation of stocks in such complex areas of overlapping jurisdictions. However, this approach has had muted success and has struggled to adopt wider ecosystem management approaches, resulting in criticism from civil society and environmental NGOs. In addition, stronger regulation, with restrictive catch quotas imposed upon the fishing industry, has been used, for example, under the EU's fisheries policy, the CFP. While this has managed the industry's capacity, such approaches have not always matched wider ecosystem needs; for example, in the North Sea, which is bordered by the UK and mainland Europe.[83] Furthermore fishing fleets are not confined to regional areas but trawl the high seas, meaning that European boats fish waters of the African coast and elsewhere. Bilateral agreements are made between the EU and individual states but this is rarely a partnership of equals. Aquaculture lacks efficient regulation and most governance is industry-led, involving HAACP-type protocols and the like.[84] The corporate sector and civil society organizations have sought to develop market-certification schemes to inform consumers and other participants in the food-supply chain of the advantages of sourcing from sustainable managed fisheries, as with Unilever and the WWF who established the Marine Stewardship Conservation (MSC) scheme (see Chapter 3). The MSC certifies catch from 4% of the world's fisheries but this includes fisheries that are depleted and so is not endorsed by environmental campaign groups such as Greenpeace.[19]

Environmental re-governance and the food-supply chain

Post-farm-gate there are three main areas of environmental impact that have been identified: water use, reduction in waste and packaging, and reduction of GHG emissions alongside greater energy efficiency. Focusing primarily on the responses generated within the UK, the supply chain's actions are shaped, for the most part, by framing legislation emerging at inter-governmental levels (global and EU, or just EU) leading to national governmental responses within these frameworks. The UK State operating at its different levels and across its different institutional remits has sought a variety of inducements to the supply chain. The policy instruments of contemporary governance have been employed. Harder regulatory standards and economic instruments (such as the Landfill Tax), have been supplemented with softer instruments of longer term target-setting, often reflecting uncertain aspirations, such as around reductions in CO_2 emissions, voluntary agreements with industry and further gathering of evidence (such as life-cycle analysis). In these ways the state has sought to mobilize the supply chain to identify with, and seek, common goals for environmental and ecosystem improvement. There has been some positive movement here, not least because the dynamics of corporate response and private governance along the supply chain have led key corporate players to take initiatives on their own, or collectively, through trade associations, such as the British Retail Consortium (BRC) or the Food and Drink Federation (FDF). Such corporate responses have signalled recognition that there is a strong business case for action, notably by the retailers as they have sought to find reliable and resilient supplies of food products. The banner of corporate social responsibility (CSR) has been unfurled to capture the wider impacts of these strategic business decisions and the importance of placing sustainability within business strategy. These actors had responded in similar ways in endorsing and promoting some of the more benign agricultural production methods, such as IFM, and in establishing them as criteria for procurement from suppliers, and in messages to their customers. In the case of resilience of supply, retailers are witnessing first-hand the vagaries of climate change upon harvests, as their opportunities for supplying customers' wishes for particular products at particular times from across the globe are becoming restricted at very short notice.

Another emerging feature of the policy response has been the consideration of how consumer and citizen support can be engaged in reaching sustainability objectives. This is reflected in the EU's Sustainable Development Strategy, which includes sustainable consumption and production amongst its key themes.[85] The puzzle remains as how to engage step changes in consumption behaviour; partly in order to send the right signals back down the supply chain to production. This has largely fallen to certification schemes and standards-setting for suppliers, and the labelling of products to inform consumers. Market-place instruments, such as labelling, have a role but they can effectively transfer decision-making responsibility back to the consumer, who often remains ignorant at worst or confused at best with their role. The need to move on to a better understanding of the consumption–production link is under-stood by policy-makers. For example, the UK Sustainable Consumption Roundtable's report *I will, if you will* highlights the problem of identifying how to motivate consumers and citizens to make step changes towards sustain ability in their behaviour.[86] Defra, at government department level, has fol-lowed this up with a detailed investigation of the characteristics of sustainable consumption habits, identities and potential barriers and drivers amongst the British public.[87] Put in ecological modernization terms, the search is on to find how to achieve the inculcation and adoption of ecological values by the public. The Roundtable report identifies the role of choice-editing as important, with the retailers amongst the key choice-editors or gate-keepers in the supply chain. Most key actors are now involved in forms of certification and labelling.

The EU has identified the greening of public procurement as a key policy instrument in achieving more sustainable consumption and production.[85] In the UK, public sector bodies serve around 3.5 million meals per weekday, spending approximately £2 billion each year with 50% of that amount spent in schools.[36] There has been an ongoing policy tension at national level over the priority for public procurement between the priority of achieving far greater savings in costs, or best value, and using it as a policy instrument for environmental objectives.[88] Defra's Strategy for Sustainable Farming and Food led to the setting up of the Public Sector Food Procurement Initiative (PSFPI) in 2003, which has sought to balance the objectives of promoting healthy food with those of improving sustainability and efficiency. The Strategy saw public procurement as a tool for sourcing good-value local produce in season, tailored to healthy-eating menus in the public sector, but evidence from the ground suggests that these goals are proving hard to realize, although there are islands of good practice in a sea of mediocrity.[89] The introduction of a range of measures under the Government's Sustainable Procurement Action Plan in 2007 aimed 'to ensure that supply chains and public services will be increasingly low carbon, low waste and water efficient, respect biodiversity and deliver wider sustainable development goals'.[90] These fine sentiments aside, a significant policy-implementation challenge remains to entrench sustainable food procurement across a wide range of public institutions, caterers and contracts in quite different sectors, from prisons to hospitals, from schools to army barracks and to government department canteens.

In the case of the UK Government, we are witnessing a hesitant state in terms of policy responses. In part, the state is caught in the dilemma of being aware that action is needed but being unsure of how best to proceed. There is policy engagement on a number of fronts, as explained above and detailed further below, but many of the actions taken to date are exploratory and so lack integration.[38] The governance tools that have been developed by the State in recent times are important but questions remain as to their effectiveness. Will the State, and the international community, need to switch to crisis mode and, if so, when? In the mean time, the environmental challenges emanating from the food-supply chain are being addressed by these mixed governance modes. There are some precautionary initiatives, some areas where problems are still being interpreted (such as embedded water) and a range of relatively unco-ordinated responses across both public and private governance, such as in relation to reducing carbon.

The incorporation of business into the national sustainability strategies included the Food Industry Sustainability Strategy (FISS) agreed between Defra and key industry stakeholders in 2006.[91] The FISS covered a wide range of areas from sustainable consumption and production to social issues like nutrition, food safety and ethical trading to science-based innovation and labour skills. Better regulation was another goal, which was defined as regulation with a lighter touch, reducing compliance costs upon industry in order to enhance international economic competitiveness. The key environmental priorities were around energy use and climate change, food transportation, waste and water use.[91] Various Champions groups were created to allow the corporate stakeholders to lead the changes in partnerships with arm's length government supported programmes or bodies, such as Envirowise and the Waste Reduction Action Programme (WRAP). LCA impacts of food products were encouraged and sponsored by both government grants and individual businesses. In the case of water, the food industry was encouraged to reduce water abstraction and use, and to enhance water-use efficiency with best practice promoted and disseminated by Envirowise. The Water Champions Group also encouraged the greater awareness of, and reduction in, embedded water.[92]

The regulatory frameworks for packaging and food waste are based on the targets set for member states under the EU Packaging and Packaging Waste

Directive and the EU Landfill Directive. The packaging targets are to increase the amount of food transit and product packaging that is recycled and the national policy response is contained in the Waste Strategy for England 2007, which includes reduction in household waste. The main elements of the strategy have been criticized by the Sustainable Development Commission (SDC), the Government's own environmental watchdog body, for being too focused on downstream measures in the waste stream and not enough on upstream.[38] The downstream measures were also criticized for relying too much on self-regulation through vague targets, and for setting insufficient cost penalties and overly weak enforcement monitoring to catalyse sufficient change in business behaviour.[38] An example of the self-regulation was the incorporation into the strategy of the Courtauld Commitment between WRAP and 13 retailers to reduce packaging and food waste.[50] Individual retailers have taken up the challenge with their own individual strategies and target-setting, for example, in phasing out the use of plastic carrier bags.[38] The UK Government had achieved some modest success, through the introduction of the Landfill Tax in 1996, in reducing the amount of waste in landfill. The EU Landfill Directive introduced much more ambitious targets, calling for a reduction of biodegradable municipal waste, mainly household in origin, by two-thirds of its 1995 level by 2020. The tax rate has been substantially raised by the Government for GHG-emitting waste to help to meet this target.[38]

In the push to reduce carbon, there are international protocols, EU-related targets and national targets, and the formulation of national actions appearing. At the international level, the Kyoto Protocol of 1997 has been a first step at legally binding international action. The UK Government has an international commitment to reduce GHG emissions by 12.5% over the period 2008–12, from baseline 1990 levels, through the Kyoto Protocol, which came into force in February 2005. The EU and its Member States agreed to an 8% target, subsequently reallocated between Member States to reflect national circumstances; this increased the UK's commitment to 12.5%. However, the GHG reductions under the Kyoto Protocol are already seen as insufficient for meeting the needs to simply stabilize climate change, let alone reduce its impacts.[28, 33] The UK also has a domestic goal to cut GHG emissions by at least 26% by 2010 and by 60% by 2050, relative to 1990 levels; these targets are in the Climate Change Bill which became law in late 2008.[93] The Climate Change Bill puts the policy more firmly at the heart of decision-making by placing a duty on the Government to assess the risk to the UK from the impacts of climate change. A Committee on Climate Change will advise the Government on the levels of carbon budgets to be set, the balance between domestic emissions reductions and the use of carbon credits, and whether the 2050 target should be increased. The Bill provided powers to establish trading schemes, following the EU's emission trading scheme, for the purpose of limiting GHGs through the Carbon Reduction Commitment.[94]

Under the FISS, a voluntary target was set with the food industry of reductions in GHG emissions of 20% by 2010, which was considered achievable under wider dissemination of current good practice and technologies.[95] Parts of the supply chain also come under other voluntary government and industry agreements, such as the Climate Change Agreements, which include bakeries but only partially covers refrigeration in the supply chain.[38] These in turn will need to merge with the new Carbon Reduction Commitment, which will authorize emissions trading and will cover targets for large emitters, such as supermarkets and their distribution centres. Defra is also co-ordinating work on standards around the use methodologies for measuring GHG impacts of food products and supply chains.[38] The food retailers have identified transport as a key contributor to GHGs but there are no government policies targeting or rewarding efficiencies made in this part of their operations.[38] Meanwhile, the large food retailers in the UK and elsewhere are setting in place innovative measures to identify and to reduce carbon use. Tesco's auditing of its carbon use across its whole operation was highlighted in Chapter 5. Other examples include: Tesco and Marks and Spencer's introduction of air miles labels; and Tesco's auditing of the carbon footprint of a range of food products in tandem with the UK Carbon Trust, which is another government-sponsored company set up in 2001.[38] The overall policy picture is one of some confusion and a high level of flux as policy seeks to respond to the changing scientific evidence concerning the rates of climate change.

The food sector is a contributor to environmental and ecosystem change. These changes are impacting directly upon the food supply in turn. An environmental re-governance is occurring along food-supply chains, reflecting some of the features of ecological modernization. This re-governance is framed by international agreements and EU regulation that is subsequently re-interpreted for implementation at the national level. From the examples given from the UK, and, within the UK, more particularly England, the re-governance is heavily reliant upon the co-operation of the key actors in supply chains, notably the retailers and food manufacturers who have the expertise and the capabilities to deliver changes. A feature of the response is the State's creation of new bodies in the form of advisory programmes, such as WRAP, or consultancies, such as Envirowise, or companies, such as The Carbon Trust. These bodies operate at arms' length from central government control and are immersed into partnership with the stakeholders, who are predominantly private corporations and their trade associations. The creation of these bodies and these governance arrangements extend the reach of the central government policy-makers but can diminish their degree of control and the accountability for the decisions made. The co-ordination and integration of this process is both complex and weak at present. This reflects a certain hesitance, particularly in the setting of appropriate targets by Government in the UK, but also within international regimes such as the Kyoto Protocol, to induce significant behaviour change along the supply chain. For food policy the demands of the environment need an integrated policy response and a prioritizing across policy sectors.

At the production end of the supply chain, EU farmers are being led to environmentally beneficial actions through the carrots of subsidies upon which they have become dependent. However, there are substantial areas of dispute over the best ways and places to apply different farming approaches, as the IAASTD process revealed. At the other end of the supply chain, great credence is given to policy instruments in the market-place, such as labelling and certification schemes, to direct the consumer to change to more sustainable consumption. Yet it is clear that there needs to be substantial changes in both production and consumption actions and behaviour to bring about such sustainability outcomes in the food supply. To these ends, policy-makers have not found many of the answers yet; but some of the right questions are beginning to be asked. Step changes are needed to ensure the health of the environment and our ecosystems, and the future quality of our food supply and human health; but these substantial step changes are still to be made. The undertaking and completion of these step changes are fundamental to food policy.

References

1. Millennium Ecosystem Assessment (Program). *Ecosystems and human well-being: synthesis.* Washington, DC: Island Press, 2005.
2. FAO. *The state of world fisheries and aquaculture 2006.* Rome: Food and Agriculture Organization, 2007.
3. Lang T, Heasman M. *Food wars: the global battle for mouths, minds and markets.* London: Earthscan, 2004.
4. Costa-Pierce BA. Use of ecosystems science in ecological aquaculture. *Bulletin of the Aquaculture Association of Canada* 2003;**103**:32–40.
5. Krkosek M, Lewis MA, Volpe JP. Transmission dynamics of parasitic sea lice from farm to wild salmon. *Proceedings of the Royal Society B* 2005;**272**:689–696.
6. Krkosek M, Lewis MA, Morton A, Frazer LN, Volpe JP. Epizootics of wild fish induced from farm fish. *Proceedings of the National Academy of Sciences* 2006;**103**:15506–15510.
7. Naylor R, Burke M. Aquaculture and ocean resources: raising tigers of the sea. *Annual Review of Environmental Resources* 2005;**30**:185–218.
8. Naylor R, Hindar K, Fleming IA, Goldburg R, Williams S, Volpe JP *et al.* Fugitive salmon: assessing the risks of escaped fish from net-pen aquaculture. *Bioscience* 2005;**55**:1–11.
9. Tacon A, Forster I. Aquafeeds and the environment: policy considerations. *Aquaculture* 2003;**226**:181–189.

10. Heller MC, Keoleian GA. Life cycle based sustainability indicators for assessment of the US. In: Arbor A (ed.) *Food system* MI: University of Michigan: Center for Sustainable Systems, 2000.

11. Weiss T. *The global food economy: the battle for the future of farming*. London: Zed Books, 2007.

12. Lang T, Clutterbuck C. *P is for pesticides*. London: Ebury, 1991.

13. Defra. *Farming and food's contribution to sustainable development: the current situation and future prospects—economic and statistical analysis*. London: Department for Environment, Food and Rural Affairs, 2002.

14. OECD. *Environmental performance of agriculture in OECD countries since 1990*. www.oecd.org/tad/env/indicators [accessed 18 June 2008]. Paris: OECD, 2008.

15. Clunies-Ross T, Hildyard N. *The politics of industrial agriculture*. London: Earthscan, 1992.

16. Environment Agency. *Agriculture and natural resources: benefits, costs and potential solutions*. http://www.environment-agency.gov.uk/commondata/acrobat/natrespt1_673325.pdf (accessed 11 June 2008). London: Environment Agency, 2002.

17. UNEP. Global Environmental Outlook 2000. Nairobi: United Nations Environment Programme, 2000.

18. AEA. *Scoping studies to identify opportunities for improving resource use efficiency and for reducing waste through the food production chain*. London: Department for Environment, Food and Rural Affairs, 2007.

19. Greenpeace International. *Eating up the Amazon*. Amsterdam: Greenpeace International, 2006.

20. Friends of the Earth. *Greasy palms*. London: Friends of the Earth, 2005.

21. FAO. *State of the world's plant genetic resources*. Rome: Food and Agriculture Organization, 1996.

22. Pretty JN, Brett C, Gee D, Hine R, Mason CF, Morison JIL *et al*. An assessment of the total external costs of UK agriculture. *Agricultural Systems* 2000;**65**(2):113–136.

23. Potts R. Cereal farming, pesticides and grey partridges in Farming and Birds. In: Pain D, Pienowski M (ed.) *Europe: The Common Agricultural Policy and its implications for bird conservation*. London: Academic, 1997:155–177.

24. Defra. *Agricultural statistics in your pocket 2007*. London: Department for Environment, Food and Rural Affairs, 2007.

25. Pretty J. *The living land*. London: Earthscan, 1998.

26. Hartridge O, Pearce D. *Is UK agriculture sustainable? Environmentally adjusted economic accounts for UK agriculture*. London: CSERGE Economics UCL, 2001.

27. Waterwise. *Hidden water and our true consumption*. London: Waterwise, 2007.

28. IPPC. *Intergovernmental Panel on Climate Change Fourth Assessment Report: climate change 2007: the physical science basis: summary for policymakers*. http://www.ipcc.ch/SPM2feb07.pdf [accessed 24 June 2008]. IPCC, 2007.

29. Tukker A, Huppes G, Guinée J, Heijungs R, de Koning A, van Oers L *et al*. *Environmental Impact of Products (EIPRO): analysis of the life cycle environmental impacts related to the final consumption of the EU-25. EUR 22284 EN*. Brussels: European Commission Joint Research Centre, 2006.

30. Garnett T. *Overall UK consumption related GHGs*. Guildford: Centre for Environmental Strategy University of Surrey, 2007.

31. FAO. *Livestock's Long Shadow—environmental issues and options*. Rome: Food and Agriculture Organization, 2006.

32. Fairlie S. A load of hot air? *The Guardian* 30 January 2008.

33. Stern SN. *The economics of climate change. The report of the Stern Review*. Cambridge: Cambridge University Press, 2007.

34. Willis R. What price carbon? *Green Futures* 2008(69):32–33.

35. World Resources Institute. *Disappearing food: how big are postharvest losses?* http://earthtrends.wri.org/pdf_library/feature/agr_fea_disappear.pdf (accessed 20 June 2008) 1998.

36. Strategy Unit. *Food: an analysis of the issues*. London: Cabinet Office, 2007.

37. Scottish Executive, AEA Technology. *Proposed plastic bag levy—extended impact assessment*. Edinburgh: Scottish Executive Waste Strategy Team, 2005.

38. SDC. *Green, healthy and fair: a review of government's role in supporting sustainable supermarket food*. London: Sustainable Development Commission, 2008.

39. Defra. *The environment in your pocket 2007*. London: Department for Environment, Food and Rural Affairs, 2007.

40. Lang T. Locale/globale (food miles). *Slow Food* 2006(19):94–97.

41. Paxton A. *The food miles report*. London: Sustainable Agriculture, Food and Environment (SAFE) Alliance, 1994.

42. Gairdner J. *Local food is miles better: the farmers weekly food campaign*. Crawley: Reed Business Information, 2006.

43. Saunders P. *A nation of home owners*. London: Unwin Hyman, 1990.

44. Williams A, Audsley E, Sandars D. *Determining the environmental burdens and resource use in the production of agricultural and horticultural commodities*. Main report. Defra project report IS0205. Bedford: Cranfield University and Defra, 2006.

45. Edwards-Jones G, Milà i Canals L, Hounsome N, Truninger M, Koerber G, Hounsome B *et al*. Testing the assertion that 'local food is best': the challenges of an evidence-based approach. *Trends in Food Science & Technology* 2008;**19**(5):265–274.

46. DFID. *Fair and accurate food pricing needed to protect environment and support poor farmers*. Press Release http://www.dfid.gov.uk/news/files/pressreleases/airfreight.asp (accessed 20 June 2008). London: Department for International Development, 2007.

47. McGregor J, Vorley B. *Fair miles? The concept of 'food miles' through a sustainable development lens. Sustaiable development opinion*. London: IIED, 2006.

48. Natural Resources Institute. *Mapping different supply chains of fresh produce exports from Africa to the UK*. Fresh Insights no. 7, DFID/IIED/NRI, 2006.

49. Allan JA. Virtual water—the water, food and trade nexus: useful concept or misleading metaphor? *Water International*, 2003;**28**:4–11.

50. WRAP. Major retailers join wrap in pledging to tackle packaging and food waste http://www.wrap.org.uk/retail/news_events/news/major_retailers.html (accessed on 22 June 2008) 26 July, 2005.

51. GlobalGAP. *Eurepgap becomes Globalgap on Sept 7 2007 at Bangkok conference*. http://www.globalgap.org/cms/front_content.php?idcat=9&idart=182 [accessed Sept 23 2007]. Cologne Germany: GLOBALGAP, 2007.

52. Weale A. *The new politics of pollution*. Manchester: Manchester University Press, 1992.

53. O'Riordon T. *Environmentalism*. London: Pion, 1981.

54. Dobson A. *Green political thought*, 2nd edn. London: Routledge, 1995.

55. Meadows DH, Meadows D.L, Randers J, Behrens WW. *The limits to growth*. London: Earth Island, 1972.

56. Naess A. The shallow and the deep, long-range ecology movement: a summary. *Inquiry* 1973(16):95–99.

57. WCED. *Our common future: the report of the World Commission on Environment and Development*. Oxford: Oxford University Press, 1987.

58. European Commission. Towards sustainability: a European Community programme of policy and action in relation to the environment and sustainable development. *Official Journal of the European Communities* 1993; C(138):5–98.

59. Baker S, Kousis M, Richardson D., Young S. (eds.) *The politics of sustainable development. Theory, policy and practice within the European Union*. London: Routledge, 1997.

60. Jacobs M. Introduction: the new politics of the environment. In: Jacobs M (eds) *Greening the Millennium? The new politics of the environment*. Oxford: Blackwell Publishing, 1997:10.

61. Mol A, Sonnenfield D. Ecological modernization around the world: an introduction. *Environmental Politics* 2000;**9**(1):3–16.

62. Hajer M. *The politics of environmental discourse: ecological modernization and the policy process*. Clarendon: Oxford, 1995.

63. Christoff P. Ecological modernization, ecological modernities. *Environmental Politics* 1996;**5**(3):476–500.

64. van Zwanenberg P, Millstone E. *BSE: risk, science, and governance*. Oxford: Oxford University Press, 2005.

65. Beck U. *Risk society: towards a new modernity*. London: Sage Publications, 1992.

66. Beck U. Politics in the global risk society. In: Jacobs M (ed.) *Greening the millennium? The new politics of the environment*. Oxford: Blackwell Publishing, 1997:18–33.

67. Lidner S. The social and political (re)construction of risk. In: Kamieniecki S, Gonzakz GA, & Voz (ed.). *Flashpoints in environmental policymaking: controversies in achieving sustainability*. Albany: State University of New York Press, 1997.

68. Barling D. GM crops, biodiversity and the European agri-environment: regulatory lacunae and revision. *European Environment* 2000;**10**(4):167–177.

69. Barling D. Regulating GM foods in the 1980s and 1990s. In: Smith DF, Phillips J (ed.) *Food, science, policy and regulation in the twentieth century: international and comparative perspectives. Routledge studies in the social history of medicine 10*. London: Routledge, 2000:239–256.

70. Barling D, Lang T, Caraher M. Joined-up food policy? The trials of governance, public policy and the food system. *Social Policy & Administration* 2002;**36**(6):556–574.

71. Barling D, de Vriend H, Cornelese J, Ekstrand B, Hecker E, Howlett J et al. The social aspects of food biotechnology: a European view. *Environmental Toxicology and Pharmacology* 1999;**7**:85–92.

72. O' Riordan T, Cameron C. *Interpreting the precautionary principle*. London: Earthscan, 2001.

73. IAASTD. *Global report and synthesis report*. London: International Assessment of Agricultural Science and Technology, 2008.

74. RSPB. *Loss of set-aside threatens farmland bird recovery*, http://www.rspb.org.uk/news/details.asp?id=term:9-182116 (accessed 18 June 2008) 2008.

75. Natural England. *The state of the natural environment in England*, www.naturalengland.org.uk (accessed 18 June 2008)2008.

76. Defra. *Climate change: rural climate change forum*, http://www.defra.gov.uk/environment/climatechange/uk/legislation/index.htm (accessed 24 June 2008) 2008.

77. FAO. *Conservation agriculture*, http://www.fao.org/ag/ca/index.html (accessed 19 June 2008) 2008.

78. CIAA. *Managing environmental sustainability in the European food and drink industries: issues, industry action and future strategy*. Brussels: Confederation of the Food and Drink Industries in the EU, 2005.

79. Lampkin N, Lampkin N, Foster C, Padel S, Midmore P. *The policy and regulatory environment for organic farming in Europe: synthesis of results. organic farming in Europe: economics and policy*. Stuttgart: Universität Hohenheim, 1999.

80. Altieri M. *Agroecology: the science of sustainable agriculture*, 2nd edn. London: Intermediate Technology Development Group Publishing, 1995.

81. Peine E, McMichael P. Globalization and global governance. In: Higgins V, Lawrence G (ed.) *Agricultural governance: globalization and the new politics of regulation*. London: Routledge, 2005:19–34.

82. Beintema N, Bossio D, Dreyfus F, Fernandez M, AGurib-Fakim A, Hurni H *et al. Global summary for decision-makers: international assessment of the role of agricultural science and technology for development*, http://www.agassessment.org/docs/Global_SDM_050508_FINAL.pdf (accessed 24 June 2008) 2008.

83. Gray TS (ed.) *Participation in fisheries governance*. Dordrecht: Springer, 2005.

84. Oosterveer P. *Global governance of food production and consumption: issues and challenges*. Cheltenham: Edward Elgar, 2007.

85. Council of the European Union. *Review of the EU sustainable development strategy (EU SDS)—renewed strategy*. Brussels: Council of the European Union,2006:10917/06.

86. National Consumer Council and Sustainable Development Commission. *I will if you will*. Report of the Sustainable Consumption Roundtable. London: Sustainable Development Commission, 2006.

87. Defra. *A framework for pro-environmental behaviours: report*. London: Defra, 2008.

88. Davis L, Dowler E, Hunter D, Lang T, Morgan K. *Food and well being: reducing inequalities through a nutrition strategy for Wales. a mid-term review (2006–7)*. Report to Food Standards Agency Wales. Warwick: University of Warwick, 2007.

89. Sustain. *Policy issues surrounding the sustainable public sector food procurement agenda in the UK: a discussion paper*. London: Sustain, 2007.

90. HM Treasury & Defra. UK Government sustainable procurement action plan. News release, 5 March http://www.defra.gov.uk/news/2007/0703056.htm (accessed 24 June 2008) 2007.

91. FISS. *Food industry sustainability strategy*. London: Department for Environment, Food and Rural Affairs, 2006.

92. FISS. *Report of the food industry sustainability strategy champions' group on water*. London: Department for Environment, Food and Rural Affairs, 2007.

93. HMG. *The climate change programme review*. London: The Stationary Office, 2006.

94. Defra. *UK legislation: taking the climate change bill forward—progress*, http://www.defra.gov.uk/environment/climate change/uk/legislation/index.htm (accessed 24 June 2008) 2008.

95. FISS. *Final submission of the Food Industry Sustainability Strategy Champions' Group on energy and climate change*. London: Department for Environment, Food and Rural Affairs, 2007.

Chapter 7

Behaviour and culture

The history of food is rich in examples of how important its social, cultural and behavioural attributes are for food policy. It is not just communities in strongly religious societies who hold to tight rules of eating. Social scientists argue that social groups have cultural rules of engagement, with norms and expectations of what 'real' food is. At its extreme, this social dimension of food can emerge when expectations are felt to be transgressed; riots can occur when norms or tolerances are trangressed. This chapter and the next explore what this socio-cultural dimension is comprised of. With the return of food's profile in public policy over recent decades, there has been a boom in attention given by social science to food. But this rich body of knowledge has long roots, which also can and should inform food policy-making. In Chapter 2 we noted the domination in formal definitions of food policy or considerations about nutrition (health) and supply chains (economic), but Chapter 4 also noted the importance of social nutrition, whose focus has been on how nutrition is shaped by social context. In this chapter we attend to what the literature and thinking among social scientists say about food culture and the meaning of food. We turn away from health, environment and economy to give full attention to food as social interaction.

The lesson that emerges for policy is that a better blend than is given at present is needed. Political attention is often shaped by urgent material matters—shortages, price rises, uncertainty of supply, market dislocation. Less attention is given to 'soft' policy matters such as what people feel about food or cultural implications. Yet in ecological public health the social dimension deserves equal weight to the biological, material, environmental and economic dimensions. Food is eaten (or not) by people in their everyday lives, so what they think about food and how they approach it in daily existence, are highly relevant. Governments have been slow and, except in times of emergency or war (see Chapter 4), reluctant to include a strong social element in policy, preferring to locate food policy, if at all, under the category of business or health or agriculture. Companies, as we saw in Chapter 5, do not make this error. There was a remarkable commercial uptake in the 20th century of social sciences' data and approaches. Companies formulated their food strategies and marketing using the social sciences.

Part of the success and rapid modern growth of Tesco, a global retailer, for example, lay with its use of consumer data derived from its use of loyalty cards.[1] This gave a picture not just of overall spending but of the minutiae and how they fit into people's life space. Harnessing modern computer power, Tesco's marketing partner, dunnhumby, could build accurate pictures of what people bought, and feed that back to the retailer, which in turn enabled it to refine and restructure supply chains and products.[2, 3] Few products come to market now without going through a screening process to check appropriateness and market fit. Buyer-driven supply chains hinge on an acute understanding of what consumers think before and as they buy. Understanding consumer lifestyles is critical when deciding where to open an outlet, as is an understanding of changing domestic divisions of labour when investing in new products. Such knowledge is critical in the increasing sophistication of business strategies. In 2005, dunnhumby created an Academy of Consumer Research with the University of Kent Business School, sharing a database on 1.2 million supermarket shoppers, a 10% sample of 12 million households (40% of UK total) covering weekly purchases from over 30,000 food products.[4] Such knowledge gives considerable power and depth alongside academic knowledge.

Public policy, of course, makes and engages with the behavioural and consumer aspects of food, and states collect spending and consumption data, but often this is done in a limited fashion and not in the hungry way that business does. Ministers will pronounce that food choice is a given, a sacrosanct pillar for food policy; the individual's right to choose food is paramount. No advertiser, however, takes such a simplistic position; marketers and the entire consciousness industry want to know what determines choice, how extensive it is and whether everyone exerts this in the same way, and how and when behaviour changes.[5] They are interested in behavioural difference, not just consistency or homogeneity. The argument underlying this and the next chapter, therefore, is that the social dimension of food is essential for any 21st century food policy. To ignore this dimension would be to distort reality and also restrict the potential for policy advance. The task of these next chapters is to show how subtle and deep social behaviour is with regard to food.

The approach taken here is that food behaviour can be located within a social process in which consumers are but one set of actors in the food system, and where contexts and social interactions may be set and inherited through wider culture, geography and history, as well as family or domestic circumstance. Policies are engaged with all these levels, factors and drivers. When preparing its new food and nutrition evidence and policy, the WHO European Region represented this multi-level engagement in the form given in Fig. 7.1.

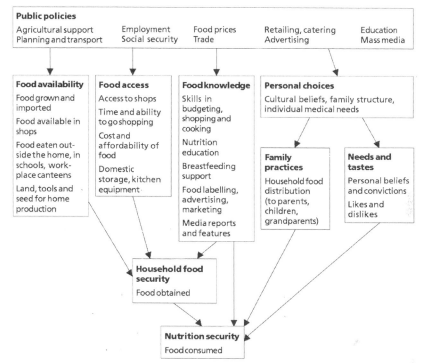

Fig. 7.1 Pathways of influence on Food Choices. Source: Robertson *et al.* (2004).[6]

This suggests just some of the ways policy affect what is consumers and their impact on public health.[6]

Food as culture

Food has deep cultural connotations and vice versa, culture shapes food behaviour and choice, but how culture is thought about and constructed is widely agreed to be in transition.[7] Some argue that change is the normal state of affairs; others that the present transition is deeper and faster than in other times. Social scientists have been leading contributors to these debates; for example, about globalization and how social networks are being laid over existing social class and demographic inheritance.[8] But they have cautioned, too, about how deep or extensive such trends are; for every modernization, there is a resistance. Some social and technical forces might be accelerating change, whiles others provide anchors and drag. They contend that change is not as extensive as its wildest exponents suggest.[9, 10] Despite this caution, few disagree that the pace and scale of change from the 20th century has been remarkable, not least in the acceleration of consumerism and mass spending power. As Mary Douglas, an acute observer of food culture, remarked in 1984:[11]

> Food policies often take no account of the ways in which the use of food is embedded in the social and cultural habits of the people whose diet it is intended to change.

Even she assumed that the policy drive is to change not retain behaviour.

Some social scientists argue that too much thinking about food policy is shaped by dominant political interests. Policy-makers implicitly accept the 'deficit' or 'empty vessel' model, which assumes that people and their food cultures are empty vessels waiting to be filled with better or correct knowledge, and that once this is achieved, they will change their attitude, behaviour and means of operation in the light of the requisite logical advice. This assumes a rational approach to food choice, and proposes that behaviour follows a rational process from information to attitudes to behaviour. It is a much rehearsed (and criticized) model of human action.[12, 13] In fact, food behaviour is subject to a range of influences, of which information and attitudes are certainly a part but only part, and influences such as taste, preferences, culture, income and food availability also play a part. As we noted in Chapter 4, health policy analysts are troubled by different nutrient intake and low fruit and vegetable consumption levels in lower socio-economic groups, but intake is not created by physiological needs alone. Behaviour is shaped by other factors such as taste, familiarity, price signals, convenience, social class, education and time.[14–17] Technology too interacts with culture and social environment, not necessarily health.[18]

In the 20th century, the social and ecological environment changed extensively. New ways of living emerged in which eating patterns altered. Snacking and 'grazing' and eating out of the home and 'on the hoof' became huge markets, serviced by caterers and pre-prepared foods. These have altered what happens in the home, too. Indeed, the shifts inside the home—changed gender roles, women being in waged employment—can contribute to the demotion of food as a household priority. When women have control over food, they tend to give it a higher priority; but when responsibility is shared with men, food assumes a lower priority in the household setting.[19] Changes in women's roles and domestic labour alter food preparation styles.[20, 21] Despite this, responsibility in Western societies is still not equally shared, with women taking the greater burden for domestic chores, particularly those associated with children. Women have eagerly and rightly adopted food technological change in the home to balance these domestic and work obligations. Time saved by women on routine domestic work and cooking is being matched by a corresponding increase in time spent on travel and shopping.[21, 22]

As economies change, domestic and family life alters. In the UK, compared to 1961, people now spend an extra 2 h and 26 min outside the home on eating-out and going-out. Thanks to pre-prepared meals and better cleaning products, people in the UK spend 2 h and 41 min less time doing domestic chores per week.[22] But they spend 2 h and 48 min per week more on shopping and associated travelling to food suppliers, largely because of the growth of out-of-town supermarkets.[23–25] Anthropologically, 'foraging and gathering' still remain an issue but what those practices mean, in the 21st century, has altered. Liberation from the kitchen and cooking has been replaced for women by a different responsibility—the gathering and assembly of food.

One of the failings of the 'empty vessel' model, if applied to food behaviour, is that it almost lends itself to conspiracy; advertising becomes depicted as all-controlling, stripping humans of volition. In this narrative, from being just a powerful input, marketing becomes omniscient.[26] It is not just inaccurate but probably patronizing to describe consumers in this way. Collectively they are partially led and enticed, of course, and on occasions more than we all like to admit; but to describe all consumer actions as wholly manipulated would be excessive. As we suggested in Chapter 5, there is a 'pull' as well as 'push' in the relationship between consumers and supply chains. Within social science there is a long tradition of debate and research on how far people are controlled by, or free from, powerful commercial or State forces, from which it is clear that the balance of power between social forces varies and is dynamic.[27] But for the present discussion of food policy, and its interest in what and how people eat, and when and why this changes, it would be a mistake to assume people are either totally free or constrained. More subtlety is required. The need to conceptualize people, as thinking and acting beings within socially created and meaningful conditions, is a more appropriate conceptual basis for thinking about food policy. This was why, for example, in his influential 1937 essay on the emergence of firms, the Nobel prize-winning economist Ronald Coase adopted the view that firms are the emergence of 'islands of consciousness power' in a particular organizational form.[28] Firms don't just exist; they are made by humans in concert, for reasons, within legal frameworks. His analysis articulated the cultural infrastructure within business. It is exactly in this vein that we propose food choice as deliberative, not only reactive. Food behaviour is no more a puppet of circumstance than is a firm. Food is a point of social interaction. This in part explains the heatedness of some debates within social science about food; as the director of a large mid-1990s UK social science programme on food said, 'the social sciences are not unitary'.[29]

In the 1980s and early 1990s, one heated social scientific debate in the UK was about whether mainstream retailers had abandoned the poor and shaped choice.[30, 31] Scottish campaigners first spoke out in the 1980s about some major cities having 'food deserts' where food availability and shops were sparse.[32, 33] Some studies showed their existence;[34, 35] others did not.[36] It is probable that food-access problems did and do exist in some locations at some times; the 1980s and 1990s were a period when big retailers were squeezing independent and small shops into closure.[37] Once they had consolidated their huge investments in out-of-town car-based hypermarkets, retailers saw growth opportunities in-town both in smaller stores and redesigning supermarkets to increase floor space.[38] This occurred not least because public policy began to close the door to further expansion. Notably this happened in France via *la loi Raffarin*, limiting hypermarkets and requiring local food-supply chain logistics.[39] The discussion on inequalities goes to the heart of food power.[40]

Food culture: a contentious concept?

To define food culture can be difficult, which has led some to caution against its uncritical use.[41] By food culture we mean the shared assumptions, meanings, social interactions, practices and mores that are exhibited in daily food behaviour. These meanings and assumptions may not always be directly related to food but to practices around food, which shape food behaviour. Food cultures are both inherited and made, via experience in families and wider society. It is not the word 'culture' that causes the difficulties, although it covers many processes, but the complexity of dissection. We retain the term, not least to guard against a reductionist and over-individualized understanding of food behaviour (see Chapter 4). The food policy lexicon has to go beyond the individual–family–society to grasp the social aspects of food. Acknowledging the social meanings associated with food, its collective and group understandings, the social practices within which social groups and households relate through food ought to be central to any policy process. After the 1980s to 1990s wave of food safety scandals in Europe, there was a rush to include 'consumers' into policy processes. This was welcomed but could, consumer organizations felt, appear tokenistic. In 2008, the UK's Food Standards Agency took a more measured step when it created a social science research committee to build a deeper engagement, a recommendation of an earlier health report.[42]

Food culture is a useful concept for policy, not least since governments are belatedly recognizing its importance, something long known, as we have suggested, by the commercial sector; why else has it invested in advertising? It was to tackle the cultural dimension of obesity that in 2008 the UK's Department of Health initiated a £75 m 'Change4Life' social marketing campaign (not all of it about food), a scale not seen since the concern about unprotected sex as a factor in the spread of HIV-aids in the 1980s.[43, 44]

Understanding food behaviour and its role in creating identities allows food policy to recognize how people act out their existence through food, not seeing their identities as fixed but as a mixture of inherited, plastic and open to change. An example is how food becomes a tension between generations, in the process of immigration, when children of first-generation migrants begin to adopt the ways of the host culture, through school or availability or willing acculturation. A mixture of cultures emerge and identities are expressed.[45] The food industry has been quick to recognize this when adapting routinized recipes to local tastes and preferences. McDonalds, for example, has altered menus to regional preferences, age and cultural groups; food advertisers have recognized different demographics and geographies; and food retailers have adapted their offer to regional tastes.[46–51] The term 'glocalization' was coined to refer to this mix.[52] In his book *Jihad vs Mcworld*, Barber showed how multinational companies can use the efficiency of global systems, while trading on the multi-culturalism and localization of food.[53]

The appropriation and incorporation of foreign cuisine by different social groups happens at differing paces and stages.[54] In socially stratified societies, the rich, urban and leisured classes appear to adopt niche cuisines as fashion borrowed from other social and cultural strata; industry mainstreams such developments. US 'french fries' originate from US soldiers bringing their newly found taste for (Belgian) 'frites'. English children now rate pizza and curries as English food just as their 19th century forebears adopted pyjamas from the colonial experience. Indeed, cuisine has been a major opportunity for poor, developing countries to influence richer, developed ones, and for rural people to link with urban areas. The growth of regional cuisine, such as Thai, Mexican and Moroccan, has been a late-20th century feature of large cities in the industrialized North. Foods are subject to the pursuit of the new, fads and tastes being changed from season to season.[55] The spread of 'burger culture' and the growth of the take-away/eat-at-home meals are examples.[56] Food transfers across the globe have happened for thousands of years, with the spread of both plants and people, but the scale of change now is unprecedented.[57] Although some past uptake was fast, most was not; the potato, for instance, was not taken up extensively for centuries.[58] Today, however, the spread of foods is much speedier. Not for nothing have sociologists taken food as a metaphor for global behaviour: 'Coca-Colonization',

'McDonaldization', 'burger culture', and cultural patterns.[59] Such terms can imply a unidirectional cultural flow when movement can be in more complex linkages.

Pizza, viewed as an 'Italian' food, was not even in Italian dictionaries in the 1920s; it was a regional rather than national speciality.[60] What made Italian food popular was emigration, particularly to the USA, and the longing of migrants for home tastes. This emigration also had a reverse effect as earnings flowed back to Italy, helping raise living standards and tastes beyond a monotonous diet. As a food cuisine develops, it can be surrounded by its own myths.[61] Morgan and colleagues have showed how modern investment by the regional government of Tuscany helped foster a rebirth of 'authentic' food culture, a deliberate policy to counteract what were perceived as destructive international-izing tendencies, and to create employment and economic diversity.[62] In 1989, the now international Slow Food movement began when some friends in Bra, in the province of Cuneo in Northwest Italy, discussed at dinner how shocked they were at the location of a US fast-food outlet next to the Spanish Steps in Rome. Their thinking moved from protest to the championing of alter-native cultural directions, and their organization is now in 132 countries with 85,000 members.[63, 64] This was a deliberate effort to reshape culture, or at least to highlight the cultural dimension of what could otherwise be seen as the grinding process of modernity. This was not fear of new food, neophobia, or pleasure in eating the familiar,[65, 66] both of which are common in human behaviour, but a political act, a pitch to confront the normalization of indus-trialized food. Such examples point to the complex dynamics beneath change. In the developed world, and for the rich in urban economies, the question is not what to eat but what to eat from numerous choices.[67, 68]

Culture, cuisine and food as metaphors

Food is on the one hand associated with routine, domestic drudgery and, on the other hand, with pleasure, comfort, exploration and fresh experiences. Changes in food preparation and consumption can become metaphors for a past that may never have existed; a bucolic haze of skills and abundance that was a reality only for the few.[69] Cooking skills can be studied for what they tell us about society and domestic roles. Interpretations vary on whether industri-alized societies experienced a decline, transition or resurgence of cooking.[70, 71] In their review of food research and theory, Mennell and colleagues point out that, despite a diverse range of research related to food, 'it is not always clear what such a point of view actually is'.[72] Food is almost a Rorschach inkblot test, where random shapes mean different things to viewers, who are projecting on to the blot their state of mind.

An argument favoured by anthropologists is that a food cuisine embodies a culture's accumulated wisdom; it is the shared body of knowledge, the commensality.[73] When he advised US readers not to eat anything not known to their grandmothers (see Chapter 4), Michael Pollan was turning that observation into a rule and trying to confront the flux of culture.[74] The argument is that in contemporary culture, like the High Street, anything goes, little is fixed. Accumulated wisdoms are being reshaped by consumer society. Yet social scientists show how food cuisines reflect geography, lifestyle (which become embodied as culture) and genes;[18, 75] they embody culture, in which case the reality of fluid food cultures might be interpreted as representing the transient nature of modernity. Yet a distinction should be made between behaviour that is ephemeral and features that are more hard-wired. Lactose tolerance, for example, is strongly associated with the spread of herding peoples, where a genetic mutation 10,000 years ago allowed adults to tolerate milk as a nutrient-rich resource; yet for some communities, such as Native Americans, milk-based products are 'the kiss of death'.[76] They had not developed a tolerance, which did not prevent some food-welfare programmes including milk and dried milk products as standard.

With technical change and complex food-processing supply chains, such intolerances have become a touchstone of how deep corporate care really goes. In the USA and elsewhere, litigation or blame can follow, hence notices on food packets such as 'this product may contain residues of nuts'. Such information assumes consumer control. The role of welfare foods and schemes such as Second Harvest based as it was on distributing over-produced foods to the US poor, cannot be taken as being operated according to the principle of choice.[77] Nor in South America is choice the key factor if stunted babies to develop into obese youngsters as the foods provided through the welfare system to combat underweight are likely to make them fat, combined with a tendency or predisposition to maintain weight gain.[78]

Yet it would be foolish to deny choice completely and to link culture directly from deep experience, over the head of volition, to social habits. The insights of social science are that such connections are networked, not causal. Culture influences food choice just as attitudes, feelings and circumstance do. Cuisines such as the Mediterranean diet—extolled for its health benefits by Ancel Keys (see Chapter 4)—may represent accumulated wisdom, with a structured range of foods and therefore micro-nutrients, but it has faded from daily existence in the Mediterranean, despite evidence that a strict adherence delivers health benefits.[53] The diet was rooted in localized knowledge; when she re-investigated Keys' work, Antonia Trichopoulou asked elderly women to cook as they did in the times when Keys studied them. This meant foraging in the fields and hills for wild herbs, which when analysed were rich in essential fatty acids and micro-nutrients. The physical activity undoubtedly helped. Such conditions are not possible in contemporary Mediterranean societies; the hills are not accessible to town dwellers; the knowledge is being lost. For many, this is an escape from drudgery; modern shopping practices, food availability and food preparation are seen as liberating and a benefit of affluence.[79]

Part of food's role as a metaphor is rooted in its role in relationships, rituals, rites of passage (marriage, divorce, bereavement), the labour process and power. Not without reason has cooking been linked to enslavement.[20, 80, 81] The relationship of women to food has been particularly studied, not just by the food and advertising industries but by clinicians, since food is such a factor in body shapes and associations. Thinness, fatness and all between are loaded with social and spiritual meanings. The ancient Maltese worshipped goddesses who would today be deemed grossly obese. Many religions have injunctions to deny food at set periods. Muslims fast during Ramadan and Catholics eschew meat for fish on Fridays or during Lent. In his outline of fat history, Stearn distinguishes between Catholic countries, such as France, where food is celebrated and Protestant societies, such as the USA and Belgium, where food has low associations with pleasure.[82] The so-called 'French paradox' of how the French could eat fatty foods in quantities not recommended by standard dietary advice yet suffer fewer dietary-related diseases, is only a paradox if portions and control, as well as pleasure, are omitted from the analysis.[73, 82] Historically, too, the French ate more greens with meals than is done today. The argument can be extended: the more instrumental and less pleasure-seeking Anglo-Saxon food cultures, such as the USA or UK, are built more on novelty and functional attributes; food is compartmentalized—for activity, for moods, for celebration. For the UK, it may be that this instrumentalism towards food was not intrinsic but shaped by the industrial revolution.[83]

In most cultures, food also has a key role in the gift relationship. Most traditional cultures link welcome to food; breaking of bread, offering drinks symbolized both welcome and care. In ancient times, the breaking of bread cakes could symbolize the start of a meal, and also its replacement. Such experiences add a different dimension to cultural tourism in pursuit of the authentic.[84] In urbanized societies, café life replaces such private-sphere formality with public space socializing, creating new forms of the public–private distinction.

Food as morality and control

When health and environmental educators appeal on the media to consumers to eat differently, they are offering new codes of conduct, different criteria from those perceived to be normal or dominant. New linkages are being proposed between routine eating or purchasing, and undesirable outcomes. Such appeals hover between offering liberation and subjugation, advantage and disadvantage. Counteracting such cultural pitches is one reason food companies employ public relations specialists, to neutralize and expose such attempts. The fragility of such exercises has been remarked, especially by analysts of the harmed. Studies of anorexia nervosa or bulimia, for example, point to the self-dislike exposed.[85, 86] A good food culture is, by implication, one free from anxiety, a demand which has been a consistent rallying cry against adulteration for centuries. The anxiety of eating is a moral problem, not just a material or microbiological one. So often, foods or ingredients are proffered to viewers or listeners as 'good' or 'bad' things to eat, creating a moral economy around food choice and consumption.[82, 87–90] Terms like 'junk food' or the French phrase *'la malbouffe americaine'* (crap American food) capture what is perceived as an essential soullessness of fast food, while acknowledging but regretting its presence.[91, 92] The world of nutrition can be seen to mimic this approach in the development of food guidelines as in food plates or food pyramids, which provide guidance on what to eat. These are guidelines of what ought to be.

For food policy, this perspective suggests the need to identify gaps in cultural knowledge and to aim to fill them from the perspective of the ordinary person, rather than assuming that expert knowledge is the correct starting point. As we have noted before (see Chapter 5), and as is testified by studies in many countries, the food industry understands and uses this perspective effectively.[93–95] The public health nutrition world lags behind in using didactic approaches to promote healthy eating.[96] In the 1970s, a now infamous health promotion campaign was aimed at the UK Asian community, which suffered a high rate of rickets in young children.[97] Rickets is a result of vitamin D deficiency, so the campaign focused on educating Asian mothers about the benefits of diet and the need to include foods high in vitamin D and to ensure children were exposed to sunlight. The underlying principle of the campaign was the mal-adaptation of 'them' to a British way of life. The indigenous population were less at risk of developing rickets since bread (white bread), margarine and cereals had been fortified with vitamin D in the period following World War II. The campaign made little attempt to understand the eating habits of Asians living in Britain, opting instead for an approach based on information concerning 'the correct thing to do'. This 'correct' approach was based on the assumptions and dominant ideologies of the host community, an assumption that good health would follow from acculturation.[97] The campaign was not a success, and was subsequently criticized as 'racist' in its conception, assuming a deficiency in behaviour on behalf of the ethnic community targeted. Like many nutrition-promotion campaigns targeting women, this one assumed that women were in control, when they were not.[98] At the time, others argued a structural approach, suggesting fortification of staples within the Asian diet. The ability of women to make choices was conceived within a deficit model of both knowledge and behaviour.

Such illustrations should not be taken to indicate they were just mistakes. The association of food with morality is probably inevitable, and should be subject to scrutiny, rather than hidden. With the current plethora of advice on healthy eating, the consumption of certain types of food assumes a value in itself and becomes a marker of 'correct' behaviour and body size. Critics have argued that the new public health—concerns with confronting NCD as population ills—have in fact focused on people's individual lives, denying almost that these ills are socially shaped.[99, 100] By demonizing such behaviour, culture is being shaped by what Foucault called governmentality by the state (see Chapter 3).[101] In the name of public health and health promotion, consumption of certain types of food are accorded a moral imperative, much in the same way that smoking as an activity has received moral approbation. A new moral architecture might be emerging in which 'good' food is healthy, slow, pure, natural, rural and so on, and being linked to high moral values associated with family, discipline, societal responsibility, and perhaps with adults, boredom and asceticism! 'Bad' food is junk (food), unhealthy and illness-related but also fun, and is often child-centred. These moral fissures may be easily exploited and reinforced by commercial interests.

Food easily establishes identity by culture, region or nation, a means for establishing boundaries between 'them' and 'us'. The Swiss and Germans called Italian seasonal railway workers 'macaroni gluttons'. The French were called by the English 'frog eaters'. Anglo-Saxons called the Germans 'krauts' (i.e. sauerkraut eaters). Yet despite such derogatory terms, the British upper classes continued to draw heavily on the French gastronomic tradition. The meal pattern associated with England and the 'proper' meal is relatively new. Until the Napoleonic wars, 'English service' consisted of all the courses appearing on the table at once; there were no courses as such. Sometimes a 'remove' dish was brought to replace a dish, usually a poultry or game dish replacing a soup or fish dish. Yet within 20 years of the battle of Waterloo, the (French) practice of serving dishes as consecutive courses was well-established among the better-off urban classes.[103, 104] This happened despite the public and political disdain for things French.[105] Such cross-cultural transfer of food and food habits has always happened. During the years of the British Empire, from the 18th century onwards, British cuisine was influenced by food from its dominions and colonies. The pace and infiltration of these foods were slow (over generations) and confined to key elements of the population (mostly the rich).

What is in a meal?

Social scientists have differed on how rational they think food consumption choices are.[105–107] Structuralists propose that all food choice is rationalized in relation to its context and that the task for social investigators is to decipher the code.[108] Psychological models, on the other hand, have focused more on the minutiae of decision-making.[109, 110] For the great French anthropologist, Claude Lévi-Strauss, food culture is a language to be translated, with the preparation and serving of food mediating cultural relations.[111] Ultimately, cooking is merely a process that transforms raw ingredients and makes them edible; but why have humans chosen this route? Rotting or degeneration of food is a natural transformation; roasting, smoking and boiling merely expand the repertoire. In this sense, food may be viewed through a series of axes: natural/cultural, raw/cooked, rapid/slow, boiled/rotten, and so on. For Lévi-Strauss, such axes were the fundamental cultural grid, into which all foods, styles and food cultures can be located. Such thinking may be represented as a culinary triangle, a model much used and adapted (see Fig. 7.2).[112, 113]

Another influential perspective has been that of Mary Douglas, who investigated the dietary consumption of working-class households in the UK. She concluded that the meal was a social occasion structured by rules.[114] Analysing different types of meal, she proposed that in all, there was one main part

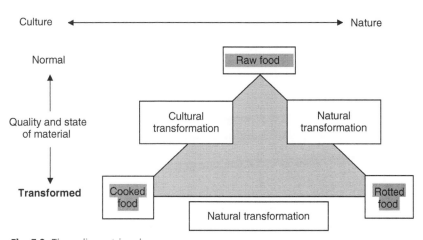

Fig. 7.2 The culinary triangle.

supported by two unsupported elements: a main meal, for example, with soup and dessert, which she expressed as an algebraic equation A+2B. She stresses that food is a symbolic system of communication and highly ordered. Even for special or symbolic meals, such as Christmas dinner, Douglas suggested that the A+2B structure was repeated but within each course. Culture and the social order can be seen in the sense of 'a proper meal', a concept further developed by Murcott in her work on families in South Wales.[115–118] A meal is seen as an occasion/event where food is consumed according to rules related to issues such as time, place, sequence of courses and so on. Snacks, on the other hand, were initially deemed to be unstructured food events without rules, but eating in fast-food outlets also has rules and structures. Fast-food service has managed to impose its own set of rules, such as self-service, the role of enjoyment and the expectation of speed.[119]

Critics have argued that the approach to the eating experience initiated by Douglas has a very English and middle-class hierarchy of structure within and between meals.[120] Italians have different structures: *antipasto*, *primo*, *secondo*, *con torno* and *dolce e caffè*.[60] The traditional Indian meal, for example, is not based on a tripartite structure but on the *thali* or platter, which focuses on a central pile of bread or rice surrounded by small containers of savoury dishes.[121] The order perceived by Douglas actually tells us little about the food itself—what it tastes like, why and how people enjoy or dislike it. The food anthropologist Sidney Mintz has proposed a different grammar of meals in developing countries, where they consist of a core food item (C), such as rice, a fringe item (F), such as a sauce, and a legume (L).[122]

With industrialization and urbanization this C+F+L has changed to M+S+2V, meat plus a staple, such as potatoes, and two vegetables. This shift may describe what happens in the Nutrition Transition (see Chapters 2 and 4). So while, on first appearances, the traditional Indian meal pattern and structure does not fit Douglas's rules, it may be that middle-class families in Delhi have more in common with her outline as globalization and urbanization take hold. As Indians have taken their various cuisines world-wide, they have been adapted to host countries. Curry is among the most common and popular foods in Britain, spawning entirely new combinations such as the tikka masala. Butlins, the UK holiday camp company, solved the problem of resistance to 'foreign' food by combining chicken chop suey with chips, maintaining the A+2B structure. John Koon, one of the foremost inventors of the Chinese take-away in Britain, pioneered the use of A, B, C, etc., on menus in the Cathay Restaurant in Piccadilly Circus, London. Children have been found to cling to this structure.[123] Such examples suggest how commerce works to, but also transforms, underlying codes. Vegetarian menus, for example, often produce a central meat substitute in order to create a 'main course'.[124, 125] The 1990s fashion in affluent countries for 'fusion food'—mixing cuisines—can be seen as a process of adaptation.[103]

A related issue is the question of manners: how to behave when eating.[126] First, people were taught that the height of manner was to use knives, then forks, then a battery of implements, laid in particular ways; then casual eating of fast-food legitimized hand use again. UK research suggests its public still holds opinions about appropriate behaviour and which foods should be served at meal occasions. Manners, too, are defined hierarchically, not just in social class but etiquette terms; refinement and income are not necessarily related. There are breaks between attitudes and behaviour, between what is thought ideal and what is actually done.[123] Psychological models of behaviour may help us to understand behaviour logically, but they do not always help explain why individuals fail to behave in predicted ways. In this sense, food culture is plastic and contextual, bending to new shapes yet retaining linkage to circumstances. There are many cultures and many rules and habits concerning food, with different manners for particular social situations. Even in the UK, there are variations across the country and in areas, between young and old, between ethnic groups and within ethnic groups.[127, 128] Gender, genes, geography and age have all been found to influence food choice.[76, 129, 130]

Cultural speed-up or lock-in?

The view that emerges from social science is that food behaviours are constructed, as well as inherited or given; they have many influences. Although these vary in importance, none is paramount; it is the whole bundle that matters. In the policy world, however, actions tend to be sought by addressing certain factors rather than others. If 'bad' food habits are not the result of commercial power, then it must be the family or parents. The policy appeals to single factors, rather than situate them within culture as a whole. Superficially, commerce looks as though it falls into this trap, too. Supermarket appeals to consumers may, for example, overtly stress the price of food—via appeals such as 'Buy-One-Get-One-Free' (BOGOF) strategies and price comparison data— but, in fact, they take a more nuanced approach. Supermarkets locate price among a welter of factors framing consumer choice. Choice is shaped by the entire shopping experience, from location, store layout, range, look, feel, not just price. Shaping the point of encounter by the shopper is a highly sophisticated skill, applied by companies to frame decisions and choice-edit to push food through and off their shelves. Success is measured against criteria such as profitability, footfall, yield per square metre of floorspace, and share value. The consumer is aware of little of that, despite being monitored by highly sophisticated market research and customer databanks.[1]

To see food culturally like this is a long road on from the process of change instituted when Marco Polo travelled to China and brought back oriental delicacies or when Venetian traders brought back spices to make European foods more palatable or when Columbus sent the potato back from the New World. In the past, such epic changes tended to occur slowly; travel was slower. Plants and animals took longer to drift across continents; not always but usually. Today, this can happen more speedily. The global reach of food-supply chains allows a family in Dublin, Paris, London or Berlin to eat food from far-off places. They can eat Italian, Japanese, Indian one moment, snack foods watching a Hollywood block-buster film the next. Food behaviours, though initially inherited, do not remain so.[131] None of this denies the importance of taste and preference, nor that they are learned as well as biologically hard-wired.[132] Coffee is an example of a learned taste; it is not innate like others that babies exhibit.[65] Despite predilections, tastes are socially determined. Some cultures do not eat horse meat; others consider offal to be a delicacy. Raw fish (sushi) is a part of Japanese culture,[133] to the extent that the Japanese Ministry of Agriculture discussed giving certificates to genuine sushi restaurants outside Japan. In part, this was mooted due to concerns beyond Japan about environmental, toxicological and supply questions, such as the danger of eating raw fish. In part, it is about identity.

The questions raised by public health and environmental evidence have not necessarily troubled early cultural analyses, but it now does. What cultural rules would be proposed by a food policy within an ecological public health framework? For decades, policy in developed countries has been driven by the need to accommodate lifestyles, and, as we saw in earlier chapters, formal policy has tended to focus on supply efficiency and quantity. Choice is for the affluent. So is a different approach to choice needed in the pursuit of ecological public health? Figure 7.3 offers a simplified conceptual model: choice as a spectrum from unbridled to restricted. It highlights the different policy foci of large-scale food retailers and current dominant neo-liberal ideology, for example, and between people with low and high disposable incomes. Progress in food policy is conventionally defined as moving from right to left, whereas for ecological public health, the rich certainly need to move from left to right.

What is strange is that in the developed world, the impact of more choice has been to limit the range of food people chose to eat; burgers are consumed every day and food marketers know that the majority of consumers only know the price of a small number of foods, known value items (KVIs). Caterers and restaurateurs have managed the uneasiness that results from this combination of belief in choice and cultural restrictions by serving strange food in a familiar manner. Grilled sushi is an example, as is the use of menu formats that allow people to choose food in meal structures with which

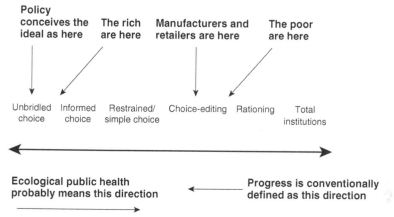

Fig. 7.3 Rethinking choice.

they feel familiar. An example already mentioned was restaurateur John Koon's allowing customers to 'customize' their choice into the familiar structure of starter, main and dessert courses. This is a strategy applied in health-education programmes such as 5-a-day. Success has been more likely when people are allowed to eat fruit juice as a part of that regime and to use fruit as a snack substitute rather than as part of the meal. Attempts to persuade people to eat more fruit or vegetables as part of their everyday meals and increase their portion sizes have been less successful. An understanding of social construction of the food plate helps explain this. Appeals to logic or information have to be tempered by fitting into existing behaviour.

Does this mean, therefore, that when faced by enormous changes needed to adapt to, let alone halt, climate change or to transform diets to reduce the toll of diet-related premature death, a food policy informed by ecological public health can only start from where people are? This is a good if highly charged question, to which we return in the final chapter. Meanwhile it must be clear that the transformation of food systems needed to address issues such as climate change, water stress, fossil fuel reliance and health costs, requires cultural change to be successful. Food policy-making must surely, therefore, include a clear and decisive commitment to understand and engage with the meanings that people bring to the table. There is a rich body of work on this cultural dimension but still a dearth of research on how and whether policy actually affects it.[97] The conventional approach is to suggest that social scientific evidence, like all evidence, merely feeds into the policy process. This is not always so, which is why academics champion the view that policy will only improve if it is based on evidence. Evidence-based policy is a fine ideal but the policy–evidence–behaviour nexus is probably inevitably messy in practice (see Chapters 1–3). The relationship is likely to be less clean, rational and uni-directional when there are so many actors involved at so many levels of governance.

A thoughtful attempt to address the issue of change was made in the UK by the Sustainable Consumption Roundtable, a joint body of the National Consumer Council and Sustainable Development Commission, both arms-length government bodies. The Roundtable conducted research that suggested a willingness of consumers to change behaviour in more sustainable directions, but only if other significant influences in government and industry did too. The report *I will if you will* suggested that the public is aware of the urgent need to act on life-determinants, such as climate change, but wants 'someone' to make the first move.[134] It proposed a triangle of change model in which actions are required to have engagement from business, government and the people, or else they are likely to fail.

This chimed with related research conducted by the British Government. In five studies of consumer behaviour—leisure, transport, finance, energy and food—the Department for Environment, Food and Rural Affairs found that consumers aspired to change but felt that if the need to do so was so important, then someone in authority, such as companies or Government, would have said so.[135] This applied for food, too.[136] Meanwhile companies, fearful of the implications of big change, put the onus on consumers to make the first step; hence the policy lock-in highlighted by the Sustainable Consumption Roundtable. The pace of change towards lower carbon footprints, for example, is painfully slow and not enough to meet the internationally negotiated Kyoto Conference carbon-reduction targets.

Old alongside new fast food

The notion of 'glocalization' proposed that food may be sold as local but is in reality creeping towards ever longer supply routes (see Chapter 5); vice versa, it has been argued that the availability of globally sourced ingredients also allows and energizes the rebirth of local food cultures.[37] Both may be true. Through cultural exchange, local interpretation and adaptation becomes possible, whether taking the form of grilled sushi or McDonalds providing mutton rather than beef burgers in India, or McCafé's in some countries. Environmentalists and health advocates tend to be judgmental about such mass cultural phenomena; this is understandable, but if there was a better recognition of why fast food has achieved its popularity and culturally iconic status, the pursuit of environmental or health gain might be more achievable too. Market analysts see a future of continued big sales for take-away and eat-out meals; so *realpolitik* probably dictates this anyway.

Some kind of fast or portable food has been part of most societies' food cultures. In medieval London, street sellers sold pies, ribs, hotcakes, and eel pie. Street or fast food (*chats*) have long been a feature of Indian society. Egypt has an established tradition of fast food including *eish baladi* (a flat bread), *falafel* (the broad bean rather than chickpea version) and pickled turnip coloured pink by beetroot.[138, 139] Today's policy concern about fast food is really due to lower costs encouraging excess consumption and the marketing of global companies. (Although McDonalds receives the limelight, others are vast too; in 2007, KFC had 11,000 outlets in 80 countries and Burger King had the same number in 69 countries.[140]) In Egypt, meanwhile, local take-away stalls always sell local traditional fast food. But while the food is traditional (kebabs and falafel), the equipment behind the counter is similar to that in McDonald's 300 m down the road. The price of similar goods is about one-third the price of food from international chains in the same street. In developing countries, the US fast-food companies tend to be located in urban areas and cater for the urban, more affluent classes. Their offer is not just the food but a lifestyle statement. Despite price differences, the international companies can threaten locally owned fast food outlets by command of supplies, lifestyle customer appeal and vast scale of operation.

It would be wrong, too, for an ecological public health approach to food policy to demean fast food for another reason. For people on low incomes, eating street food is one way of gaining time and saving money, gaining time by not cooking and saving money by not having to buy fuel or equipment and using the time thus saved to work and generate income. One study of street foods in seven countries in Asia and Africa showed that the poor spend relatively more money on street foods and have a higher calorific intake from these sources than those on high incomes.[141] Another study in Accra, Ghana found that the lowest quintile groups consumed up to 31% of their total calories outside the home. Far from being an unaffordable luxury, street and fast food is important. There are, however, food safety issues that need to be addressed. The WHO Geneva food-safety team concluded that dual safety cultures were being allowed to flourish in developing countries. Western food companies sourcing foods, such as airlines, exporters and multinational companies, were creating islands of Western-style hygiene standards with HACCP food safety regimes (see Chapter 5). WHO concluded that best practice ought to be shared with street and everyday food too, so they started a programme to improve hygiene for street sellers.[142]

Domestic labour in preparation and cooking

As we saw in Chapter 5, the labour side of food-supply chains can be a thorny issue: poor conditions, wages, and safety records. Social scientists have studied the domestic, unwaged aspects of food production, too, and have remarked on food's transition from unwaged to waged economies. This often raises a moral storm about responsibilities. One narrative depicts capacity to buy food outside of the home as social advance, particularly for women. In traditional societies, food is often depicted as playing a significant role in the division of labour and in complementary and continuity of family and work relationships. The move to eating shop-bought rather than home-cooked breads, for example, can thus change those relationships, bringing release.[20, 143–145]

The other narrative celebrates domestic skills as a core life-skill, proposing that the transfer of food skills from home to the kitchen, if not from necessity, is to de-skill and create dependencies. Many cultures codify such domestic skills in books or manuals. For the UK, the book that epitomizes this is Mrs Beeton's *Book of household management*. First produced as a part-work in the mid-19th century, with subsequent variations as a cookbook, this has never been out of print and is iconic. Isabella Beeton believed that women needed to be 'thoroughly acquainted with the theory and practice of cooking' in order to compete with the attractions of eating-out for their husbands.[46] Her cookbook was an all-round domestic management treatise. Home was where cooking occurred, controlled by a wife, for the husband and children. Edwin Chadwick, the architect of England's 1848 Public Health Act, shared this view, stating that 'ignorance of domestic economy leads to ill health by the purchase of unsuitable and at the same time expensive food'.[48]

The issue raised is not whether technical innovation is *per se* a 'good' thing but on whose terms it comes, why and who benefits—a further illustration of the debate about science and technology raised in Chapter 5. One by-product of the debate about whether cooking is or is not in decline is a relatively new question, for the UK at least, about how the skills-base of the catering industry can be maintained. It is a huge employer. Catering work is often a route into employment for migrant labour and immigrants can set up a catering business more easily than some other enterprises. The hours are long, however, and returns not necessarily great; often their children, the second generation, move more easily into other or professional employment. The catering industry may be beginning to experience the trajectory that farming has already gone through: a squeeze on labour in which there is a restriction of who actually wants to enter the food trades, resulting in a skills shortage and lock-in to migrant casual labour. This, however, can enter deeper waters: the politics of the border, nationalism, racism and fear of the outsider.

To the proponent of domestic skills, this is all academic. Cooking is about turning raw materials into a meal; the skill matters less than the confidence that the cook brings to the chopping board and stove. Cooking is the translation of an idea of the meal, plus experience and knowledge of how to plan and create it; this is what adds up to a culinary culture.[71] Fordist food production, however, allows the time-pressured to take short-cuts. Value-added products can allow 'real' food to disguise the use of pre-prepared ingredients. The image can be retained by buying ready-chopped vegetables. Cooking becomes assembly. Behind this transfer from home to waged labour (and back) is a repeated experience of low-paid work, often carried out by women from lower socio-economic groups. The celebrity chef with multiple outlets and product endorsements or TV shows and a sizeable annual income from advertising is the exception, and often a male.

This debate about what is real cooking, real food and authentic culture, is potentially endless. The insight given by social science, however, is that human relationships and the meaning of food are variable, subject to change in which humans are both passive and in control, malleable but demanding, conscious and unaware.

Does it matter for ecological public health if cooking skills are not transferred across generations? One argument is that it creates dependency; the cultural analysts argue that the loss of sociability to a community may be greater.[84] The spread and standardization of taste has, as Slow Food shows, spawned its reaction. As the first industrial nation, the British are qualified perhaps to talk. In his review of British food history, Colin Spencer argued that local, regional and national cuisines should not be romanticized; the records favour the view of food culture from the affluent.[83] Cuisines may not be worth resurrecting; in a world that needs to reduce animal production, what value boar's head? If, as the social scientists propose, all food behaviour has its rationality, and people's food choices and mores are understandable, then a food world that is highly likely to be dominated by climate change, water stress and land-use dilemmas (see Chapter 6), will throw up different food cultures, different rationalities. If, as is the case, women so often vote with their feet to enter education and to work for wages, rather than be restricted to unwaged domestic labour for men, then pressure on men to learn domestic skills will not abate but continue. This new world is highly likely to require different criteria for how to judge a good food-culture. We return to this issue in Chapter 9.

Multiple meanings: where are food cultures headed?

This entry into the social meanings of food has highlighted how food and identity are entwined. Everyone plays various roles in the food drama.

These identities may change over time or be influenced by stages in our lives—baby, child, adolescence, middle and old age—or key life events, such as marriage or parenthood. In this respect, people have food careers, with gender a key variable.[20, 99] Gender is not the same thing as sex. Gender is a social role; sex is a biological 'given'. The same food habits can originate from many backgrounds and influences. For example, vegetarians in a predominantly meat-eating culture may be choosing not to eat meat for any combination of reasons. It may be a lifestyle statement; an act of rebellion against parents or authority; for religious reasons; for concern about animal welfare; for health; or for ecological or environmental reasons. In a predominantly vegetarian culture—at home or nationally—the reasons will differ again; it may be for continuity and tradition, familiarity, pride, comfort, normality, or not for any conscious reason at all. The whole issue about culture is that it is not necessarily chosen. Cultures are not pipes demarking the inside from the outside world, restricting all and forbidding egress; only allowing ingress. The account of food culture given here is more fluid, running in various directions. This is why, like clinicians, social scientists are fascinated by the exceptional. The way new cultures emerge, articulating new priorities or combinations, is rich testament to the malleability of food culture.

What becomes clear is that food can indicate or define distinctions in our patterns of living. So, while we might eat in a 'fast-food joint' on occasions, such as a child's birthday or during the week when trying to save time in the working day, many would not consider McDonald's, Burger King or Kentucky Fried Chicken as suitable restaurants for the celebration of a major event. The association of eating-out with an event and an 'occasion' still holds strong for many. It is also true that these distinctions are breaking down. The use of McDonald's by harassed parents, of all classes, for children's birthday parties is but one example. There are still rituals associated with eating, occasions and celebration. The new distinctions are, for many of us, internal to our own lives, as opposed to differences between classes or groups. So we now eat at 'fast-food joints' and also in restaurants—the events define the appropriateness of the eating occasion. Patterns of eating out are severely constrained by macro-economic realities. Eating-out from choice of expression means something different to the affluent Westerner than to the low-waged labourer in a poor developing country.

A food policy fit for the 21st century must be alive to this complex world of food behaviour and culture. Health education, as we have shown in various examples, can be set off with good intentions but on the wrong foot, by ignoring or down-playing culture. Food policy has many examples of good intentions leading to unintended consequences, and failures due to cultural insensitivity. That happened with the health education campaigns to improve UK Asian mother and baby diets in the 1970s and 1980s.[97] Another study, of adolescent girls, showed how young women recognized that fast food was less healthy for them than home-cooked food, but chose to eat fast food for the association with friends and to escape from parental control. Health campaigns aimed at this social group would be unlikely to succeed if they demonized such food or locations.[91]

A sound and appropriate food policy requires from the social sciences good intelligence about food culture and the meanings people attach to food. Policy engagement is required, whether the goal is to speed up cultural change in particular directions, such as carbon reduction and health improvement, or just to inform about unmet needs. We have proposed that, rich though social scientific work on food cultures is, not enough work is policy-oriented. Much has been driven by the pursuit of individual, rather than population behaviour change, yet the scholarship is rich.[147] It needs to be engaged with the big challenges of the ecological public health age, yet retain its rightful focus on people, their meanings and how food expresses culture yet changes it.

What cultural rules should people eat by? Is there a 'should'? The lessons from social science are that there is a plethora of rules adding to the policy cacophony; yet environmental and health drivers suggest a vacuum needing to be filled. And to talk of 'should' locks policy into existing social dynamics of authority, order and control; yet there is good evidence of the need for leadership. Moral or cultural rules about food are an issue that should not be pigeon-holed as purely controlling or conservative. Guidance is needed about how to live and eat in an era of climate change and environmental limits. One thing is certain. The simplistic reliance on choice as the key arbiter of what drives food economies is an inadequate basis for any rational food policy. The empty-vessel model of human behaviour, with which this chapter began, is a policy blind alley. There are even suggestions that unlimited choice may inhibit behaviour and that selecting from a smaller number of options can enhance choice.[148] The next chapter explores how problems of access and inequality cut across the socio-cultural aspects of food.

References

1. Humby C, Hunt T, Phillips T. *Scoring points: how Tesco is winning customer loyalty*. London: Kogan Page, 2004.
2. Humby C. *Brand is dead, long live the consumer*. London: dunnhumby, 2006.
3. Hayward M. *Customers are for life, not just for your next bonus*. 2005. dunnhumby, London.
4. Kent Business School. *The dunnhumby Academy of Consumer Research*.

http://www.kent.ac.uk/kbs/standard.php?page_id=222 [accessed June 17 2008]. Canterbury University of Kent, 2008.

5. Davidson MP. *The consumerist manifesto: advertising in postmodern times.* London: Routledge, 1992.

6. Robertson A, Tirado C, Lobstein T, Jermini M, Knai C, Jensen JH *et al. Food and health in Europe: a new basis for action.* Copenhagen: World Health Organization Regional Office for Europe, 2004.

7. Alvard MS. The adaptive nature of culture. *Evolutionary Anthropology* 2003;**12**:136–149.

8. Castells M. *The information age: economy, society and culture, Vol. 1: the rise of the network society.* Oxford: Blackwell, 1996.

9. Held D. *Global transformations: politics, economics and culture.* Cambridge: Polity Press, 1999.

10. Gray J. *Al Qaeda and what it means to be modern.* London: Faber, 2003.

11. Douglas M. *Food in the social order: study of food and festivities in three American communities.* New York: Russell Sage Foundation, 1984.

12. Fishbein M, Ajzen I. *Belief, attitude, intention, and behavior: an introduction to theory and research.*Reading, MA: Addison-Wesley, 1975.

13. Ajzen I, Fishbein M. *Understanding attitudes and predicting social behavior.* Englewood Cliffs, NJ: Prentice-Hall, 1980.

14. Germov J and Williams L. *A sociology of food and nutrition: the social appetite.* Oxford: Oxford University Press, 1999.

15. Crotty P. Food and class. In: Germov J, Williams L (ed.) *A sociology of food and nutrition: the social appetite.* Melbourne: Oxford University Press, 1999:135–148.

16. Charles N, Kerr M. *Women, food and families.* Manchester: Manchester University Press, 1988.

17. Warde A, Martens L. *Eating out: social differentiation, consumption and pleasure.* Cambridge: Cambridge University Press, 2000.

18. Nabhan GP. *Coming home to eat: the pleasures and politics of local foods.* New York: WW Norton and Co., 2002.

19. Moir A, Moir B. *Why men don't iron: the new realities of gender differences.* London: Harper Collins, 1999.

20. Attar D. *Wasting girls' time: the history and politics of home economics.* London: Virago, 1990.

21. Gershuny J. Technical change and the work-leisure balance. In: Silberston A (ed.) *Technology and economic progress.* London: Macmillan, 1989:181-215.

22. Gershuny J, Fisher K. Leisure. In: Halsey AH, Webb J (ed.) *Twentieth-century British social trends.* Basingstoke: Macmillan, 2000:620-649.

23. Caraher M, Dixon P, Lang T, Carr-Hill R. Barriers to accessing healthy foods: differentials by gender, social class, income and mode of transport. *Health Education Journal* 1998;**57**(3):191–201.

24. Robinson N, Caraher M, Lang T. Access to shops: the views of low income shoppers. *Health Education Journal* 2000;**59**(2):121–136.

25. Reisig VMT, Hobbiss A. Food deserts and how to tackle them: a study from one city's approach. *Health Education Journal* 2000;**59**(2):137–149.

26. Barber BR. *Consumed: how markets corrupt children, infantilize adults, and swallow citizens whole*. New York: WW Norton, 2007.

27. Gabriel Y. The glass cage: flexible work, fragmented consumption, fragile selves. In: Alexander JC, Marx GT, Williams CL (ed.) *Self, social structure and beliefs*. Berkeley, CA: University of California Press, 2004:57–76.

28. Coase R. The nature of the firm. *Economica* 1937;**4**(16):386–495.

29. Murcott A. The nation's diet. In: Griffiths SAWJ. (ed.) *Consuming passions: food in the age of anxiety. Times Higher Education Supplement*. Manchester: Mandolin Press, 1998.

30. Langston P, Clarke GP, Clarke DB. Retail saturation, retail location, and retail competition: an analysis of British grocery retailing. *Environment and Planning A* 1997;**29**(1):77—104

31. Wrigley N. How British retailers have shaped food choice. In: Murcott A (ed.) *The nation's diet: the social science of food choice*. Harlow: Longman, 1998.

32. Beaumont J, Leather S, Lang T, Mucklow C. *Report on policy to Low Income Project Team of the Nutrition Taskforce*. Radlett: Institute of Grocery Distribtuion for the Department of Health Nutrition Taskforce, 1995.

33. Leather S. *The making of modern malnutrition: an overview of food poverty in the UK*. London: Caroline Walker Trust, 1996.

34. Dowler E, Rex D, Blair A, Donkin A, Grundy C. *Measuring access to healthy food in Sandwell*. Sandwell (West Midlands): Sandwell Health Authority, 2001.

35. Dowler E, Turner SA, Dobson B, Child Poverty Action Group (Great Britain). *Poverty bites: food, health and poor families*. London: Child Poverty Action Group, 2001.

36. Cummins S, Macintyre S. 'Food deserts'—evidence and assumption in health policy making. *British Medical Journal* 2002;**325**(7361):436–438.

37. Raven H, Lang T, with, Dumonteil C. *Off our trolleys? Food retailing and the hypermarket economy*. London: Institute for Public Policy Research, 1995.

38. Wrigley N, Guy C, Lowe M. Urban Regeneration, Social inclusion and large store development: the Seacroft Development in context. *Urban Studies* 2002;**39**(11): 2101–2114.

39. Fernie J, Moore C, Fernie S. *Principles of retailing*. London: Butterworth, 2003.

40. Prättälä R, Roos G, Hulshof K, Sihto M. Food and nutrition policies and interventions. In: Mackenbach J, Bakker M (ed.) *Reducing inequalities in health: a European perspective*. London: Routledge, 2002:104–124.

41. Murcott A. Epilogue: on the legacy of the politics of food. In: Lien ME, Nerlich B (ed.) *The politics of food.*. Oxford: Berg, 2004:221–234.

42. Lang T, Dowler E, Hunter D. *Review of the Scottish Diet Action Plan 1996–2005: progress and impacts*. Report 2005/ 2006 RE036. Edinburgh: NHS Health Scotland, 2006:221-234.

43. Department of Health. *Government response to report on tackling childhood obesity*. http://www.dh.gov.uk/en/Publicationsandstatistics/Pressreleases/DH_4130965 London: Department of Health, 2006.

44. Department of Health. *Healthy weight, healthy lives: a cross government strategy for England*. London: Department of Health, 2008:56.

45. Watson J., Caldwell ML. *The cultural politics of food and eating: a reader*. Oxford: Blackwell Publishing, 2005.

46. Ritzer G. *The McDonaldization thesis*. London: Sage, 1998.

47. Chadwick E. Report on the Sanitary Condition of the Labour Population and on the Means of its Improvement. London, May 1842:140.

48. Ritzer G. *Enchanting a disenchanted world: revolutionizing the means of consumption.* California: Pine Forge Press, 1999.

49. Ritzer G. *The McDonaldization of society: New Century edition.* Thousand Oaks, California: Pine Forge Press, 2000.

50. Ritzer G. *Explorations in the sociology of consumption: fast food, credit cards and casinos.* London: Sage, 2001.

51. Barber B. *Jihad VS McWorld: how the planet is both falling apart and coming together and what this means for democracy.* New York: Times Books, 1995.

52. Robertson R. Globalisation or Glocalisation. *Journal of International Communication* 1994;**1**(1):33–52.

53. Barber BR. *Jihad vs.McWorld: How the planet is both falling apart and coming together and what this means for democracy.* New York: Times Books, 1995.

54. Rodrigues SSP, Caraher M, Trichopoulou A, de Almeida MDV. Portuguese households' diet quality (adherence to Mediterranean food pattern and compliance with WHO population dietary goals): trends, regional disparities and socioeconomic determinants. *European Journal of Clinical Nutrition* 2007. Online publication: www.nature.com/ejcn/journal/v58/n3/full/1601827a.html

55. Caraher M, Coveney J. Public health nutrition and food policy. *Public Health Nutrition* 2004;**7**(5):591–598.

56. Schlosser E. *Fast food nation: the dark side of the all-American meal.* Boston: Houghton Mifflin Company, 2001.

57. Hobhouse H. *Seeds of change: five plants that transformed mankind.* London: Macmillan, 1992.

58. Salaman RN. *The history and social influence of the Potato.* Cambridge: Cambridge University Press, 1949.

59. Ritzer G. *Explorations in the sociology of consumption: fast food, credit cards and casinos.* London: Sage, 2001.

60. Dickie J. *Delizia! The epic history of the Italians and their food.* London: Hodder and Staunton, 2007.

61. Rozin P, Fischler C, Imada S, Sarubin A, Wrzesniewski A. Attitudes to food and the role of food in life in the USA, Japan, Flemish Belgium and France: possible implications for the diet-health debate *Appetite* 1999;**33**(2): 163–180.

62. Morgan K, Marsden T, Murdoch J. *Worlds of food: place, power and provenance in the food chain.* Oxford: Oxford University Press, 2006.

63. Petrini C. *Slow food nation.* New York: Rizzoli, 2006.

64. Petrini C, Padovani G. *Slow food revolution: a new culture for eating and living.* New York: Rizzoli, 2008.

65. Drewnowski A. Taste preferences and food intake. *Annual Review of Nutrition* 1997(17):237–253.

66. Drewnowski A. Energy density, palatability and satiety: implications for weight control. *Nutrition Reviews* 1998;**56**(12):347–353.

67. Pollan M. *The omnivore's dilemma; the search for the perfect meal in a fast-food world.* London: Bloomsbury, 2006.

68. Mason J, Singer P. *Eating: what we eat and why it matters*. London: Arrow Books, 2006.

69. Murcott A. The lost supper. *The Times Higher* 31 January 1997:15.

70. Lang T, Caraher M. Is there a culinary skills transition? Data and debate from the UK about changes in cooking culture. *Journal of the Home Economics Institute of Australia* 2001;**8**(2):2–14.

71. Short F. *Kitchen secrets: the meaning of cooking in everyday life*. Oxford: Berg, 2006.

72. Mennell S, Murcott A, Otterloo AHv, International Sociological Association. *The sociology of food: eating, diet and culture*. London: Sage, 1992.

73. Rozin P, Fischler C, Imada S, Sarubin A, Wrzesniewski A. Attitudes to food and the role of food in life in the USA, Japan, Flemish Belgium and France: possible implications for the diet-health debate. *Appetite* 1999;**33**(2):163–180.

74. Pollan M. *In defence of food: the myth of nutrition and the pleasures of eating*. London: Allen Lane, 2008.

75. Flannery T. *The future eaters: an ecological history of the Australasian lands and people*. Sydney: Reed New Holland, 2005.

76. Nabhan GP. *Why some like it hot; food: genes and cultural diversity*. Washington: Island Press, 2004.

77. MacDonald M. *Food, stamps, and income maintenance*. New York: Academic Press, 1977.

78. Pena M, Bacallao J. *Obesity and poverty: a new public health challenge*. Washington: Pan American Health Organization, 2000.

79. Trichopoulou A, Costacou T, Bamia C, Trichopoulos D. Adherence to a Mediterranean Diet and Survival in a Greek Population. *New England Journal of Medicine* 2003;**348**(26):2599–2608.

80. Mason L. *Food and the rites of passage*. Devon: Prospect Books, 2002.

81. Short F. *Kitchen secrets: the meaning of cooking in everyday life*. London: Berg, 2006.

82. Stearns P. *Fat history: bodies and beauty in the modern west*. New York: New York University Press, 2002.

83. Spencer C. *British food*. London: Grub Street, 2002.

84. Graca P, Jopanaz S, Graca E. Traditional cuisine as a cultural tourism project. In: Edwards JSA, Hewedi MM (ed.) *Culinary arts and sciences III: Global and national perspectives*. Bournemouth: Worshipful Company of Cooks Centre for Culinary Research, Bournemouth University, 2001.

85. Orbach S. *Fat is a feminist issue*. London: Hamlyn, 1978.

86. Orbach S. *Hunger strike: the anorectic's struggle as a metaphor for our age*. London: Faber and Faber, 1986.

87. Caplan P. *Food, health and identity*. London: Routledge, 1997.

88. Coveney J. *Food, morals and meaning*. London: Routledge, 2006.

89. Lien ME. Dogs, Wales and Kangaroos: transnational activism and food taboos. In: Lien ME, Nerlich B (ed.) *The politics of food*. Oxford: Berg, 2004.

90. Lupton D. *Food, the body and the self*. London: Sage, 1996.

91. Chapman G, Maclean H. 'Junk food' and 'healthy food': meanings of food in adolescent women's culture. *Journal of Nutrition Education* 1993(**25**):108–113.

92. Bové J, Dufour F. *The world is not for sale: farmers against junk food*. London: Verso, 2001.

93. Lawrence M. Folate fortification: public health policy making in a food regulation setting. In: Lin V, Gibson B (ed.) *Evidence-based health policy: problems & possibilities*. Sydney: Oxford University Press, 2003:110–126.

94. Nestle M. *What to eat*. New York: North Point Press (Farrar, Straus and Giroux), 2006.

95. Nestle M. Food industry and health: mostly promises, little action. *The Lancet* 2006; **368**:564–565.

96. Caraher M, Landon J. The impact of advertising on food choice: the social context of advertising. In: R. Shepherd MR (ed.) *The psychology of food choice*. Wallingford, Oxfordshire: CABI, 2006:227-245.

97. Pearson M. Racist notions of ethnicity and culture in health education. In: Rodmell S, Watt A (ed.) *The politics of health education: raising the issues*. London: Kegan Paul, 1986:38-56.

98. Crawford R. You are dangerous to your health: the ideology and politics of victim blaming. *International Journal of Health Services* 1977;**7**(4):663–680.

99. Lupton D. *The imperative of health: public health of the regulated body*. London: Sage Publications Ltd, 1995.

100. Patel R. Stuffed and Starved: Markets, Power and the Hidden Battle for the World Food System. London: Portobello, 2007.

101. Foucault M. *The archaeology of knowledge and the discourse on language*. New York: Pantheon Books, 1972/1991.

102. Goody J. *Cooking, cuisine and class: a study in comparative sociology*. Cambridge: Cambridge University Press, 1982.

103. Oddy DJ. *From plain fare to fusion food: british diet from the 1890s to the 1990s*. Suffolk: Boydell Press, 2003.

104. Rogers B. *Beef and liberty: roast beef, John Bull and the English nation*. London: Vintage books, 2004.

105. Mennell S, Murcott A, van Otterloo AH. *The sociology of food*. London: Sage, 1993.

106. Beardsworth A, Keil T. *Sociology on the menu*. London: Routledge, 1997.

107. Wood RC. *The sociology of the meal*. Edinburgh: Edinburgh University Press, 1995.

108. Douglas M. Deciphering a meal. In: Douglas M (ed.) *Implicit meanings: essays in anthropology*. London: Routledge, 1975:179–192.

109. Shepherd R. *Handbook of the psychophysiology of human eating*. Chichester: Wiley, 1989.

110. Shepherd R, Raats MM (ed.) *The psychology of food choice*. Wallingford (Oxon): CABI Publishing, 2007.

111. Lévi-Strauss C. *The raw and the cooked: introduction to a science of mythology: 1*. Harmondsworth: Penguin, 1966.

112. Lehrer A. Semantic cuisine. *Journal of Linguistics* 1969;**5**:39–56.

113. Beardsworth A, Keil T. *Sociology on the menu: an invitation to the study of food and society*. London: Routledge, 1997.

114. Douglas M. Deciphering a meal. *Daedalus* 1972;**101**:61–82.

115. Murcott A. On the social significance of the 'cooked dinner' in South Wales. *Anthropology of Food* 1982;**21**(4/5):677–696.

116. Morgan E, Purvis Dhj, Taylorson D (ed.). 'It's a pleasure to cook for him': food, mealtimes and gender in some South Wales households. *The public and the private*. London: Gower, 1983:78-90.

117. Murcott A. 'It's such a pleasure to cook for him': food, mealtimes and gender in some South Wales households. In: Jackson S, Moores S (ed.) *The politics of domestic consumption*. Hemel Hempstead: Prentice Hall/Harvester Wheatsheaf, 1995:89-99.

118. Murcott AI. Is it still a pleasure to cook for him? Social changes in the household and family. *Journal of Consumer Studies and Home Economics* 2000;**24**(2):78–84.

119. Ritzer G. *The McDonaldization of society: an investigation into the changing character of contemporary social life*. London: Pine Forge Press, 1993.

120. Mitchell J. The British main meal in the 1990s: has it changed its identity? *British Food Journal* 1999;**101**(11):871–883.

121. Davidson A. *The Oxford companion to food*. Oxford: Oxford University Press, 1999.

122. Mintz S. Tasting food, tasting freedom: excursions into eating, culture and the past. Boston: Beacon Press, 1996.

123. Caraher M, Baker H, Burns M. Children's views of cooking and food preparation. *British Food Journal* 2004;**106**(4):255–273.

124. Gvion Rosenberg L. Why do vegetarian restaurants serve hamburgers? Towards an understanding of a cuisine. *Semiotica* 1990;**80**(61–79).

125. Holm L, Mϕhl M. The role of meat in everyday food culture: an analysis of an interview study in Copenhagen. *Appetite* 2004;**34**(277–283).

126. Visser M. *Much depends on dinner*. Harmondsworth: Penguin, 1989.

127. Hartley D. *Food in England*. London: Macdonald, 1954.

128. Mason L, Brown C. *Traditional foods of Britain*. Devon: Prospect Books, 1999.

129. Lupton D. The heart of the meal: food preferences and habits among rural Australian couples. *Sociology of Health and Illness* 2000;**22**(1):94–109.

130. Dixon J, Bannell C. Heading the table: parenting & the junior consumer. *British Food Journal* 2004;**106**(3):181–193.

131. Keane A, Willetts A. Factors that affect food choice. *Nutrition and Food Science* 1994; **4**:15–17.

132. Bourdieu P. *Distinction: a social critique of the judgement of taste*. London: Routledge, 1984.

133. Bestor TC. How sushi went global. In: Watson J, Caldwell ML (ed.) *The cultural politics of food and eating: a reader*. Oxford: Blackwell Publishing, 2005:13–20.

134. National Consumer Council and Sustainable Development Commission. *I will if you will*. Report of the Sustainable Consumption Roundtable. London: Sustainable Development Commission, 2006.

135. Defra. *Understanding and influencing pro-environmental behaviour. research programme 2006/07 theme 3*. London: Department for Environment, Food and Rural Affairs, 2007.

136. Defra. *Public understanding of sustainable food*. London: Department of the Environment, Food and Rural Affairs, 2007.

137. Cook I, Crang P. The world on a plate: culinary culture displacement and geographical knowledge. *Journal of Material Culture* 1996;**1**(2):131–153.

138. Roden C. *A new book of Middle Eastern food*. London: Viking, 1985.

139. Zubadia S, Tapper R. *A taste of thyme*. London: IB Tauris, 2000.

140. Millstone E, Lang T. *The atlas of food: who eats what, where and why*. London/Berkeley: Earthscan/University of California Press, 2008.

141. Tinker I. *Street foods: urban food and employment in developing countries*. New York: Oxford University Press, 1997.

142. Barling D, Lang T. *Codex, the European Union and Developing Countries: an analysis of developments in international food standards setting. Report to Department for International Development*. London: Centre for Food Policy City University, 2003.

143. Symons M. *The pudding that took a thousand cooks: the story of cooking in civilisation and daily life*. Australia: Viking, 1998.

144. Symons M. *One continuous picnic: a history of eating in Australia*. Adelaide: Penguin, 1998.

145. Pendergast D. *Virginal mothers, groovy chicks & blokey blokes: re-thinking home economics (and) teaching bodies*. Brisbane: Australian Academic Press, 2001.

146. Hope A. *A Londoners' larder. English cuisine from Chaucer to the present*. Edinburgh: Mainstream Publishing, 1990.

147. Anderson EN. *Everyone eats: understanding food and culture*. New York: New York University Press, 2005.

148. Gigerenzer G. *Gut feelings*. London: Allen Lane, 2007.

Chapter 8

Inequality, poverty and social justice

This chapter resumes a discussion about food poverty and hunger, topics which have generated policy action throughout the 20th century and before (see Chapters 2, 4 and 6). A moral commitment to tackle them has united diverse interest in food policy, whether from a social, technocratic, nutritional, economic or environmental starting point. Hunger and poverty alleviation have long been core issues defining what food policy is about, giving it a moral sense of purpose. Yet, as the 20th century came to a close, that moral purpose was fractured by different health and environmental pressures. The food system needs to gear up to feed 7 billion people today and 9 billion people in a few decades' time, when its internal workings are already under considerable stress from socio-cultural, environmental and health challenges. The 21st century food policy task is not just feeding people but feeding them appropriately, sustainably and equitably.

The stark facts are that, measured by mal-nourishment and premature diet-related deaths, the post-World War II food policy project has not been a complete success, despite honourable intentions and actions. The pessimists can opine that medical progress has enabled populations to grow too fast and that, despite plant and animal breeding, management, mechanical techniques, waste-reduction, improved storage, refrigeration and so on, the capacity to make the quantum leap needed to feed 9 billion by mid-21st century is not likely. The success of the 1960s and 1970s Green Revolution relied on oil for fertilizers and energy. Now, when oil is approaching or at 'peak', this cannot be repeated. The pessimists—whether citing Malthus or the earth's carrying capacity—can paint a dire picture.

This is a delicate policy situation, requiring clarity about what the problem is here. As so often, one heading—'hunger' or 'food poverty'—covers a multitude of foci. These range from extreme hunger (famines) to routine under-consumption; from mass to localized market failure; from seasonal to all-year-round unmet need; from absence of food altogether to inappropriate eating due to poverty; from failures of crops to those of distribution; from absence of rights to being victims of events beyond control; from poor world to rich world.

The manifestation of lack of food takes different forms, as do proffered solutions and terminology. Terms used include: food poverty, food insecurity, malnutrition, underconsumption, social injustice, market failure and lack of food rights, citizenship or sovereignty, each coming with particular nuances and interpretations. This chapter does not exhaustively cover those variations; instead our focus is on how food policy, informed by an ecological public health perspective, might interpret the problem. For the present purposes we use famine to refer to extreme events and food poverty to persistent underconsumption. There is hunger and injustice in both. Both reflect challenges and failings of contemporary food systems.

What's the problem?

Poverty and hunger have been persistent and harrowing themes for the literary world. Steinbeck's portrayal of migrant US farm workers in the dustbowl of the 1930s is justly celebrated, as is the pioneering photo-journalism of Dorothea Lange, Walker Evans and Gordon Parles in the US Farm Security Administration, which ran from 1935-1944 as part of the President Roosevelt's New Deal programme. Maharidge and Williamson did a follow-up in the 1980s, reminding US readers of continuing problems living at agriculture's edge.[1] Fewer people beyond Norway, however, read the equally brilliant and sober account of despair in the 1890 novel *Hunger* by Knut Hamsun, winner of the Nobel Prize for Literature in 1920. Scholarly and political analyses have also been spawned by periods of intense food crisis and hunger. Examples range from Engels' classic study of mid-19th century Manchester, which informed his understanding of class politics, to Woodham-Smith's study of the 1845–47 Irish famine or Sen's of the 1943 Bengal famine or those in Ethiopia in the 1970–80s.[2–5] Alongside these studies of famine, another tradition has explored under-consumption and ill-health due to poor diet, the subject of inquiries by Rowntree and Pember Reeves in the early 20th century, right up to those by modern researchers such as Riches and Leather.[6–8] Some studies of rich society hunger have emphasized nutrient intake.[9, 10] Others have focused more on the social meaning.[6, 11–14] The point is that there is a continuity between novelists, economists, social reformers and nutritionists. They share a view that hunger and food poverty hold up a mirror to mainstream society.

Despite such apparent unity of moral and social concern, the formulation of policy response—if there is one—can be a murky and tough business, far from the neat model of evidence feeding into policy and practice in Fig. 1.2 (see Chapter 1). An illustration from the UK, rather than a developing country, is given by the infamous example of the Black Report. This was an inquiry into inequalities in health by three academics, Douglas Black, Jerry Morris and Peter

Townsend, under a Labour Government in the late-1970s. Its publication was buried by an incoming Conservative Government, which did not want to 'hear' the evidence in 1980. The report was published independently subsequently but ignored by official policy.[15] Considered unfinished business, a follow-up inquiry into inequalities and health was one of the first acts of the re-elected Labour Government in 1997.[16] This Acheson Report like the Black Report 20 years earlier and similar reports world-wide provide a cumulative documentation of food poverty as a significant factor on health, shaped by wider social determinants such as income, education and social status, the mantle championed by the 2006–08 WHO global Commission on the Social Determinants of Health.

Within this discourse, the notion of food security has been a key concept for health and agricultural strategies since World War II (see Chapter 4). It is used as shorthand for the challenge of feeding people adequately, by ensuring sufficient food production, affordability and access. FAO states that:[17]

> [f]ood security exists when all people, at all times, have access to sufficient, safe and nutritious food to meet their dietary needs and food preferences for an active and healthy life.

Like all simple terms, its meaning can be taken in different directions. Community food security is almost a proxy for anti-poverty work with an environmental and sustainability focus, while, for others, food security can be interpreted in national terms as 'self-sufficiency' or 'self-reliance'—whether a country can meet its own food needs. The OECD has stated that it sees the term as a slippery slope to economic protectionism or autarky. It formally defines food security as a[18]

> [c]oncept which discourages opening the domestic market to foreign agricultural products on the principle that a country must be as self-sufficient as possible for its basic dietary needs.

Recognizing the malleability of the term, UK Government economists summarized food security as having[19]

> common themes [which] are: availability of food; access of consumers to affordable, nutritional and safe food; resilience of the food system to significant disruptions, and public confidence in that system'.

From this book's perspective, we could shorten the definition of food security to a state where everyone is fed well, sustainably and healthily, and able to choose culturally appropriate food. The criteria by which to judge those terms then becomes the problem for policy.

Even defining the term illustrates the sensitivities of food failures due to poverty. Definitions and foci of food security, for instance, have changed with the policy times.[20] It has shifted from a collective or societal focus in the 1970s, to an individualized notion of responsibilities in the 1990s, and from being about access to food as a direct benefit and as a material and public good, to one where income—the means for buying food—has been the focus of policy, alongside those of more information and more choice (see Chapter 6). In the late-1990s, a gathering of European poverty researchers almost despaired at the popular belief that poverty and food poverty were a feature of Third World economies only, or that rich countries' welfare systems were in place to save only the unfortunate few individuals, but that extensive welfare was being abused and was unnecessary.[21] Food poverty goes to the heart of modern conceptions of the world and social progress.

Reasons for policy involvement

In response to the fatalists, then, a number of reasons for food policy involvement and interest in food poverty and hunger can be given. Few policy positions call upon each of these, but few deny at least one.

The first is *realpolitik*. Social movements for centuries have had rallying cries about food poverty, prevention of hunger, and demands for land to feed people. In late-20th century Brazil, for example, the hunger movement had millions of active members, altering its country's politics. Food prices are always politically troublesome, a touchstone of how successful an economy is, with the relationship between income (wages) and the price of food highly sensitive. Food prices are a high-profile factor in the cost of living.[22–24] Wage demands are frequently couched in terms of the cost of existence, and food's role can be taken as an indicator of the condition of a state.[25]

The second reason to take this issue seriously in food policy is that the absence of food and responses to that situation can be overt political actions, where food is a means of social control. Using food as a political weapon is a tactic with a harsh history; many a siege was won, not militarily but by starving defenders into submission. Using access to food as a weapon was a policy infamously modernized for President Nixon by Earl Butz, his Secretary of Agriculture in the 1970s. He argued that US farmers should 'get big or get out' and is remembered for re-articulating US foreign policy around huge grain deals, first with the 'enemy' the Soviet Union and then refining the use of US grain surpluses as a political weapon on countries the administration wished to influence.[26, 27] Such policies are overt, but food philanthropy can also be a more subtle mode of control on the poor. Charles Dickens, for example, endlessly probed beneath the veneer of Victorian charitable 'good works'. The critics of food-aid point out how aid rarely comes without strings attached.[28, 29] Scepticism can greet good will, questioning the terms and conditions and the equality of the donation. In the 2000s, Zambia, Zimbabwe and Mozambique were all offered, but refused, GM stocks as food-aid, arguing that they were being used as a dumping ground or as experiments.

The third reason for food policy interest is that poverty in general and food poverty particularly expose decisions about the allocation of resources. Even today, when there are unprecedented billions of inhabitants, there is enough food, measured calorifically, to feed the world; everything depends on distribution and who eats which sort of diet. [30, 31] Peter Townsend, one of the authors of the 1980 Black Report, wrote previously that:[32]

> [i]n all societies, there is a crucial relationship between the production, distribution and redistribution of resources on the one hand, and the creation of sponsorship of style of living on the other hand. One governs the resources which come to be in the control of individuals and families. The other governs the 'ordinary' conditions and expectations attaching to membership of the society, the denial or lack of which represents deprivation.

A fourth reason for policy interest is that adequacy of feeding and levels of food supply are indicators of 'national efficiency'. Not to feed or educate its people well opens a state to the charge of a loss of potential. This was the patrician view of Bismark in newly unified Germany in the late-19th century and is the view still of otherwise industrialized countries like the USA and France, giving them advantage when world prices are high.[33] The notion of human capital (championed by the economist Pigou) proposes that good economies optimize their human capital, ensuring their people have the skills to perform effectively within an efficient division of labour. The social consequences of not doing this is a theme emerging from many studies of food poverty.[34–36] In the 1990s and 2000s, countries with rising high-growth, such as China and India, were liberalizing their economies but seeing a slowing of progress in reducing childhood mortality. In China, the restructuring of the food supply was judged to have raised the relative cost of food, slowing progress in tackling infant mortality.[37, 38] Meanwhile, Vietnam and Bangladesh, with lower national income but who continued to invest money from taxation in public services, were more successful in lowering childhood mortality rates.[39] Vietnam and Bangladesh invested in food programmes for schools and communities, reaping rewards in the medium and, they hope, the long term.

Fifthly, there are financial (as opposed to social or health) advantages in investing in food-poverty reduction, and costs in not doing so. Tackling inequality or poverty makes financial sense. A 2006 report from the UK's Rowntree Foundation calculated that the cost of halving UK childhood poverty by 2010 would be a £4 bn saving to the national economy. If this were to be reduced to 5% over the ensuing decade, there would be a further £28 bn savings.[40] The reports on health by the banker Sir Derek Wanless to the UK Treasury and the 1990s World Bank/WHO methodology for calculating disability-adjusted life-years (DALYs) have been further examples of winning central government attention to the value of ill-health prevention using cost arguments.[41, 42]

The sixth reason is pragmatic, that famines and food poverty create pools of discontent and political trouble, which cascade down the decades. Greater understanding of how famines and food poverty are socially manufactured exposes both short and long term impacts.[43, 44] The fact that food was exported, such as butter, wheat and other select products, which the Irish poor could not afford, throughout the 1840s Irish famine, shocked people then and still today.[3, 45] Debates about the great famine at its 150th anniversary played a part in the Irish Government initiating a new social exclusion policy, with food as a key indicator.[46] In 2002, Argentina continued exporting significant amounts of foodstuffs, while it had a problem of child hunger and malnourishment.[47]

The final reason for food policy interest is that how hunger or food poverty are addressed, not just manifest, betrays a society's values. Whatever their politics, people have a conception of what sort of society they deem to be decent. Notions of social justice may vary but they exist. The poor are in this respect like miners of old, who used live canaries to test whether the air in the mine was safe to breathe. If the bird died, the miners ran. Food crises almost always hit the poor worst and first. The more affluent can side-step problems but the poor lack such flexibility. Ultimately, food poverty is a matter of human concern and care, the recognition that one's fellow citizen—whether this word is defined in planetary, regional, national or local terms—is not too dissimilar to oneself. The need for food from a healthy, sustainable food supply is common even if its achievement is not.

How to measure food poverty?

There are many indices of poverty. The Jarman index, for example, was designed to estimate how heavy the demand for medical services would be.[48] The Townsend Deprivation Index was developed to look at material circumstances.[49] Generally indices are developed to research whether deprivation is a factor affecting other manifestations, such as health or longevity. From the late-1890s, Atwater in the USA calculated how much and which foods workers, performing different tasks, needed to maintain health. Such findings became the benchmarks for estimating different welfare levels.[50–52] Rowntree and Bowley took a different route in the UK, defining in 1902 what they termed the 'primary' poverty line as the threshold at which a minimum standard, necessary for physical health, could be maintained.[53] Subsequently, in 1941 Rowntree added a higher threshold allowing for 'social participation', not just the bare minimum of dietary needs; this was an acknowledgment that social interaction is intrinsic to a decent, dignified existence.[54]

Nutrition and food intake are almost always used as measures of poverty, if not as the main focus (as for Rowntree), then as a part (as with Townsend). This is why many nutritionists prefer to measure what people actually eat, rather than to set a socially framed threshold of what they ought, might or minimally could eat. At its most extreme, the ultimate threshold is death from starvation or mal-nutrition but there can be confusion for statisticians about the final cause of death. For food policy, however, the questions that matter are which conditions engender or prevent hunger, and which indicators best predict outcomes. Measurements are delicate policy matters. The British Office of National Statistics (ONS) and its forerunners have been accurately measuring British diets since 1940.[55] Its data shows that in 1975–2000 the gap between rich and poor, in consumption of fresh fruit, increased.[56] That is fact but, politically, did it matter? That is a policy not just a scientific question.

One approach to this problem is to define the requirements necessary to meet basic human needs, but such 'scientific' standards can be criticized as social judgements masquerading as science. Scientific standards for whom and what? Policy arguments revolve around the process of setting those standards. Are they arbitrary? Socially loaded? Too high or too low? Where the budget level is pitched becomes a highly sensitive issue, even in affluent countries like the USA, UK, Australia and Canada.[57] But trying to do measurements can keep attention on at risk social groups, which otherwise slip beneath the societal and political radar. UK research in the 1980s and 1990s found the following social groups at food risk: families with dependent children,[58] young single men paid at or below the minimum wage,[59] and older people living on state pensions.[60] Dowler showed that lone parents living for long periods on low incomes were unable to afford to purchase sufficient basic, appropriate food for a healthy life, particularly if they were living on means-tested state benefits for more than a year.[61] Neo-liberals could interpret this as failure to budget sensibly or as family failure, but critics argued that it showed how the gradually high welfare standards, won from the late-1940s to the late-1970s, had been eroded by the neo-liberal erosion of welfare. In 1980–2000, low-income households increased in numbers in the UK, generating the widest gap between rich and poor for 40 years.[62] At the turn of the century, one in five children in the UK lived in families with income below the poverty line.[40 59, 63] Even in the mid-1990s, Leather could show the evidence that a significant proportion of the population could not afford to eat a healthy diet in line with UK recommended standards.[6]

In response to findings such as these, the newly created Food Standards Agency, of which Leather had been deputy chair, set out to do a 'proper' study which would end arbitary standards and get a clear picture of UK food poverty today. The Low Income Diet and Nutrition Survey (LIDNS) study found that the poor ate worse than others, but not to the extent anticipated.[9] The FSA narrative to the press was that all the British failed to eat adequately, not just the poor. In fact, the detailed findings showed a more complex picture, with the sample exhibiting high levels of obesity and overweight, low exercise, excess calorific intake, and low fruit and vegetable consumption.[64] Far from grounds for complacency—the impression given by the government's media managers—there was much to be troubled by: 39% of LIDNS respondents said they had been worried they would run out of food before more money came in; 36% said they could not afford to eat balanced meals; 22% reported reducing or skipping meals; 5% reported not eating for a whole day because they did not have enough money to buy food. Yet the FSA took the view that 'this study did not identify any direct link between dietary patterns and income, food access or cooking skill' and that the findings from the study will be used 'to help inform their policy making in areas of diet, nutrition and health—in particular those departments with responsibility for lifestyle issues such as smoking and drinking'.[65] Food poverty became a 'lifestyle' issue.

Meanwhile, in the early 1990s, the Family Budget Unit at the University of York had found that, in order to eat a healthy diet that was 'modest but adequate', which admittedly lacked variety and options, those living on benefits would have to increase their food spending by between 6 and 13%.[66] This was expenditure that families living on benefits could not afford. The most immediate concern of families living in poverty, according to other research, is less their long-term health, than the immediate satisfaction of hunger and filling up children.[67] It is not that families in poverty are unaware of the health benefits of eating certain types of foods; just that that these assume a lower priority than the immediate concern of filling stomachs.[6, 11, 68]

Although average spending on food dropped to historic lows—about 10% of household income by the 2000s—meeting government guidelines for a nutritionally sound diet required more expenditure than is usually given. A 1996 study found that basic foodstuffs cost 24% more in local shops than in supermarkets and that a household on benefits would have to spend 25% of its income on food to achieve some semblance of a nutritionally sound diet.[69] The conclusion sent a signal to policy-makers that supermarkets were not just good value for the poor but the answer. Making food cheap, rather than making a health-enhancing diet affordable became the policy yardstick. The distinction is crucial. Another study of local access costed a food basket that would give a young UK male 2,550 kcal, while meeting dietary recommendations. It found a big gap between the money available in welfare benefits and the amount it would actually cost to eat healthily.[70] Such studies suggest that food intake follows income rather than long-term health needs. People on low incomes are financially driven—whatever other reasons exist—to eat more processed foods and lower amounts of healthy enhancing nutrients. Cost and culture are locked in.

Another approach to measurement is relativist. There is ample evidence of how relative inequalities within a society can have a powerful effect on health.[71-75] Perhaps the simplest relativist system of measuring was that developed by Mack and Lansley in the mid-1980s, who asked people to judge what they thought were necessary needs. From this they produced a 'people's definition'.[76] Rather than seeking absolute, scientific or objective measures, they argued that it is more socially meaningful to build in expectations and social values. In 2008, Bradshaw and colleagues refined this approach by both asking 'ordinary' people to define what they deemed necessary for existence in modern society and refining this against specialist scientific assessment. This produced a minimum income standard with budgets based on consensus about social norms in modern society but tested these against expert knowledge and research.[77] This methodology, they argued, could produce assessments of how people in different circumstances—individuals or in multi-person households, elderly or young—could feed themselves appropriately.

The EU takes a relativist approach. In practice, it and member states set 60% of median income as a proxy for the poverty line. It defines as poor those

> [p]ersons, families and groups of persons whose resources (material, cultural and social) are so limited as to exclude them from the minimum acceptable way of life in the Member State to which they belong.

In 1997, Ireland's Office for Social Inclusion adopted a socially relativist definition:[78]

> People are living in poverty if their income and resources (material, cultural and social) are so inadequate as to preclude them from having a standard of living which is regarded as acceptable by Irish society generally. As a result of inadequate income and resources people may be excluded and marginalised from participating in activities which are considered the norm for other people in society.

Along with an income standard, the Irish National Anti-Poverty Strategy uses comparative expectations of foods and meals (rather than just nutrients) as part of its measure of 'consistent' poverty. It has a composite deprivation index of eight items, three of which relate to food: having a meal with meat, fish or chicken every second day; having a roast or its equivalent once a week; not having gone without a substantial meal in the last 2 weeks.[46]

In truth, both absolute and relative approaches are valuable. They show the absolute characteristics, such as lack of resources and physical health outcomes, alongside relative aspects of food poverty and inequality, such as feeling isolated, not being able to eat what you feel necessary. From whichever quarter, studies have shown policy-makers that there are consistently large groups of people experiencing food deficits, even in developed countries. A study of Londoners may show different food problems to those experienced in sub-Saharan Africa but, for Londoners, that is their reality. Indeed, one study in the Greater London area, with its over 7-million population and then booming economy, showed huge disparities in income and living standards. It estimated that 20% of respondents could be defined as food insecure and 6% food insecure with hunger.[79]

The many studies that have mapped access to shops and relative cost of food for different social groups in affluent societies are actually documenting how people live and make sense of their lives.[80–82] A consistent finding from such research is how people on low incomes can feel isolated from the cultural norm; they may have food options way above crisis points but within their own culture they are disadvantaged and diminished.[70] A family may be well-nourished from a calorific perspective but experience deprivation through lack of access to valued foods, preferred foods or consistent amounts of food.[83] This can result in making decisions about food, not on the basis of cost or health but to meet social objectives, as when parents on low incomes buy more costly branded foods for their children in order not to let them feel at odds with their peers. To be censorious about such actions is to misunderstand how everyone brings their values to the table (see Chapter 7).

Policy questions arising

A number of policy issues arise from the above. The first is whether food poverty and inequalities are special and warrant specific rather than macroeconomic policy responses. Generally, governments take the latter course, seeing little special about food poverty that 'ordinary' macro-economics and policy levers cannot resolve. In times of crisis such as the rocketing prices of 1971–74 or 2007–08, food poverty does receive more attention.[84] Generally, however, food needs and poverty have been subsumed within macro-economics. An example is the UK's pursuit of 'cheap food policies' from the 19th century. This was not philanthropy but central to a deliberate economic goal, of keeping wages under control; cheap food, low wages. Today, cheap food is under attack for externalizing environmental, as well as social, costs (see Chapters 5 and 6). Behind cheap food may lie uncosted or under-costed externalities in the form of threats to the environment, healthcare bills, distant workers on low wages and other social dislocations. This raises moral questions of general economic policy, but also specific ones for food policy.[85] Rather than polarizing understanding—and therefore policy—between the general and specific, macro-economic and food policies, it is more sensible to accept that the two foci are related. David Gordon has captured this connection between overall policy and specific food policy in policies common in Europe over the last four centuries (see Table 8.1).

Another debate concerns whether better policy follows a structural or an individualized approach.[86] If the former, policy attention is more distal and systemic, concerned about the determinants of issues such as access, affordability, availability and income. If the latter, attention is more proximal and concerned with issues such as choice, awareness and acceptability. Both see the matter of responsibility as crucial for policy. Does it lie with state, companies or people? The commercial sector's low profile on poverty and hunger does not signal disinterest. The State is frequently the arbiter of last resort about poverty, and the entity with power to alter the terms on which markets operate. Setting a minimum wage puts an onus on employers, for instance, as do labour regulations on health and safety, or the setting of welfare rates funded by taxes.

Another issue arising is whether food poverty illustrates a shift in social stratification. In the 19th century, working people would not have imagined that their low-income descendents might be troubled by inappropriate diets amidst what, to them, would have looked like abundance. In the late-20th century,

Table 8.1 Aims of European anti-poverty policies and food policy for the poor, 17th to 21st centuries

Century	Purpose of Anti-poverty Policy	Food Policy for Poor
17th and 18th	Relief of indigence	Prevent starvation but setting minimalist standards.
19th and early 20th	Relief of destitution	Economic production/physical efficiency. Prevent idleness.
20th	Alleviation of poverty	Nutritious diet for subsistence. Prevent hunger.
21st	Eradication of poverty	Inclusive diet. Prevent exclusion.

Source: modified from Gordon D. *Child poverty*. Presentation to conference 'Poverty, food and health in welfare: current issues, future perspectives'. July 1-4, 2003. Lisbon, Portugal. www.bristol.ac.uk/ sps/downloads/spsnews/gordonppt_cpsj.doc [accessed June 19 2008]. Bristol, Townsend Centre for International Poverty Research.

some theoreticians argued that globalization meant the end of old class structures and that a new era had emerged with wide and unprecedented opportunities and choice.[87] In fact, inequalities within and between societies never went away, although the fortunes of some countries improved. Vietnam, China, India and Brazil moved from being poor, post-colonial countries to vibrant economies with a growth of overall wealth and the emergence of new middle classes, but this cannot disguise the astonishing inequality of wealth, nor the emergence of a super-rich global élite. A much cited statistic, produced by the UNDP at the height of the celebration of the supposed end of the 'old' class stratification, showed that the income gap between the fifth of the worlds' people living in the richest countries and the fifth in the poorest, doubled from 1960 to 1990, from a ratio of 30:1 to 60:1. By 1998, the gap had jumped to 78:1.[88]

Food-consumption patterns illustrate the existence of old harsh inequalities with new faces. New consuming class structures have been grafted on to, rather than replacing, existing systems of social stratification, such as gender, religion, caste or socio-economic status. To capture this, Durning proposed the global existence of three consuming classes.[89] He painted a picture of 'over-consumers' eating meat and dairy, pre-processed packaged food, a diet that is both wasteful and that would now be judged to be with high carbon and deep ecological footprints. They assuage thirst with soft drinks and use cars to get to shops. The 'middle class' bikes and buses to shops, eats grain and drinks water. And the 'under-consuming' or poor class has insufficient food, unsafe water and is restricted to walking, if it goes anywhere. This typology resonates with the complex dietary data from studies of the nutrition transition.[90] Those suggest, not just that there is a shift from under- to over- or mal-consumption, but that the nature and quality of the foods changes at the same time, meshing three related transitions: socio-cultural, nutritional and economic.[91] In this process the meaning of poverty alters, as the significance of food changes from being a source of human motor power (eating to have energy) to being shaped by psychological motives (assuming energy). Food shifts from being a physiological need to a cultural want.

This is the new context for food poverty and hunger. There is calorific surplus and a deleterious move to a diet dominated by energy-dense foods in which fat and sugar are cheap. The poor consume inferior diets, both in terms of amounts and quality. Meanwhile, role models and other dietary ramifications also change. Whereas in past eras, the poor were thin and the rich able to be fat; now it is the poor of Western societies who are overweight, while the affluent of developing countries are the fatter within their societies. A new typology of food poverty emerges from the ecological public health perspective (see Table 8.2).

Table 8.2 'Old' and 'new' forms of food poverty

	'Old' food poverty	'New' food poverty
Availability	Lack of food	Over-abundance of processed foods
Nutrition problem	Under-nutrition	High-calorie intake and overall lack of balance
Nutrient profile	Nutrient light	Energy/calorie dense
Nutrition problem	Under-nutrition	Lack of balance
Availability	Lack of food	Food in abundance but 'warped' choices
Meal occasions	Few	Continual 'grazing'
Food expenditure	High % of household spending	Low % of household spending
Price Implications	Absolute cost of food	Relative cost of food
Social implication	Removal from the norm	Social and cultural isolation
Work	Manual	Sedentary
Easiest mode of Access	Walk or bike	Car
Fuel	Food	Fossil fuel
Drink	Water	Carbonated drinks
Price pressures	Cost of food	Cost of food relative to other demands
Social implication	Removal from the norm	Social and cultural isolation
Appearance	Thinness	Obesity
Fantasy role model	Plump/fat royalty	Thin celebrities

There is no single factor that determines food poverty and inequalities; no 'magic bullet' that can transform it. The literature suggests a complex interplay of factors for which there is unlikely to be a single social or technical fix; understandably, researchers thrive on proposing, debunking and downgrading single factors. The vehemence with which some researchers dismissed the arguments about the impact of retail restructuring on the poor is a case in point. In the 1980s, for example, Scottish anti-poverty campaigners argued that health education homilies urging the poor to consume more wisely were omitting the realities of the difficulties of healthy shopping in areas that lacked good shops. The argument was that retail geography could be a barrier to behaviour.[92–94] Others countered that there was no such evidence in places such as Glasgow or Brisbane.[95] A study that monitored the impact of the opening of a new hypermarket into one low income city area found that access to a reasonable range of cheaper fruit and vegetables when did not radically change the purchasing patterns or intakes in low income households in the area.[96, 97] However, such research is probably too restrictive, in that it does not interweave cultural alongside price and physical geography.[59, 60] A study of food shopping in Newcastle in north-east England found that retail-related factors were not important predictors of food patterns for the majority of the population, who shopped at larger supermarkets where the range of 'healthier' food, including quality fruit and vegetables, was better than in smaller 'convenience' stores. There were, however, some areas of the city where it was hard to obtain reasonably priced fresh fruit and vegetables in local shops or supermarkets. Another study, in a deprived area of London, showed marked variation in availability and price of fruit and vegetables.[70] In short, what started as a simple 'food deserts' argument, brought out complex linkages. Access to where food is cheaper can depend on access to a car. A study showed that of the poorest 30% of households, more than half had no car. In a society that gives priority to cars as the main means for mobility, not to have one is to be restricted.[98] The conclusion from this welter of important data is that single factors are unlikely to be the sum of the situation.

Another issue raised by food poverty is the question of institutional appropriateness. Most hunger institutions are focused on developing countries with the UN's food crisis bodies, the World Food Programme and the FAO, having the highest profile. But there has been a remarkable growth of local initiatives too in both rich and poor countries. In Canada, the city council created the Toronto Food Policy Council, in part to monitor food poverty. In the UK, the NGO alliance Sustain has had a 20-year project on food poverty. In Brazil, the Movimento Sem Terra has been a leading social force for justice around land and food. The growth of civil society campaigns has put strong pressure on state and corporate institutions to change and tackle deficiencies. Civil society bodies have been remarkably inventive in generating international networks to share experience. They focus on giving voice to those at the bottom of society, rather than liaising with the élite. Table 8.3 illustrates how different stakeholders conceive of food poverty at different levels of governance.

Solutions: who should do what?

Generally, across the whole range of food poverty issues, from extreme famine to 'softer' wants, the discourse tends to be between the state and civil society. Food companies seem to be embarrassed by food poverty. Privately, one magnate from a large UK food company has many times said to one of the present authors that this is a matter for the State and the welfare system to resolve. Recently, however, food corporations have begun to support charitable

Table 8.3 Illustrative positions on food poverty, inequality and social justice issues by governments, supply chains and civil society, global, regional, national/local

Level	Statements on...	...by Government	...by Companies	...by Civil society
Global				
	Anti-poverty goals	UN Declaration of Human Rights. Millennium Development Goals.	n/a	Jubilee 2000.
	Example of mode of working/ approach	Commission on Social Determinants of Health (WHO).	World Economic Forum (Davos).	World Social Forum.
	Child health and breastfeeding	Unicef /WHO Baby Milk Marketing Code.	Some ignore the Code.	International Baby Foods Action Network (IBFAN). La Leche League
	Control over food availability	WTO trade and agricultural agreements. World Food Summits.	Buyer networks. Standards Product development GlobalGAP and CIES-GFSI food standards.	World Social Forum. International Council on Social Development (Commission on Social Development).
	Information and education	UNESCO. Science programmes. Codex Alimentarius.	Lobbies at Codex Alimentarius meetings. International Advertising Association.	Consumers International. International Association of Consumer Food Organizations.
	Obesity policy	World Health Assembly 2004 resolution 57.17.	Codes of conduct. Product reformulation.	International Obesity Taskforce.
Regional (e.g. EU)				
	Anti-poverty goals	EU policy on social exclusion. Structural Funds. European Year against Poverty 2010.	Corporate responsibility.	European Anti-Poverty Network.
	Example of mode of working/ approach	European Foundation for the Improvement of Living and Working Conditions. EU Free fruit scheme.	Buyer networks to lower prices.	Food Banks (restaurants du Coeur).

Continued

Table 8.3 (continued) Illustrative positions on food poverty, inequality and social justice issues by governments, supply chains and civil society, global, regional, national/local

Level	Statements on...	...by Government	...by Companies	...by Civil society
Regional (e.g. EU)				
	Child health and breastfeeding	WHO-E resolutions and support programmes.		IBFAN. La Leche League.
	Control over food availability	EU Health Policy Forum.	CIAA.	European Public Health Alliance. European Public Health Association.
	Information and education body	Food labelling. Research programmes. Communications policy, e.g. EU Television Without Frontiers Directive.	Advertising and lobbying for 'free' market in marketing. Company helplines and websites.	Campaigns and Coalitions.
	Obesity policy	EU Platform for Action on Diet, Physical Activity and Health. WHO-E Istanbul Declaration.	CIAA labelling project. European Technology Platform 'Food for Life'.	European Heart Network. European Public Health Association.
National and Local				
	Anti food poverty statement of goals	Irish Govt national anti-poverty strategy.	Fare Share (company charity).	eg. UK.Children's Food Campaign Zaccheus 2000 Trust.
	Example of mode of working/ approach	Income support and welfare schemes.	In-store price competition.	Anti poverty alliances eg. UK. Child Poverty Alliance.
	Child health and breastfeeding	National programmes on maternal and child health.	Special children products.	Parenting groups, e.g. UK National Childbirth Trust.
	Control over food availability	Community food schemes. Cooking skills.	Food price competition.	eg. UK Sustain's Food Access Network.

Table 8.3 (continued) Illustrative positions on food poverty, inequality and social justice issues by governments, supply chains and civil society, global, regional, national/local

Level	Statements on...	...by Government	...by Companies	...by Civil society
National and Local (UK)				
	Information and education body	School food education. Policies on TV advertising for children.	Sponsorship and marketing.	Campaigns and use of media.
	Obesity policy	National campaigns, e.g. UK *Better Weight, Healthier Lives* National programmes, e.g. MEND.	Marketing. Product reformulation. Corporate sports sponsorship.	NGO campaigns on food and physical activity.

systems and have helped institutionalize the donation of surpluses or unsellable food. North American Food Bank, Fare Share and Second Harvest schemes, which take left-overs from shops and restaurants, have been aided by tax breaks. In Canada, for example, which used to have a strong welfarist societal ethos, such schemes grew as welfare was restructured, and some argue that such schemes provide a basis for that process.[8, 99] Corporate responsibility initiatives rarely make overt links to anti-poverty but company corporate relations departments are open for opportunities to strengthen brands by 'community engagement'.

Economic

In practice, however, much economic debate about food poverty centres on whether market solutions are possible or whether intervention is required via taxation and other fiscal measures. Taxation provides funds that the state may direct to ends as it sees fit. Throughout the 20th century, taxation and state insurance schemes softened the harsh edges of high industrial capitalism, when charity and philanthropy were the only alternatives to family support. Different policy mixes emerged, including insurance-based systems (Bismarckian) and universalist provision (Beveridge). The high point was probably the triumph of Keynesianism in the mid-20th century, which yielded real gain, but by the 21st century the onus had shifted back from state or collective provision to private provision and responsibility.[100] Variations exist between countries, even at the same level of wealth, with some placing emphasis on market-based social insurance and other being more overtly redistributive.[101] Using taxation for redistributive purposes has been the implied solution for inequalities in health; individual responsibility cannot replace societal signals.[102] Average incomes may rise but there may be more people who are relatively poor.[103, 104] The link between inequalities in income and population mortality could also be an artefact of the curvilinear relationship between income and health.[105]

Despite the broad connections, few governments openly espouse the need to reduce inequality of income distribution, for fear of sending anti-market signals.[106] As a result, in food policy, the options have been narrowed to a generally ameliorative approach and concerns about the implications of giving benefits in cash or in kind, and via which channels. Giving money directly to people invites accusations of encouraging easy living off the backs of others less indigent; giving benefits in the form of actual food, as is done in the US through food stamp schemes, for example, retains control. Many societies have a patchwork of measures that lack coherence. Ideas are borrowed; small schemes tried. Incrementally a labyrinthine welfare structure emerges. In the 1990s, for example, UK policy was to raise children out of poverty but tax receipts were used to fund welfare reforms while encouraging disadvantaged groups or long-term unemployed back to work.[40] Extra vouchers for low-income pregnant mothers might be provided but the fundamental issue of benefit levels not being related to minimum food intake levels necessary for a healthy diet was not addressed, nor was the question as to whether the employment was environmentally sustainable.[107] The model assumed parents would be working but could not address parents who might choose not to return to work but to look after their children.

Does it make economic sense for a society to ensure that all citizens are fed well? An argument has emerged that resolving food poverty could be conceived as a 'public good for health' drawing on the parallel notion of environmental goods and 'public goods'.[108] The assumption is that human well-being requires both public and private goods and that the pursuit of each has value. Public goods have in the past tended to be outside the market place. They are 'goods' that are accessible to the public and with universal value, even if they are privately owned in whole or in part. For economists to accept something as a public good, it must meet at least two criteria. The benefits must be public and not open to rival bids, thus being 'non-rivalrous', and 'non-exclusive' in the sense that no-one should be excluded from having access to it. Within this terminology, to view food welfare and poverty alleviation through the lens of public goods might be championing a return to seeing food as a common right, or it might signify a new twist in its commodification.[100]

Education and information

Education and information are the default anti food poverty strategy, with many initiatives targeted at the poor. For example, weight-reduction programmes show signs of doing this, since overweight and obesity in rich countries are associated with lower income groups, the reverse for poorer countries. The purpose of information and education srategies are to change behaviour. They fit psychological analyses locating the reasons for poor nutritional intake primarily at the level of behaviour and attitudes, rather than the societal or economic level.[109, 110] Yet individual preferences are, in fact, a complex of factors ranging from the physiological to cultural (see Chapter 7). This is why the policy focus on individual behaviour, lifestyle and 'healthy choices' has been so contentious, and resisted by civil society organizations.[111]

Technical intervention

Harnessing technical change to deliver dietary improvements for the poor has been another policy approach. The goal of improving nutrient availability has been pursued since von Liebig's day. Infrastructural improvements, such as refrigeration and storage, have been highly effective in reducing waste and spoilage throughout the food-supply chain, and have increased supply.[112] Besides infrastructure, other important technical measures are supplementation and fortification. Supplementation refers to the addition of foods, compounds or specific supplements to ensure at-risk groups receive required nutrients over and above their normal dietary intake. WHO and Unicef, for example, have followed a supplementation strategy for vitamin-A deficiency in children for 10 years, which affects an estimated 127 million pre-school children world-wide. The strategy has been broadly judged to be effective in both health and cost terms,[113] although there have been calls to renew its focus.[114]

Fortification, on the other hand, is the addition of nutrients missing in a diet to existing foods, usually staple foods.[115] Folic acid, for example, is added to bread to reduce neural tube defects.[116, 117] Fortification works if there is a specific or a limited number of nutrients absent from diet or needing to be boosted for at-risk populations. Its impact can be quick. In its World Health Report 2002, the WHO gave a sober account of the global situation with regard to child and maternal underweight, causing an estimated 3.4 million deaths in 2000, 1 in 14 deaths globally. About 1.8 million of these were in Africa. About 138 million DALYs, 9.5% of the global total, were due to under-nutrition, over half of all child deaths in developing countries. The solution to this dire effect of poverty, recommended by WHO, was supplementation and fortification, arguing that it combines preventive and curative interventions, and is the 'most cost-effective strategy to reduce under-nutrition and its consequences'. Micro-nutrient supplementation and fortification of vitamin A, zinc and iron is 'very cost-effective', WHO states, but should be combined with maternal counselling to continue breast feeding, and targeted provision of complimentary food, as necessary. While effective, such approaches are fixes for outcomes rather than causes of food poverty.

The attractions of fortification and supplementation to policy-makers are easy to see. In 2002, the Bill and Melinda Gates Foundation made a $50 million donation via the Global Alliance for Improved Nutrition (GAIN) over 5 years for a new fortification effort to tackle micro-nutrient deficiencies.[118] But can fortification and supplementation work for the more complex health profile now emerged world-wide? Different technical directions tend to be favoured by the three nutritions (see Chapter 4). The life sciences, for instance, have attracted significant funding for functional foods, while ecological approaches, have tended to favour low-tech technical solutions, such as sustainable agriculture projects utilizing different modes of cultivation to deliver improved food security.[119] Functional foods are much more expensive and, so far, of little proven population effect.

Supporters of genetic modification argue that this can provide the new green revolution, taking hundreds of millions of people again out of poverty and hunger. Experience suggests that technical approaches on their own can be problematic and that they need to be located within, not replacements for, social strategies.[120] Although GM crops have grown dramatically in developing countries, it is there that the rising need is most acutely felt. There is always the danger that social needs are a rationale for technologies looking for a market.

Public welfare schemes

The highest profile policy response to food poverty and hunger is the systematic use of food-aid, welfare and relief programmes. Famine-relief and emergency food-aid are the ultimate crisis interventions,[121] involving a formidable co-operation between governmental and non-governmental bodies. The World Food Programme is the overarching UN food crisis alleviation programme (see below for a longer account). It is designed to fill immediate needs and provide emergency nutrition as part of crisis management and humanitarian relief. Less high-profile, but also within the welfare mode, are programmes such as school feeding schemes (food and milk), focused on mothers and children,[122] and 'food for work' programmes.[123] The latter are where food welfare is tied to work programmes. They are a form of food control but proponents argue that they are a response to critics of 'hand-outs'. Their use in India in the 1970s was highly contentious but the World Food Programme still has projects with a food-for-work title.

Welfare programmes frequently refer to food needs in their rationale. The Five Giants, which Beveridge's 1942 plans for a UK national insurance scheme set out to slay, were: want, squalor, idleness, ignorance and disease. The US war on poverty under President Lyndon B Johnson, as part of his Great Society set of programmes, included projects like Headstart, which is still regarded as having been successful.[124, 125] Such programmes became hate objects to the US neo-conservative movement, which argued that they were a waste of money. Globally many welfare programmes focus on children, young people and mothers; for example, breastfeeding support, school meals, cooking skills classes and milk. The latter was strongly favoured by 1940s nutritionists like Boyd Orr, whereas today, health organizations and academics more strongly support proposals to increase fruit and vegetables. In the EU, for instance, there was pressure to introduce a fruit scheme in the EU in the late-2000s.[126] England introduced such a scheme for key groups of 4-7 year olds in the mid-2000s. Public health advocates had noted how schemes such as US Second Harvest had been dogged by the criticism that it appeared to be responding more to farmers' interests—seeing the poor as a market for foods such as dairy products in surplus—than on the health needs of people on low incomes. In Europe, the case for improving fruit consumption is over-whelming; production and distribution need to be improved.[127]

Globally, the WHO has a strong international programme of support for school feeding programmes but school meals schemes can be dogged by politics.[122, 128, 129] In the century since they were created in 1906 English school meals have gone through a roller coaster of policy shifts. The scheme received (1944) and lost funding (1980); operated to nutrition standards then saw them removed to aid privatization, only to return as 'guidelines' (2006); went from being only for the poor (1906) to becoming a universal service (1940s), achieving market penetration of three-quarters of all children by the late-1970s, only to fall to a third by the 2000s, when privatization added costs; operated under a family service system (1950s), sitting at tables with crockery (to teach manners), then went to self-service to fit fast-food times (1980s), and then had little guidance on social behaviour at all; went from being cooked on site to being frozen or chilled and 'regenerated' on site; and so on. The history of school meals in the UK is in fact a microcosm of how food poverty can be a political football in multiple respects—technology, business, nutrition, culture, class and family responsibilities.[130–133] Despite this policy flux, public health analyses world-wide have continued to favour school feeding systems as a direct welfare service 'in kind' not 'in cash', which feeds children to adequate nutrition standards. Environmental criteria, however, have not featured highly so far, although they are emerging, particularly in

Nordic countries and in pioneering schools with championing headteachers or cooks.[134]

Food-aid and the World Food Programme

The World Food Programme (WFP) is the UN's umbrella organization for emergency food welfare. It is a donation system under which rich countries either give cash to enable local purchases or, in the case of surplus-producing countries, in the form of food. Despite donations being given in times of crisis, the system is remarkably smooth and efficient. In the 2000s, however, levels of donations declined, but at a meeting in Rome in June 2008, promises of increased donations (an extra $1.2 bn) were made. With world food-stocks having dropped to long-term lows, the WFP was entering a difficult period.[135] Just-in-time systems might be the favoured supermarket model but on a world scale carry considerable risks. (Even for supermarkets their effectiveness depends on controlling all variables.)

The birth and working of the WFP has been well-documented by John Shaw, a worker for decades in the World Food Programme.[136] Unlike the slow, patient generation of legal food rights, the WFP was created in the space of a few days in 1961, largely due to opportunistic leadership by George McGovern at a conference on behalf of US President John F Kennedy. This conference was reviewing slow progress on use of food surpluses, a matter of concern to US agriculture. McGovern was clearly frustrated by the lack of movement and seized the chance to propose a fully fledged programme. In a flurry of international telephone calls, he got Kennedy's approval that he could suggest this on behalf of the US Government and a 3-year temporary World Food Programme was approved. At the end of its first term, it was re-endorsed and the WFP is now an embedded element in the UN institutional architecture. Table 8.4 provides a summary outline of key events in the creation of the current system.

It would be inappropriate to leave the narrative about the WFP and its role in crisis food-aid there. Behind a curtain of humanitarian sentiment and apparent success in crises can sit some dubious practices and less than altruistic motives. Food-aid has been criticized for being corrupt, too tied to Western interests, linked to agency interests, dominated by local élites and failing to get to those who most need it. For critics, the archetype 'bad' food-aid is probably still that given by the US under its 1954 Agricultural Trade Development and Assistance Act, Public Law 480. PL-480, as it was known, was the key law of the US 'food for peace' programme. It subsidized donations to politically sympathetic regimes.[26, 137] Critics argue that aid has become routinized, an industry not a solution. These are views the big aid organizations take seriously. NGOs, for instance, have championed structural reform, as a result. Others counter

Table 8.4 The institutionalization of food relief programmes, 1940s to 2000s

Date	Event	Comment
1943	International Conference on Food and Agriculture, Hot Springs, USA	Begins planning for post-World War II policy on agriculture
1945	United Nations created (June)	Attempt to create a stronger international institution than the pre-War League of Nations (which had begun to forge a multilateral position on food needs[a]
1945	Food and Agriculture Organization created (October)	This had been flagged in World War II
1954	FAO Principles of Surplus Disposal written	Enshrines argument that surpluses be used for emergencies
1954	US passed Agricultural Trade Development and Assistance Act (Public Law 480)	Signals that food aid is linked to US foreign policy
1955	Pilot FAO investigation of use of project food aid in India	
1958	FAO proposed emergency food reserve; rejected by governments	
1960	UN General Assembly backed use of UN to transfer surpluses to 'food-deficient peoples'	Resolution 1496 (XV)
1961	President John F Kennedy created Office of Food for Peace in the White House, USA	George McGovern appointed first director
1961	World Food Programme created for 3 years only	Decision to continue it made at 1964 UN Conference on Trade and Development
1967	1st Food-Aid Convention	
1974	World Food Conference, Rome	Established World Food Council, FAO Committee on World Food Security; and Committee on Food Aid Policies and Programmes
1975	Global information and early warning system established	Monitoring system received huge attention and technical development
1986	Review by McKinsey and Co of World Food Programme secretariat	Arrival of 'efficiency' criteria
1993	World Bank conference on Overcoming Global Hunger, Washington DC	Symbolises the World Bank's close involvement in social goals and the end of its 'narrow' economistic approach

Continued

Table 8.4 (continued) The institutionalization of Food Relief programmes, 1940s to 2000s

Date	Event	Comment
1996	World Food Summit, Rome	Summarises the conventional approach that under-nourishment is the key social challenge for food policy
2002	World Food Summit + 5, Rome	Reiterates the above position
2008	High-Level Conference on Food Security, Rome	Raised $1.2 billion extra funding for the World Food Programme to address rising need caused by commodity price rises 2006–08

Sources: Shaw (2001).[121]

[a] Although rarely acknowledged, part of the passion for creating a new international institutional system in the UN 'family'—WHO, FAO, Unicef, UNCTAD, etc.—was the experience of the failed League of Nations. This failed in the sense that it did not prevent either Europe's war or the hardships that preceded it. Yet the League did begin to be a location in which international experience on food insecurity and food and health could be shared. League of Nations. *The problem of nutrition: interim report of the Mixed Committee on the Problem of Nutrition, Vol. 1.* A.12.1936.II.B. Geneva, League of Nation, 1936.

that aid provides vital support when development processes hit difficulties. US Senator George McGovern argued that food-aid could be a winner all round. Food-aid helped, firstly, the American farmer by disposing of surpluses (therefore raising commodity prices); using those surpluses for good ends fed people; and delivering this through the United Nations, rather than bilaterally, promoted the value of internationalism and inter-governmental institutions.[121] In truth, food aid inevitably reflects wider market conditions. Before the WFP was created in the 1960s, over 90% of food-aid was American, but by the 1980s, the European Union had emerged as a big donor. Like the US this was largely due to subsidized surpluses, with the EU giving around one-third of world donations, the USA over 40% and 11% from Japan. The latter gave cash to purchase grains on world markets.[138]

Politically, there are a number of broad positions on food aid:

- Food-aid is no substitute for decent livelihoods and equitable food systems. This requires re-adjustment of international trade relations. Pursuit of trade justice and, internationally, more open markets should be priorities. Aid is fine in the right place but should not deviate political attention from these wider, long-term goals of fair trade.[139, 140]

- Food-aid will always be needed as a crisis-management system and food-welfare safety net, just as some kind of global food stocks are needed. A decent and just world demands that the world has a system of international co-operation for crises.[121]

- Judicious use of food-aid is appropriate but should not be given for too long as it creates a dependency food culture and undermines local food systems. Food-aid should be linked with other social and economic regenerative goals. For social democrats this means routes such as fair trade.[138] For neo-liberals, this means market reform to promote growth to serve the individual.[141]

- Food-aid is a modern form of imperialism. Over-producing countries use the under-nourished as a convenient 'sink'.[28, 44] Aid rarely comes without conditions attached.

Measuring food insecurity

One outcome of the UN's role in food-aid has been the development of food (in)security monitoring. Today, the FAO and agencies have access to global monitoring systems, which predict where problems will emerge, collating weather, crop assessments and other data. Both the EU and USA have their own projects but the global network is currently co-ordinated by the FAO through its Food Insecurity and Vulnerability Information and Mapping Systems (FIVIMS).[142] The rationale for FIVIMS is simple: 'that improved information can be actively used to produce better results in efforts to reduce the number of under-nourished and achieve food security for all'. Figure 8.1 presents FIVIMS' conceptual framework for understanding the possible causes of low food consumption and poor nutritional status. The focus is clearly on the proximal dynamics, rather than the wider socio-economic context. The task of FIVIMS is to aid micro-management of crisis prevention and to help those in charge of aid distribution to get resources to where it is most needed. No measurement system, however, can replace proper political processes.

Globally, the figures generated by the FAO annually are sobering. The annual State of Food Insecurity (SOFI) reports catalogue the picture.[143, 144] After decades of reducing the number of under-nourished people (from the 1970s to the mid-1990s), absolute numbers of the under-nourished began to creep back up. Despite commitments made at the 1996 World Food Summit, again at the WFS+5 2002 conference, let alone measured against the ambitious targets set by the Millennium Development Goals, the picture is not rosy (see Fig. 8.2). The FAO continues to argue that there is ground for optimism and that more investment in agriculture would resolve nutrition problems in developing countries.[144] FAO (see Fig. 8.3) pointed to how China, South-East Asia and South America have significantly reduced their numbers of people experiencing under-nourishme nt (but Central Africa, the near East and East Africa's situations have worsened); and to how Southern/East and West Africa and China have reduced the proportion of under-nourishment (whereas Central Africa, East Asia and Central America have not).

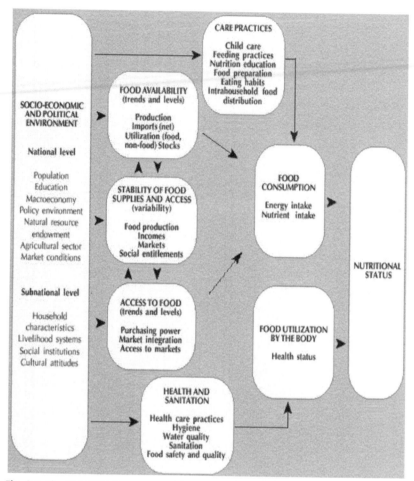

Fig. 8.1 The FAO/FIVIMS conceptual framework for understanding the possible causes of low food consumption & poor nutritional status

Food movements and food democracy

Social movements on poverty and hunger have taken many forms, ranging from mass liberation struggles to specific campaigns and civil society engagement. An illustration of the former are the land movements in Latin America, Asia and the Far East, demanding land redistribution and/or fairer distribution of wealth public.[145–148] An illustration of the latter might be the modern phenomenon of consciousness-raising and mass lobbies, such as the 1984 Band Aid concerts raising money for relief of the Ethiopian famine or the Jubilee 2000 global campaign calling on the G8 rich nations to back debt relief.[149]

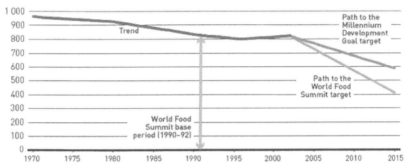

Fig. 8.2 Number of undernourished people in the developing world (millions)

Source: FAO State of Food Insecurity in the World 2006 pg 5(FAO, 2006)

Although modern campaigning has access to hugely powerful tools in the form of media reach and internet communications, solidarity actions are not new. The anti-slavery and emancipation movements of the 18th and 19th centuries were able to organize internationally too. Modern campaign tools are no guarantor of success, which is why many campaign groups combine public consciousness raising with lobbying and policy intervention at the national and inter-governmental level. One illustration is the long-running 'make poverty history' by Oxfam.[150]

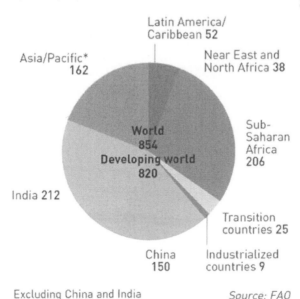

Fig. 8.3 Number of undernourished people in the world, 2001-03 (millions)

Source: FAO State of Food Insecurity in the World 2006 pg 8(FAO, 2006)

The right to food: from abstract to statutory?

One offshoot of the increasingly sophisticated analysis of food poverty and hunger since the 1960s has been a decades-long, international movement to create an international legal or statutory right to food.[151, 152] Table 8.5 summarizes some key events in this long process. The 1948 Universal Declaration on Human Rights, a key international document on general rights, located the right to food within the right to livelihoods. The language was general, saying less about how this should be judged or delivered. Article 25 (1) stated:[153]

> Everyone has the right to a standard of living adequate for the health and well-being of himself and of his family, including food, clothing, housing and medical care and necessary social services, and the right to security in the event of unemployment, sickness, disability, widowhood, old age or other lack of livelihood in circumstances beyond his control.

By the mid-1960s, 20 years into the post-war effort to expand food output mainly by technical means, it was already clear that hunger was not being beaten. As already noted, neo-Malthusian perspectives emerged suggesting too many mouths, not enough food. In 1966, the UN Committee on Economic, Social and Cultural Rights toughened the 1948 Declaration, expressing the right to food in four paragraphs, passed on 19 December 1966.[154] These commitments were due to come into force a long time ahead, 9 years later, on 3 January 1976, but by then the 1974 World Food Conference had been held in Rome, at which acknowledgment was made that, despite technical advances, hunger was still a major threat to developing countries. Although the green revolution was underway, its technocratic approach was being questioned by new analyses. These came from various quarters: egalitarian and social justice perspectives,[43, 44] environmentalism,[155, 156] and civil society appeals to act and eat differently.[157] Informed by these analyses, in the 1980s a new network was created by academics, lawyers, politicians and NGOs, intent on delivering food security as a legal right. Key among the academics were Asbjørn Eide, Wenche Eide, Arne Oshaug and George Kent. Active NGOs included Food First Information and Action Network (FIAN),* the World Alliance for Nutrition and Human Rights (WANAHR)** and the Institut Jacques Maritain International. They produced and promoted an International Code of Conduct

---

* This was an offshoot of the San Francisco think-tank created by Jo Collins and Francis Moore Lappé, from their big-selling books *Diet for a small planet* (1971) and *Food first* (1980).

** The World Alliance for Nutrition and Human Rights (WANAHR) is a network of individuals and institutions focusing on advocacy and outreach work in the promotion of a human rights approach to food and nutrition problem.

Table 8.5 The evolution of food rights in the United Nations, 1948–2008

Date	Event	Relevant article or action	Obligation and focus
1948	Universal Declaration of Human Rights.	Article 25 (1) (one sentence).	States that food is a basic human right.
1966	International Covenant on Economic, Social and Cultural Rights.	Article 11 (four paragraphs).	Calls on governments to (1) 'improve methods of production, conservation and distribution of food', using science, technology, nutrition and sound utilization of natural resources; (2) take into account 'the problems of both food-importing and food-exporting countries, to ensure an equitable distribution of world food supplies in relation to need'.
1974	World Food Conference.	States 'every man, woman and child has the inalienable right to be free from hunger and malnutrition in order to develop their physical and mental faculties'.	Created World Food Council to deliver this goal; disbanded in 1993. WFC asked each country annually to set out its needs, supply chain demands, etc. The WFC was closed in 1996 and its functions transferred to the FAO.
1989	UN Study 'Right to adequate food as a human right'.	Study Series No. 1, United Nations publication, Sales No. E.89.XIV.2.	Proposes 3 levels of right to food: 'to respect, protect and assist/fulfil' the right to Food.
1999	NGOs complete a Code of Conduct on the Human Right to Adequate Food.	Signed/supported by many NGOs in an international campaign following World Food Summit 1996.	Proposed to UN bodies.
1999	Committee on Economic, Social and Cultural Rights.	General Comment 12 (10 page document).	Obligation to respect, to protect and to fulfil the right to food (which includes the obligations to facilitate and to provide).
2000	UN Millennium Development Goals.	Goal 1: eradicate extreme poverty and hunger.	Target is to 'halve, between 1990 and 2015, the proportion of people who suffer from hunger'.

Continued

Table 8.5 (continued) The evolution of food rights in the United Nations, 1948–2008

Date	Event	Relevant article or action	Obligation and focus
2000	UN Commission on Human Rights Resolution 2000/10.	Recommends the appointment of a Special Rapporteur on Right to food.	(1) To 'receive information and highlight violations of the right to food.' (2) To 'co-operate with UN agencies, international organisations and NGOs to put the right to food into practice around the world'. (3) To 'identify emerging issues related to the right to food.'
2004	Voluntary Guidelines to Support the Progressive Realization of the Right to Adequate Food in the Context of National Food Security.	Whole document (19 specific Guidelines in 126 paragraphs).	Agreed voluntary guidelines on enabling: National measures on environment, assistance and accountability; International measures, actions and commitments.
2008	Declaration of the High-Level Conference on World Food Security: the Challenges of Climate Change and Bioenergy, June 3–6 2008.	Whole document (9 clauses).	Re-asserting importance of 2004 Voluntary Guidelines when addressing the rocketing of oil and food commodities on world markets, leading to a 'food vs. fuel' clash over land use.

on the Human Right to Adequate Food. This was widely circulated among civil society organizations and the development lobby following the 1996 World Food Summit. This combination of internal and external pressure succeeded. In 2002 the FAO Council set up an Inter-governmental Working Group, which 2 years later steered through the FAO policy-making processes a set of *Voluntary guidelines to support the progressive realization of the right to adequate food in the context of national food security*.[158] These voluntary guidelines proposed six core responsibilities that governments should deliver: an enabling environment; suitable policies and strategies; legal frameworks; adequate food, which is safe and nutritious quality within food markets; knowledge of vulnerable populations; and actions in the event of emergencies or disasters. Although not international statutes, the guidelines lay down how and when governments should act. The main onus is on National Governments. 'States have the primary responsibility for their own economic and social development, including the progressive realization of the right to adequate food in the context of national security'. But the guidelines acknowledge the importance of having an enabling international environment. UN bodies are 'urged to take actions in supporting national development efforts for the progressive realization of the right to adequate food in the context of national food security'.

This transition from an implicit 'right' in 1948 to 126 paragraphs of obligations grouped under 19 over-arching guidelines, ranging from general legal rights, frameworks and institutions to advice on markets, strategies, economic environments and safety nets in the 2004 voluntary guidelines, is at one level a testament to persistence and good international campaigning. The 2004 voluntary guidelines are a triumph of incrementalism within food policy. Supporters argue that the guidelines have at last put flesh on to the 1948 Universal Declaration's bare bones. At the 2008 High-Level Conference on Food Security, they were used to provide a moral compass and were referenced in the final declaration. A number of reservations remain, however. Firstly, the jury is still out on whether this right makes a difference at the national or local level. Proponents of the voluntary guidelines argue, understandably, that food rights provide a point of leverage on governments. Secondly, the food rights movement has, again understandably, focused on the State as the point of moral entry for tilting power over food supply in favour of the poor. In fact, in the late-20th century, as was shown in Chapter 5, food multinationals have emerged as the key location of modern food power.[29, 159–163]

Food democracy

Effective though the food rights movement has been, one of the lessons of food history is that rights are only valuable if they are used and incorporated into demands by the people and at-risk populations themselves. On their own, rights do not feed people any more than food being available ensures that all are fed. The key factor is whether people actively demand and pursue those rights, as Sen showed. The struggle to enshrine food rights has been an important rallying cry for decency within food policy, a set of criteria against which governments and the food system can be held to account. Yet at the time of writing, few National Governments have translated those rights into national laws, let alone celebrate how this right is an entitlement. Only two countries— Brazil and South Africa—have placed the 'right to food' in their constitutions. The South African Constitution contains three references to food and nutrition rights and requirements to legislate such rights. At his inauguration in 2003, Brazilian President Luiz Inácio 'Lula' da Silva launched *Fome Zero* (Zero Hunger), a national hunger eradication policy, now institutionalized at both national and programme policy levels. Such programmes and approaches to food poverty or insecurity are rare and it is a testament to the long mobilization in which Brazilian social movements held governments and societal values to account.

Fome Zero illustrates how improvements require struggle, dedication and hard work. There are powerful social forces unhappy to lose control and for whom charity may be less threatening than redistribution or resource reallocation. The modern Brazilian experience is particular to that country's politics, culture and history, but in the West too hunger and poverty were major national issues in the 20th century, a rallying cry for progressive groups. In the early 20th century, for instance, the dietary consequences of poverty brought together an alliance of women campaigners, medical interests and unemployed workers.[164, 165] They worked hard to build a political consensus around the value of welfare reforms, food safety nets and the need to give ordinary people more dignified lives. The indignity suffered by poor people due to cash shortages and poor quality diets was a persistent theme,[166, 167] in contrast to the emphasis on efficiency and national, military and morale factors being articulated at governmental level.[168] The term 'food democracy' has been proposed to articulate this citizens perspective, and the need for struggle and engagement.[169] Table 8.6 gives some key moments in the long English process of food democracy, with the ups and downs of progress.

One result of the ceaseless change in the world of food is that new social movements constantly emerge. Some are spawned protesting *against* something. Others emerge to *promote* something. Most quickly adopt both modes. Campaigns against adulteration have always become movements to improve food, moving from 'clear out' to 'clean up' mode, from protection to promotion. Campaigns evolve. They have developed for example from hunger to land rights; from labelling to advertising controls; and from rural to urban agriculture. Access to soil is limited in cities, yet NGOs like RUAF and UN research groups like CGIAR see urban agriculture as important policy directions for tackling food poverty.[170] Such thinking bridges the chasm between developed and developing countries, in that the needs are similar—for land, skills and tools— but projects can be developed on a human scale.[171] Urban agriculture is the antithesis of intensive, profit maximizing agriculture, celebrating rather than dispensing with labour, exchanging rather than replacing skills and knowledge of the at times tortuous process of nurturing food out of the earth.

The growth of community-led anti food poverty movements around the world shows remarkable inventiveness. Some are project-based, localized and environment-led like the VicLANES project in Melbourne.[86] Some have evolved from anti-poverty into pro-food justice campaigns such as Sustain's 20-year project the Food Access Network in the UK, believing that a food system

Table 8.6 Some events on the (long) English food democratic road

Date	Event	Actors/issue
1381	Peasants' Revolt	John Ball, Wat Tyler, Jack Straw led peasants in a march on London; almost succeeded but were tricked and defeated
17th C. & 18th C.	Sporadic outbursts about land rights	e.g., resistance to drainage of Fens and wetlands, and about other common spaces from which people fed themselves.
1770s–19th C.	Enclosure Acts	Latest of long bout of annexation of common lands by land-owners; an early example of privatization sanctioned by law.
1795–1830s	Speenhamland	A system of poor relief run at the local level to compensate if grain prices went high. Paid for by landowners. Culminated in 1834 Poor Law Amendments Act which set up workhouses instead, trapping the poor into grinding poverty. Object of mass unrest.
1819	'Peterloo' massacre	15 protesters killed by troops at a mass rally in Manchester on 16 August calling for right to vote, and angered by hunger following the end of Napoleonic Wars and introduction of Corn Laws designed to keep food prices high. Led to mass protests.
1832	Tolpuddle Martyrs deported to Australia	Earlier bans on trades unions and workers organising to improve wages had been lifted but six farmworkers in Dorset were arrested for forming a Friendly Society in protest against dropping wages. Their deportation led to massive outcry and they were reprieved in 1836.
1830s	'Captain Swing' riots	Luddism—an outbreak of violent breaking of new agricultural machines (e.g. threshers) judged (rightly) to be a threat to employment.
1846	Repeal of Corn Laws	Repeal of the 1815 Importation Act, which kept cheap food out of England by imposing tariffs. Subject to mass meetings. Spawned long tradition of UK state policy commitment to cheap food.
1820–70s	Anti Adulteration Campaigns	Long struggle to clean up food and ensure that food should be 'of the nature, quality and substance demanded'. Began with Accun's 1820 expose of food frauds and only finally won with a legal amendment in 1895. Process renewed in 1980s (see below).
1906	Education (Provision of Meals) Act	Enabled local authorities to levy a small sum from householders (rates) to create a school meals system in each Borough. Few did till women were wanted for waged work in World War I. Not made a universal benefit till 1944. Nutrition standards repealed in 1980 and returned in 2002.

Continued

Table 8.6 (continued) Some events on the (long) English food democratic road

Date	Event	Actors/issue
1905	Royal Commission on Supply of Food and Raw Material in Time of War	Reported on an inquiry into threats to food supply exposed in part by poor malnourished state of recruits for the Boer war in South Africa. Exposed risks of Imperial supply routes, as well as poor diets exposed by the Departmental Committee on Physical Deterioration Report (1904).
1930s	Hunger Marches	Organized by working class and trades union movements in protest at lack of jobs, welfare and food.
1930s	Co-operative Women's Guild investigation into hunger	Concluded that incomes were so low that it was nigh impossible to eat adequately.
1947	Agriculture Act	Popular agitation played its part in encouraging post-war Labour Government to rebuild food production, not least since the Empire had gone.
1955	End of rationing	As deeply unpopular after World War II as it had been accepted as just and fair in it. Health had been improved by more equitable distribution and rights. Particularly benefited the poor, but resented as 'top-down' control.
1990	Food Safety Act	Result of food campaigns from the 1970s and 1980s about new adulteration and safety standards.
2000	Food Standards Act	Created a new Food Standards Agency after campaigners—with public backing—argued for need for independent scientific body not influenced by food industry lobbies.
2002	Abolition of Ministry of Agriculture, Fisheries and Food	First created in 1879, popular outcry against perceived 'agency capture' led to MAFF being replaced by a new Dept for Environment, Food and Rural Affairs.
2006	School food nutrition standards reintroduced	New standards introduced, 25 years after they were removed in 1980 and after decades of campaigning to get new ones back.

should not penalize people for their birth or circumstances. In this respect the pursuit of food democracy is a ceaseless task, involving many interest groups, professions, trade unions, faith groups, voluntary organizations and community groups. The new language is of food citizenship, with rights and responsibilities. Citizens have capacities beyond those of consuming goods and services, they are active in society, which is more than simply a marketplace.

The analysis of food inequality, poverty and social justice presented here suggests a complex policy situation. Food poverty and inequality mean different things to different interest groups. This is a situation not just of facts but of interpretation and politics. The policy lexicon lengthens as movements articulate their demands. What began as food security has spawned: *food democracy*, to stress full social engagement; *food capacity*, stressing the capabilities and infrastructure necessary for sustainable production and consumption; *community food security*, stressing the need for local delivery by food systems to be meaningful; *food sovereignty*, pointing to the rights of small producers with more equitable social distribution; and *food citizenship*, suggesting active, knowledgeable participation. These actions express a common reluctance to abandon food poverty to the whims of the State or to the vagaries of markets and thoughtless commercial actions. In the evolving policy debates about food poverty, inequality and rights, civil society movements have been important in voicing the interests and experiences of those suffering food insecurity.[172] They have confronted the easy language of partnerships, so often offered in stakeholder perspectives on food poverty and hunger. Partnerships are beguiling but can be preferred as deviations from tackling fundamental inequalities of resource and power between state, commerce and civil society.[173] Among the many challenges for proponents of 21st century ecological public health is to ensure that voices for social rights and justice are not drowned out by the pressing health and environmental demands to protect the planet and physiological health. Policy-making needs to ensure that the evidence of societal inequalities' impact on food, and food's reinforcement of social inequalities, are at the heart of the 21st century food policy project.

References

1. Maharidge D, Williamson M. *Journey to nowhere: the saga of the new underclass*. New York: Hyperion, 1995.
2. Engels F. *The condition of the working class in England in 1844*. London: Penguin Classics, 1987 (1845/1892).
3. Woodham Smith CBFG. *The great hunger: Ireland, 1845–9*. London: Hamish Hamilton, 1962.
4. Sen A. *Poverty and famines*. Oxford: Oxford University Press, 1981.
5. Franklin T. *Cleft stick: the Ethiopian famine* London: Pluto Press, 1990.
6. Leather S. *The making of modern malnutrition: an overview of food poverty in the UK*. London: Caroline Walker Trust, 1996.
7. Riches G. *First world hunger: food security and welfare politics*. London: Macmillan, 1997.
8. Riches G. Food banks and food security: welfare reform, human rights and social policy. *Social Policy and Administration* 2002;**36**(6):648–663.
9. Nelson M, Erens B, Bates B, Church S, Boshier T. *Low income diet and nutrition survey*. Vol.1, 2 & 3. London: The Stationery Office/Food Standards Agency, 2007.
10. Nelson M, Naismith D. The nutritional status of poor children. *Journal of Human Nutrition* 1979;**33**:33–45.

11. Dowler E. Nutrition and poverty in contemporary Britain: consequences for individuals and societies. In: Köhler BM, Feichtinger E, Barlösius E, Dowler E (ed.) *Poverty and food in welfare societies*. Berlin: WZB, 1997:84-96.

12. Dowler E. Food poverty and food policy. *IDS Bulletin: Poverty and Social Exclusion in North and South* 1998;29(1):58–65.

13. Dowler E. Food and poverty: the present challenge. *Benefits* 1999;24:3–6.

14. Dowler E, Leather S. 'Spare some change for a bite to eat?' From primary poverty to social exclusion: the role of nutrition and food. In: Bradshaw J, Sainsbury R (ed.) *Experiencing poverty*. Aldershot: Ashgate, 2000:200–218.

15. Townsend P, Davidson N, Whitehead M. *Inequalities in health: the Black Report & the health divide*. Harmondsworth: Penguin, 1988.

16. Acheson D. *Independent inquiry into inequalities in health*. London: The Stationery Office, 1998.

17. FAO. *Special programme on food security*. http://www.fao.org/spfs/en/ [accessed June 19 2008]. Rome: Food and Agriculture Organization, 2008.

18. OECD. *OECD glossary of statistical terms: food security*. http://stats.oecd.org/glossary/detail.asp?ID=5006 [accessed June 19 2008]. Paris: Organization for Economic Co-operation and Development, 2008.

19. Defra. *Food security and the UK: an evidence and analysis paper. Food Chain Analysis Group*. London: Department for Environment, Food and Rural Affairs—Food Chain Analysis Group. http://statistics.defra.gov.uk/esg/reports/foodsecurity/foodsecurity.pdf [accessed 22 Dec 2006], 2006:96.

20. Maxwell S. The evolution of thinking about food security. In: Devereux S, Maxwell S (ed.) *Food security in Sub-Saharan Africa*. London: ITDG Publishing, 2001:13–31.

21. Köhler BM, Feichtinger E, Barlösius E, Dowler E (ed.) *Poverty and food in welfare societies*. Berlin: WZB, 1997.

22. Rowntree BS. *The human needs of labour*. London: Longmans, 1921.

23. International Labour Office. The worker's standard of living. *Studies and Reports Series B (Economic Conditions)* Geneva: International Labour Office of the League of Nations, 1938.

24. Kuczynski J. *A short history of labour conditions in Great Britain 1750 to the present day*. London: Frederick Muller, 1942.

25. Hartwell RM, Mingay GE, Boyson R, McCord N, Hanson CG, Coats AW *et al. The long debate on poverty: eight essays on industrialisation and 'the condition of England'*. London: Institute of Economic Affairs, 1974.

26. Morgan D. *Merchants of grain*. London: Weidenfeld and Nicolson, 1979.

27. Solkoff J. *The politics of food*. San Francisco CA: (Sierra Club Books, 1985.

28. Hayter T. *Aid as imperialism*. Harmondsworth: Penguin, 1971.

29. Wisner B. *Power and need in Africa*. London: Earthscan, 1988.

30. Dyson J. *Population and food: global trends and future prospects*. London: Routledge, 1996.

31. Smil V. *Feeding the world: a challenge for the twenty-first century*. Cambridge, Mass.; London: MIT, 2000.

32. Townsend P. *Poverty in the United Kingdom: a survey of household resources and standards of living*. Harmondsworth: Penguin, 1979.

33. Ernst and Young. *Food for thought: how global prices will hit UK inflation and employment*. Report of the Item Club, May. London: Ernst & Young, 2008:10.

34. Deveraux S, Maxwelll S. *Food security in sub-Saharan Africa*. London: ITDG Publishing, 2001.

35. Pena M, Bacallao J. *Obesity and poverty: a new public health challenge*. Washington: Pan American Health Organization, 2000.

36. Pena M, Molina V. *Food based dietary guidelines and health promotion in Latin America*. Washington DC: Pan American Health Organization, 1999.

37. Oxfam. *In the public interest: health, education and water and sanitation for all*. Oxford: Oxfam, 2006.

38. French H. Wealth grows but health care withers in China. *New York Times* 14 January 2006.

39. United Nations Development Programme. *Human Development Report 2005: International Cooperation at a Crossroads; Aid, Trade and Security in an Unequal World*. New York: United Nations Development Programme, 2005.

40. Hirsch D. *What will it take to end child poverty? Firing on all cylinders*. York: Joseph Rowntree Foundation, 2006.

41. Murray CJL, Lopez AD (ed.) *The global burden of disease: a comprehensive assessment of mortality and disability from diseases, injuries and risk factors in 1990 and projected to 2020*. Cambridge MA: Harvard School of Public Health on behalf of the World Health Organization and the World Bank, 1996.

42. Wanless D. *Securing our future health: taking a long-term view*. London: H M Treasury, 2002.

43. Tudge C. *The famine business*. London: Faber and Faber, 1977.

44. George S. *How the other half dies: the real reasons for world hunger*. Harmondsworth: Penguin, 1976.

45. Kinealy C. *The great Irish famine: impact, ideology and rebellion*. Basingstoke: Palgrave, 2002.

46. Government of Ireland. *Building an inclusive society. Review of the national Anti-Poverty strategy under the Programme for Prosperity and Fairness*. Dublin: Department of Social and Family Affairs, 2002.

47. Vernon J. *Hunger: a modern history*. Cambridge: Harvard University Press, 2007.

48. Jarman B. The identification of underprivileged areas. *British Medical Journal* 1983;**286**:1705–09.

49. Townsend P. *The international analysis of poverty*. Hemel Hempstead: Harvester Wheatsheaf, 1993.

50. Atwater WO. *Methods and results of investigations on the chemistry and economy of food. US Department of Agriculture Bulletin 21*. Washington DC: Department of Agriculture, 1895.

51. Atwater WO. *Foods, nutritive value and cost. US Department of Agriculture Bulletin 23*. Washington DC: US Department of Agriculture, n.d.

52. Atwater WO, Woods CD. *Investigations upon the chemistry and economy of foods*. Connecticut (Storrs): Agricultural Experimental Station, 1891.

53. Rowntree BS. *Poverty: a study of town life*. London: Macmillan, 1902.

54. Rowntree BS. *Poverty and Progress*. London: Longmans, 1941.

55. Ministry of Agriculture (FaF). *Loaves and fishes: an illustrated history of the Ministry of Agriculture, Fisheries and Food, 1889–1989*. London: Ministry of Agriculture, Fisheries and Food, 1989.

56. Office for National Statistics. *Social inequalities*, 2000 edn. London: The Stationery Office, 2000.

57. Fisher GM. *An overview of recent work on standard budgets in the United States and other anglophone countries.* Washington DC: US Department of Health and Human Services, 2007.

58. Parker H (ed.) *Low cost but acceptable: a minimum income standard for the UK: families with young children.* Bristol: The Policy Press and the Zacchaeus 2000 Trust, 1998.

59. Morris JN, Donkin AJM, Wonderling P, Wilkinson P, Dowler EA. A minimum income for healthy living. *Journal of Epidemiology and Community Health* 2000;**4**:885–889.

60. Morris J, Dangour A, Deeming C, Fletcher A, Wilkinson P. *Minimum income for health living: older people.* London: Age Concern England, 2005.

61. Dowler E. *Factors affecting nutrient intake and dietary adequacy in lone-parent households.* London: MAFF, 1995.

62. Joseph Rowntree Foundation. *Poverty and wealth across Britain 1968 to 2005.* www.jrf.org.uk/KNOWLEDGE/findings/housing/2077.asp York: Joseph Rowntree Foundation [accessed November 3 2008], 2007.

63. Donkin A, Dowler E, Stevenson SJ, Turner SA. Mapping access to food at a local level. *British Food Journal* 1999;**101**(7):554–564.

64. Lobstein T. *Low income diet and health—next steps after the report of the Low Income Diet and Nutrition Survey (LIDNS).* London: Sustain, 2007.

65. Food Standards Agency Press Release. *FSA publishes findings of the low income diet and nutrition survey.* Sunday 15 July 2007. http://www.food.gov.uk/news/pressreleases/2007/jul/lidns 2007.

66. Family Budget Unit. *Modest but adequate food budgets for six household types.* York: York University, 1992.

67. Dowler E, Rushton C. Diet and poverty in the UK: contemporary research methods and current experience. *Department of Public Health and Policy Publication No. 11.* London: London School of Hygiene and Tropical Medicine, University of London, 1994.

68. Dobson B, Beardsworth A, Keil T, Walker R. *Diet, choice and poverty: Social cultural and nutritional aspects of food consumption among low income families.* York: Joseph Rowntree Foundation Family Policy Studies Centre, 1994.

69. Piachaud D, Webb J. *The price of food: missing out on mass consumption.* Suntory and Toyota International Centre for Economics and Related Disciplines. London: London School of Economics and Political Science, 1996.

70. Donkin A, Dowler E, Stevenson SJ, Turner SA. Mapping access to food at a local level. *British Food Journal* 1999;**101**(7):554–564.

71. Marmot M. *The social determinants of health.* Oxford: Oxford University Press, 1999.

72. Marmot M. *Inequalities in health: the role of nutrition.* London: The Caroline Walker Trust, 2001.

73. Marmot M. *Status syndrome: how your social standing directly affects your health.* London: Bloomsbury, 2005.

74. Marmot MG, Wilkinson RG (ed.) *Social determinants of health.* Oxford: Oxford University Press, 2006.

75. Wilkinson RG. *The impact of inequality: how to make sick societies healthier.* London: Routledge, 2005.

76. Mack J, Lansley S. *Poor Britain*. London; Boston: G Allen & Unwin, 1985.

77. Bradshaw J, Middleton S, Davis A, Oldfield N, Smith N, Cusworth L *et al*. *A minimum income standard for Britain: what people think*. York: Joseph Rowntree Foundation, 2008.

78. Office for Social Inclusion. *What is Poverty?* http://www.socialinclusion.ie/poverty.html [accessed June 19 2008]. Dublin: Office for Social Inclusion, Department of Social and Family Affairs, Government of the Republic of Ireland, 2008.

79. Tingay RS, Tan C.J, Tan NCW, Tan S, Teoh PF, Wong R *et al*. Food insecurity and low income in an English inner city. *Journal of Public Health Medicine* 2003;25(2):156–159.

80. Robinson N, Caraher M, Lang T. Access to shops: the views of low income shoppers. *Health Education Journal* 2000;59(2):121–136.

81. Kavanagh A, Thornton L, Tattam L, Thomas A, Jolley D, Turrell G. *Place does matter for your health*. A report of the Victorian Lifestyle and neighbourhood Environment Study (VicLANES): University of Melbourne, 2007.

82. Bowyer S, Caraher M, Duane T, Carr-Hill R. *Shopping for food: accessing healthy affordable food in three areas of Hackney*. Centre for Food Policy: City University London, 2006.

83. Crotty P. Food and class. In: Germov J, Williams L (ed.) *A sociology of food and nutrition: the social appetite*. Melbourne: Oxford University Press, 1999.

84. Cabinet Office Strategy Unit. *Food: an analysis of the issues*. http://www.cabinetoffice.gov.uk/strategy/work_areas/food_policy.aspx. London: The Strategy Unit of the Cabinet Office, 2008:113.

85. Lawrence F. *Eat your heart out: why the food business is bad for the planet and your health*. London: Penguin, 2008.

86. Kavanagh A, Thornton L, Tattam A, Thomas L, Jolley D, Turrell G. *VicLANES—Place does matter*. A Report of the Victorian Lifestyle and Neighbourhood Environment Study FOR YOUR HEALTH. Melbourne: University of Melbourne, VicHealth and Key Centre for Women's Health in Society, 2007.

87. Fukuyama F. *The end of history and the last man*. New York: Free Press, 1992.

88. UNDP. *Human Development Report 1999*. New York: Oxford University Press & United Nations Development Programme, 1999.

89. Durning AT. *How much is enough?: the consumer society and the future of the earth*, 1st edn. New York: Norton, 1992.

90. Popkin BM. An overview on the nutrition transition and its health implications: the Bellagio meeting. *Public Health Nutrition* 2002;5(1A):93–103.

91. Lang T, Rayner G. Overcoming policy cacophony on obesity: an ecological public health framework for policymakers. *Obesity Reviews* 2007;8(Suppl.):165–181.

92. Beaumont J, Leather S, Lang T, Mucklow C. *Report on policy to Low Income Project Team of the Nutrition Taskforce*. Radlett: Institute of Grocery Distribtuion for the Department of Health Nutrition Taskforce, 1995.

93. Hitchman C, Harrison M, Christie I, Lang T. *Inconvenience food*. London: Demos, 2002.

94. Dowler E, Rex D, Blair A, Donkin A, Grundy C. *Measuring Access to healthy food in Sandwell*. Sandwell (West Midlands): Sandwell Health Authority, 2001.

95. Cummins S, Macintyre S. Food environments and obesity—neighbourhood or nation? *International Journal of Epidemiology* 2006;35:100–104.

96. Wrigley N. Food deserts' in British cities. *Policy Context and Research Priorities Urban Studies* 2002;39(11):2029–2040.

97. Wrigley N, Guy C, Lowe M. Urban regeneration, social inclusion and large store development: the Seacroft development in context. *Urban Studies* 2002;**39**(11):2101–2114.

98. Carley M, Kirk K, McIntosh S. *Retailing, sustainability and neighbourhood regeneration*. York: Joseph Rowntree Foundation, 2001.

99. Canadian Association of Food Banks. 'Something has to give': food banks filling the policy gap in Canada. *HungerCount 2003*. Toron to: Canadian Association of Food Banks, 2003.

100. Caraher M, Carr-Hill R. Taxation and public health: 'sin taxes' or structured approaches. In: Galea AaP, S (ed.) *Macrosocial determinants of population health*. New York Springer Science and Business Media Publishers, 2007:211–231.

101. Cochrane A, Clarke J. *Comparing welfare states: Britain in international context*. Milton Keynes: Open University Press and Sage, 1997.

102. Commission on the Social Determinants of Health. *Achieving health equity: from root causes to fair outcomes*. Interim Statement from the Commission. http://www.who.int/social_determinants/resources/interim_statement/en/index.html. [accessed November 3 2008] Geneva: World Health Organization, 2007.

103. Carr-Hill RA. The inequalities in health debate: a critical review of the issues. *Journal of Social Policy* 1987;**16**(4):509–542.

104. Carr-Hill RA. Being statistical with the truth. *Radical Statistics Newsletter* 1990;**47**: 18–20.

105. Gravelle H. How much of the relation between population mortality and unequal distribution of income is a statistical artefact? *BMJ* 1998;**316**:382–385.

106. Stewart-Brown S. What causes social inequalities: Why is this question taboo? *Critical Public Health* 2000;**10**(2):233–242.

107. Carr-Hill RA, Lintott J. *Consumption jobs and the environment*. London: Macmillan, 2003.

108. Kaul I, Grunberg I, Stern MA. Defining global public goods. In: Kaul I, Grunberg I, Stern MA (ed.) *Global public goods: international cooperation in the 21st century*. Oxford: Oxford University Press/United Nations Development Programme, 1999.

109. Dibsdall L, Lambert N, Frewer L. Using interpretative phenomenology to understand the food related experiences and beliefs of a select group of low-income UK women. *Journal of Nutrition Education and Behaviour* 2002;**34**(6):298–309.

110. Dibsdall LA, Lambert N, Bobbin RF, Frewer LJ. Low income consumers' attitudes and behaviours towards access, affordability ad motivation to eat fruit and vegetables. *Public health Nutrition* 2003;**6**(2):159–168.

111. National Food Alliance. *Myths about food and low income*. London: National Food Alliance, 1997.

112. Robinson DH. *The new farming*. London: Thomas Nelson & Sons, 1938.

113. UNICEF. *Vitamin A supplementation: a decade of progress*. Geneva: UNICEF, 2007.

114. Dalmiya N, Palmer A, Darnton-Hill I. Sustaining vitamin A supplementation requires a new vision *The Lancet* 2003;**368**(9541):1052–1054.

115. Allen L, de Benoist B, Dary O, Hurrell R (ed.) *Guidelines on food fortification with micronutrients*. Rome: World Health Organization and Food and Agriculture Organization, 2004.

116. Lawrence M. Folate fortification: public health policy making in a food regulation setting. In: Lin V, Gibson B (ed.) *Evidence-based health policy: problems & possibilities.* Sydney: Oxford University Press, 2003:110–126.

117. Lawrence M. Synthetic folic acid vs. food folates. *Public Health Nutrition* 2007;**10**(5):533–534.

118. Gates Foundation. *Food fortification promises improved health and productivity in developing nations.* http://www.gatesfoundation.org/GlobalHealth/Pri_Diseases/ Nutrition/Announcements/Announce-020509.htm. Seattle: Bill & Melinda Gates Foundation 2002.

119. Pretty J, Hine R. *Reducing food poverty with sustainable agriculture: a summary of new evidence.* Colchester: Centre for Environment and Society, University of Essex, 2001:http://www.essex.ac.uk/ces/esu/occasionalpapers/SAFErepSUBHEADS.shtm.

120. Evans S, Partidário PJ, Lambert J. Industrialization as a key element of sustainable product-service solutions. *International Journal of Production Research* 2007;**45**(18–19): 4225–4246.

121. Shaw DJ. *The UN World Food Programme and the development of food-aid.* Basingstoke: Palgrave, 2001.

122. Berger N. *The School Meals Service: from its beginnings to the present day.* Plymouth: Northcote House, 1990.

123. Tarrant JR. *Food policies.* Chichester, UK; New York: J. Wiley & Sons, 1980.

124. Fitchen JM. Hunger, malnutrition, and poverty in the contemporary United States. In: Counihan C, Van Esterik P (ed.) *Food and culture: a reader.* New York: Routledge, 1997:384–401.

125. Pressman J, Wildavsky A. *Policy implementation: how great expectations in Washington are dashed in Oakland; or, Why It's amazing that Federal Programs work at all.* Berkeley: University of California Press, 1973.

126. Danish Cancer Society. *Submission to the expert hearing on the school fruit scheme,* 24 September 2007, DG AGRI Brussels. http://ec.europa.eu/agriculture/markets/ fruitveg/sfs/expert/pederson_en.pdf [accessed June 20 2008]. Copenhagen: Danish Cancer Society, 2007.

127. Pomerleau J, Lock K, McKee M. The burden of cardiovascular disease and cancer attributable to low fruit and vegetable intake in the European Union: differences between old and new Member States. *Public Health Nutrition* 2006;**9**(5):575–83.

128. Lang T. *Now you see them, now you don't: a report on the fate of school meals and the loss of 300,000 jobs.* Accrington: The Lancashire School Meals Campaign, 1981.

129. Webster C. Government policy on school meals and welfare foods, 1939–1970. In: Smith DF (ed.) *Nutrition in Britain: science, scientists and politics in the twentieth century.* London: Routledge, 1997:190–213.

130. Lang T. The school meals business. *Critical Social Policy* 1983;**3**:117–128.

131. Caraher M, Dixon P, Lang T, Carr-Hill R. Barriers to accessing healthy foods: differentials by gender, social class, income and mode of transport. *Health Education Journal* 1998;**57**(3):191–201.

132. Lang T, Caraher M. Food poverty and shopping deserts: what are the implications for health promotion policy and practice? *Health Education Journal* 1998;**58**(3): 202–211.

133. Reisig VMT, Hobbiss A. Food deserts and how to tackle them: a study from one city's approach. *Health Education Journal* 2000;**59**(2):137–149.

134. Morgan K, Sonnino R, *The School Food Revolution*. London: Earthscan, 2008.

135. World Food Programme. *Food-aid flows 2007*. Rome: World Food Programme of the United Nations, 2008.

136. Shaw DJ. *World food security: a history since 1945*. London: Palgrave Macmillan, 2007.

137. Wessel J, Hantman M. *Trading the future: farm exports and the concentration of economic power in our food system*. San Francisco CA: Institute for Food and Development Policy, 1983.

138. Barraclough S. *An end to hunger? The social origins of food strategies*. London: Zed Books & UN Research Institute for Social Development and the South Commission, 1991.

139. Barratt Brown M. *Fair trade: reform and realities in the international trading system*. London: Zed Press, 1993.

140. Oxfam. Food-aid or hidden dumping? Sorting the wheat from the chaff. *Oxfam Briefing no.71*. Oxford: Oxfam publications, 2005:37.

141. American Enterprise Institute. *Food and agricultural policy: papers from a conference*. Washington DC: American Enterprise Institute for Public Policy Research, 1977.

142. FAO. *What is FIVIMS? The Food Insecurity and Vulnerability Information and Mapping Systems*. http://www.fivims.net [accessed July 24 2007]. Rome: Food & Agriculture Organization, 2007.

143. FAO. *The state of food insecurity in the world 2004: monitoring progress towards the world food summit and millenium development goals*. Rome: Food and Agriculture Organization, 2004.

144. FAO. *The state of food insecurity in the world 2006: eradicating world hunger—taking stock ten years after the world food summit*. Rome: Food and Agriculture Organization, 2006.

145. Barrington Moore Jnr W. *Social origins of dictatorship and democracy*. Harmondsworth: Penguin, 1969.

146. Stavenhagen R (ed.) *Agrarian problems and peasant movements in Latin America*. New York: Doubleday Anchor, 1970.

147. Lehmann D (ed.) *Agrarian reform and agrarian reformism: studies of Peru, Chile, China and India*. London: Faber and Faber, 1974.

148. Paige JM. *Agrarian revolution: social movements and export agriculture in the underdeveloped world*. New York: Free Press/Collier Macmillan, 1975.

149. Greenhill R, Pettifor A, Northover H, Sinha A. *Did the G8 drop the debt? Five years after the Birmingham Human Chain, what has been achieved, and what more needs to be done?* London: Jubilee Research @ NEF, CAFOD and Jubilee Debt Campaign, 2003.

150. Oxfam. *Rigged rules and double standards: trade, globalization and the fight against poverty*. Oxford: Oxfam, 2002.

151. Eide WB, Kracht U (ed.) *Food and human rights in development. Volume I: legal and institutional dimensions and selected topics*, 1st edn. Antwerp (NL): Intersentia, 2005.

152. UN Economic and Social Council. *The right to food*. Report of the Special Rapporteur on the right to food, Commission on Human Rights, Sixty-second session, Item 10 of the provisional agenda: Economic and So 16 March 2006, 2006:23.

153. UN. *Universal declaration of human rights*. Adopted and proclaimed by General Assembly resolution 217 A (III) of 10 December 1948. Geneva: United Nations, 1948.

154. UN Committee on Economic SaCRU. *International Covenant on Economic, Social & Cultural Rights Adopted by General Assembly resolution 2200 A (XXI) of 16 December 1966*. Entry into force 3 January 1976 in accordance with article 17. Geneva: UN Committee on Economic, Social and Cultural Rights, 1966.

155. Ward B, Dubos RJ. *Only one Earth: the care and maintenance of a small planet—an unofficial report commissioned by the Secretary-General of the United Nations Conference on the Human Environment*. Harmondsworth: Penguin, 1972.

156. Brown LR, Finsterbusch GW. *Man and his environment: food*. New York: Harper and Row, 1972.

157. Lappé FM. *Diet for a small planet*. New York: Ballantine Books, 1971.

158. FAO. *Voluntary guidelines to support the progressive realization of the right to adequate food in the context of national food security*. Adopted by the 127th Session of the FAO Council November 2004. Rome: Food and Agriculture Organization, 2004.

159. Bonanno A, Busch L, Friedland W, Gouveia L, Migione E (ed.) *From Columbus to ConAgra: the globalization of agriculture and food*. Lawrence: University Press of Kansas, 1994.

160. Tansey G, Worsley T. *The food system: a guide*. London: Earthscan, 1995.

161. Lang T, Heasman M. *Food wars: the global battle for mouths, minds and markets*. London: Earthscan, 2004.

162. Krebs AV. *The corporate reapers: the book of agribusiness*. Washington DC: Essential Books, 1992.

163. UK Food Group. *Hungry for power*. London: UK Food Group, 1999.

164. Spring Rice M. *Working class wives: their health and conditions*. Harmondsworth: Penguin, 1939.

165. Brockway AF. *Hungry England*. London: Victor Gollancz, 1932.

166. Hannington W. *Unemployed struggles 1919–1936*. London: Lawrence & Wishart, 1977 (1936).

167. Paulus I. *The search for pure food*. Oxford: Martin Robertson, 1974.

168. Curtis-Bennett N. *The food of the people*. London: Faber, 1949.

169. Lang T. Towards a food democracy. In: Griffiths S, Wallace J (ed.) *Consuming passions: food in the age of anxiety*. Manchester: Manchester University Press, 1998.

170. Pretty J. *Agri-culture*. London: Earthscan, 2002.

171. Funes F, Garcìa L, Bourque M, Pérez N, Rosset P. *Sustainable agriculture and resistance: transforming food production in Cuba*. Oakland CA: Food First Publications, 2002.

172. Prättälä R, Roos G, Hulshof K, Sihto M. Food and nutrition policies and interventions. In: Mackenbach J, Bakker M (ed.) *Reducing inequalities in health: a European perspective*. London: Routledge, 2002:104–124.

173. Yach D, Hawkes C, Epping–Jordan J, Galbraith S. The World Health Organization's framework convention on tobacco control: implications for global epidemics of food-related deaths and disease. *Journal of Public Health Policy* 2003;**24**(3/4):274–290.

Chapter 9

On what terms ecological public health?

Tectonic plates shifting

We began this book with an analogy that the tectonic plates of food policy are shifting and an argument that new fundamentals on which food policy should be based have emerged (see Chapter 1). Responses to the new terrain are emerging. Food policy has again become a high-profile 'hot' topic. This augurs well in some respects. Investment and attention are likely to flow but the outcomes are less certain. Competing positions have come to the fore: high tech versus low tech; social justice versus market; more trade versus maximization of domestic production; health through diet based on food from agriculture versus health through supplements via pill bottles; environmental protection by informing the consumer of each food item's carbon load versus reducing entire food system's ecological footprint; and so on.

A remarkable array of features, dimensions and options is emerging in food policy discourse. The entire terrain is characterized by vibrant debate, with passionate appeals to address this or that factor. Some argue that the 'answer' lies in GM foods and massive investment in large-scale agriculture. Others that food systems need to be re-localized around urban settlements, a latter day return to the city state with a modernized system of urban agriculture. Some argue that animal production needs to be reduced, since they now consume a huge proportion of available water and grain. Others remind policy-makers that in many regions, animals are a source of wealth. Some argue that population control, for all its authoritarian and Malthusian overtones, has to be factored into public policy more effectively. Others argue that since population levels off with rising income, it is more effective to alter what people eat and that there is plenty of land to feed people but not if they eat a North American diet.

Such divergence of opinion, policy direction and emphasis as to which evidence ought to take priority in shaping food policy, is neither surprising nor to be dismissed as 'experts being unable to agree'. It is testament to the complexity and seriousness of the food-policy challenge and to that project's inevitable ideological positioning. Food policy is not and cannot be neutral. Of course not, it is framed by assumptions, informed by values. It is about what people eat on a daily basis, and whether and how they do.

The book has also indicated where significant barriers and tensions lie. It has pointed to tensions between sectoral interests and to fragmentation of policy influence between the state, the corporate sector and civil society. It has suggested that food policy can be disaggregated and compartmentalized into discrete issues but that the consequences may be dire, with the poor and socially marginalized almost always receiving the brunt end of rough change. In policy, some compartmentalization is probably bureaucratically inevitable; policy cakes have to be cut up somehow (if we want to eat them). At the same time, the intellectual case for a more integrated, coherent food policy is also unanswerable, not least since consumers eat food as social, health and environmental acts simultaneously, whether consciously or not.

The review of the terrain given in preceding chapters has suggested that food policy is entering a new, important phase, characterized by the need for what we term ecological public health. We have pointed to where progress in that direction is being seen. The health impact of different diets is a case in point (see Chapter 4). Campaigns for food justice are another (see Chapter 8). Food waste is yet another (see Chapter 6). Undoubtedly, greater awareness of food's environmental impact has been a breakthrough feature for ecological public health, although the connections to human health have tended to be less well articulated. An innovative project championed by WWF, the international conservation NGO, has suggested a promising point of connection.[1] Taking the notion of 'one planet living', WWF calculated the footprint of different diets, from existing average diets (which consume as though there were many planets) to ultimate local, healthy, organic and vegetarian (the 'simplest' in its modelling).[2] Such studies suggest that there might be win-wins for both health and environment if diet shifts away from the conventional to the simplest. But equally, it is known, for example, that a 'local' diet is not always the best environmentally. A tomato salad in mid-winter, grown in a coal-heated greenhouse, may provide nutrients but at considerable cost of greenhouse gas emissions, while a tomato grown in the sun but transported long distance by lorry may have a lower ecological footprint.[3, 4]

Such studies need to be done on a systematic footing, at the national and international levels. Good life-cycle assessments point to the complexity of measuring food's environmental footprint. Yet, pending methodological refinement, it looks likely that some foods, notably meat and dairy, carry more weight than others. But some caution is in order. Meat from an intensive indoor system may emit more GHGs and use more hectares than an extensive system. A sheep that lives on Welsh hills and lambs outdoors in the spring, rather than indoors fed on rations, may or may not be less carbon-intensive than a cow kept indoors and fed on imported grain in Malta. The point is that broader criteria are needed to judge food than just price or whether it is local or 'healthy'. This suggests the need to work out a more subtle and complex way of judging what an adequate diet is, one that integrates not just nutrition and carbon but also issues such as place, time and mode of production.[5] In the place of single issue standards, which can be traded off against each other, an integrated system is required in which the goal is improvement on all factors. This will be complex and suggests that future food policy will not be of a 'one size fits all' variety. Different outcomes and approaches may be suitable for one policy issue but not for another. An appropriate diet in one region might be not appropriate elsewhere, just as nutrient intake should vary according to physiological need. Ecological appropriateness can inform health rules not just environmental ones.

Given such complexity, policy-makers might be forgiven for despairing at receiving any clear messages and advice from evidence gatherers. Reality is messier than the neat, logical ideal model we outlined in Fig. 1.2 (see Chapter 1). Faced by this, politicians are quick to justify inaction by pointing to uncertainties in science. But uncertainty is not an excuse for policy drift, and politicians should be saluted when they do make moves without being prompted by a crisis or other urgencies and when there are still uncertainties. What matters is the level of uncertainty and the consequences of not acting. This realization has motivated pioneering efforts to shift official and commercial thinking on food policy. Pressure from scientists, for instance, has had some effect in reducing food-industry reluctance to address the issue of hidden fats, excessive sugar and salt in foods. The campaign to reduce population salt intake, for instance, by the World Action on Salt and Health (WASH), an international coalition of blood pressure specialists, epidemiologists and public health advocates, has begun to be effective in alerting governments as to the health advantages of getting food companies to take their responsibilities seriously; but there is a very long way to go before unnecessary salt intake is reduced.[6]

Part of the challenge ahead is to persuade institutions that are nominally and democratically responsible to address the complexity of ecological public health. There are some encouraging signs of movement. In 2000, for example, a WHO European Region process that began in the nutrition division, and which took 3 years to develop, came to fruition in Copenhagen at its 5-yearly continental meeting. The 51 member states of the WHO European Region debated and approved an ambitious new food and nutrition policy.[7] The resolution proposed that nutritional variations needed to be tackled but alongside safety and sustainability. A long debate convinced member states' senior health officials and ministers that nutrition needed a higher priority but that this had to be addressed in an integrated fashion. Nutrition advance was unlikely to happen unless it engaged the entire food supply chain. Nutrition could not, nor should be, 'bolted on' as a health appendage. Equally, it needs to be linked to efforts to make food supply more sustainable. Because the WHO, like much in the UN system, can only advise rather than require its member states to act—unlike the WTO or EU, whose strictures can be binding agreements with the force of law—this 2000 resolution merely requested them to act more strongly and on the grounds of diet-related ill-health. The model used by the WHO-E was innovatory.[8] Knowing that governments tend to approve policies that are incremental, this model placed nutrition within a structure whose pediment was the existing WHO-E overall health commitment Health 21,[9] and to sustainable development through the 1992 UNCED 'Rio' Declaration commitment to local and community action for sustainable development.[9, 10] The 2000 Resolution depicted nutrition as one of three pillars, alongside sustainability and food safety, built on a pediment of those existing policies. It won overwhelming political approval and paved the way for subsequent more integrated thinking on obesity in Istanbul in 2006. There was no need to argue that tackling obesity meant reshaping the environment as well as diet. There was no false either/or policy distinction; member states agreed that they needed to act on both fronts.[11]

Another example of emerging, more integrated thinking was at the global level when in 2003, the WHO and FAO combined to issue a strongly worded statement on the case for better integration of food supply with public health. Their joint report saw the rising toll of NCDs as directly connected to the commodification of food and food products. Entire lifestyles have been serviced by oil-based cultures—'motorized transport, labour-saving devices at home, the phasing out of physically demanding manual tasks at work, and leisure time that is preponderantly devoted to physically undemanding pastimes'—alongside increased consumption of energy-dense diets high in fat, particularly saturated fat, and low in unrefined carbohydrates. The net effect was to place 'additional burdens on already overtaxed national health budgets.'[12] This language would have been unthinkable a decade earlier.

Although such initiatives are very much to be welcomed, some caution is also in order. WHO and FAO are advisory bodies responsible to member states whose actions are needed to deliver on their recommendations. These may be strong but encounter the reality check of other policies which promote consumer choice, commercial priorities and economic competitiveness. These may point in different directions, and politicians might privately agree that radical change in food systems is needed but fear confronting consumers, who are also their electorate, in so doing. While this classic political stand-off continues, pressure on core elements of 20th century food-policy legacy inexorably mounts. As the climate-change specialists now state, if action is not taken now—costly and awesome though it will be—the difficulties and cost of doing so later will be all the greater.[13] With food policy, the political difficulties of change towards sustainable food systems are not just economically costly but deeply personal, as well as cultural. They call into question a particular 'Western' 20th century notion of progress—greater individual freedom, choice and disposable income.

The 21st century food policy is likely to have to face some fundamental questions: how much choice do people actually need or require, and believe they need? And how much is fair? How much oil or embedded water can humanity afford to expend on its food system? What exactly is a sustainable food system? And what institutions, politicians and political processes might take responsibility to lead changes that seem to be required? So often, these big picture questions fall between ministerial 'boxes' and divisions of responsibility. As a result, there can be policy drift and conflict, even as evidence mounts of the need for action. On top of that, there are hard political realities. Powerful commercial interests can be against change, as well as consumer buy-in to business-as-usual. Thus a 'perfect storm' of contrary positions can cumulatively hold back integration. Urban–rural relations, for example, are not helped if agriculture thinks of nutrition as something it delivers through *quantity*, when agriculture has a major impact on which nutrients are produced (and consumed) and in what ratios. If nutrition remains fragmented in three traditions—as a life science (food as biochemical components), social nutrition (food as social relations) and eco-nutrition (food as environment)—when all have much to offer ecological public health, how can policy improve? The three traditions have gradually separated just when they need to be together.

The policy terrain for future food policy looks bound to be complex. Nevertheless, this book has presented grounds for both pessimism and optimism. Shocks, such as the rapid oil and food commodity price rises of 2006–08, might have worried political élites and brought suffering for people on low incomes but they might turn out to be overdue triggers for change. The implications of the rapid emergence and costs of obesity is another such set of signals. Obesity is to health what climate change is to the environment.[14, 15]

What is a sustainable food system?

The argument from this book is that sustainability is not just a matter of the environment. Health and social dimensions are intrinsic too to the new policy picture. Gradually, it transpires that if food is looked at through the lens of ecological public health, the need for a different range of criteria by which to judge it emerges. We term this the omni-standards problem: by what criteria can anyone judge whether a food warrants being called sustainable? Let us return to the example of fish outlined earlier (see Chapter 4). Nutrition science strongly advises as to the benefits of eating fish, yet equally, environmental advice is either sceptical or hostile to following that advice and seeks drastic action to conserve fish stocks. A compromise position suggests that the eater should eat more discriminatingly: not eat cod but eat fish from aquaculture (unless it too is fed from the seas). Each position—'eat more', 'eat less', 'eat differently'—has good data, focuses on an equally important issue and can cite impeccable sources.

The fish question becomes even more thorny if viewed from a labour or international framework. Jobs are at stake. Valuable seashore ecosystems have been altered to develop export seafood farming in some areas of Asia, for instance. There thus appears to be no simple advice to give to consumers, other than the medical rule of 'first do no harm'; but not eating fish and not consuming the omega 3s they contain may be harmful, which is why nutrition advice recommends it.[16] If the omega 3s are not from fish, as governments advise almost world-wide, from where should they be derived? Reviewing British fish available for discriminating consumers, Sustain, an alliance of 100 plus UK NGOs, found just five fish to which it was able to give a clear and positive seal of approval when evaluating consumer choice against just three criteria: health, sustainable stocks and contamination.[17]

And what if our average European consumer follows advice to consume ample amounts of green vegetables? Should s/he buy Kenyan green beans in mid-winter to support this burgeoning trade for a developing country or be concerned about its embedded water? Each stem of a green bean has 4 litres of potable water embedded—this from a water-scarce country. Should policy support the export trade for bringing welcome income back to a developing country? Worry about who actually gets the money? Or shift attention to the labourers' working conditions? Or just approve the nutrient flow? Or see it as new international division of labour and demand a reciprocal right to allow Western banks in?

The process of trying to map what a sustainable food system might look like is complex, and policy needs improved methodologies for weighing up competing demands. Some indicators of sustainability are less clear and 'softer' than others. Quality, for instance, might include freshness, local-ness, seasonality and authenticity, but these can be difficult to define. Quality issues are socially prized, however, as are social justice and moral and ethical issues, such as animal welfare, fair trade and working conditions, which have fairly robust criteria already existing. Some issues are intrinsically tricky, such as cost internalization. The notion is clear but the implications for low income consumers or low cost developing nations might be threatening. No wonder indicators are not yet agreed, despite preliminary costings at the national level (see Chapter 5 and 6). Generally environmental criteria for defining sustainable food systems, however, are beginning to be firmed up within existing policy processes, which are beginning to recognize the need to slow down, if not reverse, climate change. Policy has barely begun to recognize how to audit embedded water, however, while indicators for land use and biodiversity are stronger but still contentious. Health criteria are reasonably robust with regard to safety and nutrition. All are subject to constant debate and new research.

The net effect of all this is that while a composite approach to ecological public health might be creeping up the policy agenda, the precise mechanics and criteria for policy objectives are still too unclear. These issues are not just academic. They pose real complexities for politicians. Interestingly, food companies are alive to this 'omni-standard' issue and are beginning to develop their own partial criteria already through systems of commercial or private standards, such as GlobalGAP, GFSI and the Sustainable Agriculture Initiative (see Chapter 5). The need for comprehensive policy has to be filled, particularly in relation to social and cultural criteria. The modern reality is one of competing systems of standards—public, commercial and civil society—adding to policy cacophony. Policy-makers therefore need to engage in an open task of trying to agree what criteria might be applied to food systems: what are the criteria by which we may judge whether a food system is or is not sustainable? Clarification of this question would help to refine the direction for policy and enable concerted, rather than fragmented, efforts to be made. At present there is no level playing field, no international shared set of goals, yet there needs to be one, and one that is, and can be, ratcheted up to meet tougher goals, while taking all food systems with that process.

The 'elephant in the room' for ecological public health might well turn out to be consumer values as we argued in Chapter 7. Companies and governments, which have power to shape policy, both worship but are held back by fear of the 'consumer', this person who apparently wants to consume without recognizing the health or environmental consequences of her/his actions. At one level, this sensitivity to ordinary people can be interpreted as evidence of the advance of food democracy (as outlined in Chapter 8), but it also suggests a policy lock-in. Consumers might be contradictory, in which case they need to be helped out of, rather than trapped in to, particular patterns of consumption.[18] A shift from judging food policy effectiveness by whether it delivers 'value-for-money'—defining food by price, quality, regularity, availability, etc.—to judging it by a broader compilation of 'values-for-money'—integrating social, environmental and health criteria alongside point-of-sale criteria—is overdue.

Accountability: the political issue

At the heart of the ecological public health perspective we have outlined here, has to be a commitment to improve food democracy and accountability. If we want to behave as citizens and ensure that food's impact on the environment, public health and society is improved, democratic accountability is critical. Food accountability is currently split in three directions: to governments through the ballot box and electability; to companies through channels such as market share, share-holdings, pension funds and private stock-holdings; and to civil society in the form of consumer purchasing patterns at the check-out till. In each of these channels, pressure to deliver ecological public health has been building up. A new wave of public campaigns since the 1980s has begun to push governments and politicians to take health, environment and social justice more seriously in relation to food. Refining and using the power of public procurement is one strategy that has emerged in that process.[19] Shareholders and companies have also been held more to account by the emergence—small but noisy—of ethical and environmental investment holdings. These are made stronger by the arrival of serious health audits by banks and financiers.[20] Methods have been designed to judge companies across health, environmental and societal performance.[21, 22] Civil society and consumers, too, need to be helped to change behaviour rapidly.

Methodologies, such as deliberative democracy and citizens' juries, keep new ideas coming into public discourse and engagement.[23] And the vibrant NGO world is never short of advice and thoughts as to what needs to happen. But there is a danger of governments and companies putting the onus on consumers to change by applying the thinnest of policy measures, such as labelling. A plethora of food labels does not amount to an integrated food policy. As we suggested in Chapter 7, choice is too often presented as what consumers do, while down-playing the choice-editing made 'upstream' in food-supply chains by contracts and specifications from farm to shop. That is not to say that consumers do not need, and would not welcome, new cultural 'rules' for, and advice on, choosing and eating food in a world that tries to address the ecological public health challenge. If the food system inherited from the 20th century now needs to change for the 21st, part of that change process must be the cultural recognition of the limits of consumer power. The ecological impact of consumerism might be great, but that is not the same thing as building policy process on a myth that consumers are in charge.

Ultimately, food policy is likely to come of age in this ecological public health era if it is constantly informed by vibrant and open debate and pressure to link health, environment and social justice. The role of civil society organizations over recent decades has shaken complacency within 'inside track' food-policy thinking in governments and boardrooms. NGOs may be quick to put issues on to the agenda but they alone cannot resolve food policy's challenges. The grounds for policy change are strong but the gaps between evidence, policy and practice are often frustratingly wide. Yet food policy history teaches us that progress is possible. Pursuing that requires all of us.

References

1. Frey S, Barrett J. *Our health, our environment: the ecological footprint of what we eat.* International Ecological Footprint Conference 'Stepping up the Pace: New Developments in Ecological Footprint Methodology, Applications'; 8–10 May 2007; Cardif. http://www.brass.cf.ac.uk/uploads/Frey_A33.pdf.

2. Frey S, Barrett J. *The footprint of Scotland's diet. The environmental burden of what we eat.* A report for Scotland's Global Footprint Project. York: Stockholm Environment Institute, 2006.

3. Smith A, Watkiss P, Tweddle G, McKinnon PA, Browne PM, Hunt A *et al. The validity of food miles as an indicator of sustainable development.* Report to DEFRA by AEA Technology. London: Department for the Environment, Food and Rural Affairs, 2005.

4. Saunders C, Barber A, Taylor G. *Food miles—comparative energy/emissions performance of New Zealand's agriculture industry.* Research Report 285. Christchurch NZ: Agribusiness and Economics Research Unit, Lincoln University, 2006.

5. Edwards-Jones G, Milà i Canals L, Hounsome N, Truninger M, Koerber G, Hounsome B *et al.* Testing the assertion that 'local food is best': the challenges of an evidence-based approach. *Trends in Food Science & Technology* 2008;**19**:265–274.

6. WASH. *Introduction to world action on salt and health.* London: World Action on Salt and Health. http://www.worldactiononsalt.com/ [accessed on November 30 2008], 2008.

7. WHO Regional Office for Europe. WHO (2000). *Resolution: the impact of food and nutrition on public health: the case for a food and nutrition policy and an action plan for the European Region of WHO 2000–2005.* Regional Committee for Europe, Fiftieth session, Copenhagen, 11–14 September 2000. EUR/RC50/R8. Copenhagen: World Health Organisation Regional Office for Europe, 2000.

8. Robertson A, Tirado C, Lobstein T, Jermini M, Knai C, Jensen JH *et al. Food and health in Europe: a new basis for action.* Copenhagen: World Health Organisation Regional Office for Europe, 2004.

9. WHO European Region. Health 21: health for all in the 21st century—an introduction. *Health for All series no. 5.* Copenhagen: World Health Organisation Regional Office for Europe, 1998.

10. UNCED. *Rio Declaration, made at the UNCED meeting at Rio de Janeiro from 3 to 14 June 1992.* Rio de Janeiro: United Nations Conference on Environment and Development, 1992.

11. WHO European Region. *European Charter on Counteracting Obesity, agreed at WHO Ministerial Conference on Counteracting Obesity, Istanbul Turkey November 15–17 2006.* EUR/06/5062700/8. Copenhagen: WHO European Region, 2006.

12. WHO/FAO. *Diet, nutrition and the prevention of chronic diseases.* Report of the joint WHO/FAO expert consultation. WHO Technical Report Series, no. 916 (TRS 916). Geneva: World Health Organisation & Food and Agriculture Organisation, 2003.

13. Stern SN. *The economics of climate change. The report of the Stern Review.* Cambridge: Cambridge University Press, 2007.

14. Foresight. *Tackling obesities: future choices.* London: Government Office of Science, 2007.

15. Woodcock J, Banister D, Edwards P, Prentice A, Roberts I. Energy and transport. *The Lancet* 2008;**370**(9592):1078–1088.

16. Food Standards Agency. *Eat well, be well: fish and shellfish.* http://www.eatwell.gov.uk/healthydiet/nutritionessentials/fishandshellfish/ [accessed January 9, 2008]. London: Food Standards Agency, 2008.

17. Sustain. *Like shooting fish in a barrel.* www.sustainweb.org *Food facts.* London: Sustain, 2005.

18. National Consumer Council and Sustainable Development Commission. *I will if you will.* Report of the Sustainable Consumption Roundtable. London: Sustainable Development Commission, 2006.

19. Cabinet Office Strategy Unit. *Recipe for success: towards a food strategy for the 21st century.* London: Cabinet Office, 2008.

20. Langlois A, Zuanic PE, Faucher J, Pannuti C, Shannon J. *Obesity: re-shaping the food industry.* London: JP Morgan Global Equity Research, 2006.

21. Lang T, Rayner G, Kaelin E. *The food industry, diet, physical activity and health.* A review of reported commitments and practice of 25 of the world's largest food companies. London: City University Centre for Food Policy, 2006.

22. Nestle M. Food industry and health: mostly promises, little action. *The Lancet* 2006;**368**: 564–565.

23. Kass G. *Open channels: public dialogue in science and technology.* London: Parliamentary Office of Science and Technology, 2001.

Index